Microbiology & Immunology

Microbiology & Immunology

An Illustrated Review with Questions and Explanations

Second Edition

David J. Hentges, Ph.D.
Professor and Chairman
Department of Microbiology and Immunology
Texas Tech University Health Sciences Center School of Medicine
Lubbock, Texas

Little, Brown and Company
Boston   New York   Toronto   London

Library of Congress Cataloging-in-Publication Data

Medical microbiology & immunology : an illustrated review with questions and explanations /
    edited by David J. Hentges. — 2nd ed.
        p.   cm.
    Includes bibliographical references and index.
    ISBN 0-316-35784-7
1. Medical microbiology — Outlines, syllabi, etc.   2. Medical
microbiology — Examinations, questions, etc.   I. Hentges, David J.
    [DNLM: 1. Microbiology — examination questions.   QW 18 M489   1995]
QR46.M472   1995
616'.01'076 — dc20
DNLM/DLC
for Library of Congress   94-29942
                                                              CIP

Printed in the United States of America

SEM

Editorial: Evan R. Schnittman, Rebecca Marnhout
Production Editors: Kellie Cardone, Marie A. Salter
Copyeditor: Libby Dabrowski
Indexer: Nancy Newman
Production Supervisor/Designer: Louis C. Bruno, Jr.
Cover Designer: Michael A. Granger
Cover Illustrator: Peg Gerrity

Contents

Preface

Microbiology and Immunology, Second Edition, like the first, presents an overview of medical microbiology and immunology. It is designed to serve as a guide for students either taking a formal course in medical microbiology or preparing for board or graduate level examinations. The objective is to provide a means whereby students can master the basic information essential for a thorough understanding of the subject matter. The material contained in this book is the same as that presented to medical and graduate students taking our course in medical microbiology at Texas Tech University Health Sciences Center—these students consistently perform well on the microbiology subtest of the National Board Medical Examination.

The book is organized into chapters discussing immunology, general bacteriology, microbial genetics, pathogenic microbiology, virology, mycology, and parasitology; the final summation chapter groups microorganisms according to the region of the human body in which they produce infections. Self-test multiple choice questions similar to those used on the board or other comprehensive examinations supplement the book's first seven chapters. Answers to these questions are accompanied, when appropriate, by brief explanations.

D.J.H.

Acknowledgments

We gratefully acknowledge the efforts of Rose Williford-Smith, who typed the manuscripts, and Kelle Fralick, who prepared the excellent illustrations found throughout the text.

Contributing Authors

Thomas C. Butler, M.D.
Professor, Departments of Internal Medicine and Microbiology and Immunology, Texas Tech University Health Sciences Center School of Medicine; Physician, Department of Internal Medicine, University Medical Center, Lubbock, Texas

W. LaJean Chaffin, Ph.D.
Associate Professor, Department of Microbiology and Immunology, Texas Tech University Health Sciences Center School of Medicine, Lubbock, Texas

Joe A. Fralick, Ph.D.
Associate Professor, Department of Microbiology and Immunology, Texas Tech University Health Sciences Center School of Medicine, Lubbock, Texas

David J. Hentges, Ph.D.
Professor and Chairman, Department of Microbiology and Immunology, Texas Tech University Health Sciences Center School of Medicine, Lubbock, Texas

Terence M. Joys, Ph.D.
Associate Professor, Department of Microbiology and Immunology, Texas Tech University Health Sciences Center School of Medicine, Lubbock, Texas

Stanley S. Lefkowitz, Ph.D.
Professor, Department of Microbiology and Immunology, Texas Tech University Health Sciences Center School of Medicine, Lubbock, Texas

Danny B. Pence, Ph.D.
Professor, Departments of Pathology and Microbiology and Immunology, Texas Tech University Health Sciences Center School of Medicine, Lubbock, Texas

Earl M. Ritzi, Ph.D.
Associate Professor, Department of Microbiology and Immunology, Texas Tech University Health Sciences Center School of Medicine, Lubbock, Texas

Rial D. Rolfe, Ph.D.
Associate Professor, Department of Microbiology and Immunology, Texas Tech University Health Sciences Center School of Medicine, Lubbock, Texas

David C. Straus, Ph.D.
Associate Professor, Department of Microbiology and Immunology, Texas Tech University Health Sciences Center School of Medicine, Lubbock, Texas

Microbiology & Immunology

Immunology

Terence M. Joys

Introduction

The concept that humans have some kind of immune mechanism arose from the ancient observation that individuals who recovered from an epidemic disease were often no longer susceptible during further outbreaks of the disease. Although Edward Jenner developed an empirical method of stimulating this mechanism to prevent smallpox infection in 1796, the basis of immunity has only been elucidated during the past 100 years. The cells and molecules responsible for immunity constitute the *immune system,* and their collective and coordinated responses to foreign substances comprise the *immune response* (Fig. 1-1). The primary concern is maintenance of the body against invasion by both external agents and its own unregulated cells, and immunity now is defined as a reaction to foreign substances without implying a physiologic or pathologic consequence of such a reaction.

All animals have *nonadaptive* (also called natural, native, or innate) systems that act as a first line of defense against foreign invaders. In humans these include the epithelial surface, phagocytic cells, a class of lymphocytes called natural killer (NK) cells, and circulating factors such as lysozyme, C-reactive protein, and properdin. Four types of defensive obstacles are involved. Anatomic barriers include intact skin, which prevents penetration and has local fatty acids to provide a low pH environment and various mucous membranes that have secretions and cilia to wash away potential pathogens. Physiologic barriers consist of temperature, pH, oxygen tension, and soluble factors (lysozyme, interferon, complement) and endocytic and phagocytic barriers that result in removal of the foreign material by ingestion into a cell. Inflammation is also part of the normal response to injury and invasion. Endocytosis involves macromolecules and occurs by pinocytosis (nonspecific membrane invagination) and receptor-mediated endocytosis (molecules are internalized after binding to specific receptors). In both, the molecules are enclosed in endocytic vesicles that fuse with endosomes (which have an acid environment that cleaves off any receptors) and then fuse with primary lysosomes to form secondary lysosomes. Primary lysosomes are derived from the Golgi apparatus and contain large numbers of degradative enzymes (proteases, lipases, nucleases, and others). These break down the macromolecules into smaller pieces, which are eliminated. Phagocytosis involves specialized cells, which can engulf particulate matter to form phagosomes (10–20 times larger than endosomes). These fuse with primary lysosomes and then follow the same degradative pathway. Some bacteria can survive this attempted digestion. Vertebrates have evolved an additional *adaptive* (acquired, specific) system that takes time to respond, is exquisitely specific, and increases in magnitude with successive exposures (to a maximum). This adaptive system can *remember* an exposure (the anamnestic response) so that subsequent encounters result in an increasingly effective defense response and *amplify* the protective mechanisms of natural immunity to focus them on the site where the natural immunity broke down. It is dual in nature and involves both a humoral (liquid) and a cellular response. Agents that cause an immune response are called *antigens.*

Fig. 1-1 Summary of the immune response. Ag, antigen; APC, antigen presenting cells; Ig, immunoglobulin; MHC, major histocompatibility complex.

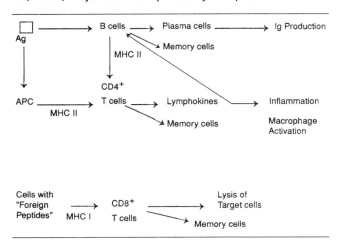

Substances that appear in serum as a result of antigen exposure are called *antibodies*. The immune system reacts in a highly selective manner that is very *specific*, and this specificity is determined by lymphocytes.

Lymphocytes are morphologically similar but can be divided on physiologic, developmental, and functional grounds into two major classes, the T cells and the B cells. B cells are responsible for the humoral response and may differentiate into plasma cells when activated by recognition of foreign material. Plasma cells secrete antibodies, which bind specifically to such material and initiate a variety of elimination responses. Humoral immunity can be transferred by plasma to give passive immunity. The T cells also recognize foreign substances and differentiate into a variety of cells that either mediate the cellular response, cause cytotoxic effects, or influence the B-cell response. This cellular response can only be transferred by cells. An individual lymphocyte in either class is highly specific in its recognition ability and will respond to only one or a few closely related foreign substances. Following recognition, these cells must reproduce and differentiate to generate an immune response. The clonal selection theory proposes that each lymphocyte expresses on its surface one of a large library of recognition molecules. In addition to the lymphocytes, several other types of cells are essential to the immune system, and their functions include processing of the foreign material for presentation to the T cells, scavenging of foreign material after its reaction with the immune system, and mediation of physiologic changes that occur in the immune response. These accessory cells include blood monocytes, macrophages, polymorphonuclear leukocytes, and dendritic reticular cells.

In addition to its obviously beneficial property in aiding in defense against pathogens and unregulated host cells, the immune response can be modulated not to respond (that is, a state of tolerance is induced) or to respond in a manner that is deleterious because of hypersensitivity. Disease states that influence the immune system can result in the breakdown of the ability to distinguish "self" from "nonself," and an immune response can be generated against host material.

Immune responses are self-limited and wane with time. They consist of a *cognitive phase*, in which the foreign antigens bind to preexisting specific receptors on mature lymphocytes; an *activation phase*, in which the lymphocytes proliferate; and an *effector phase*, in which cells and mediators (phagocytes, complement, mast cells, cytokines, and leukocytes that are involved in inflammation) that can function in the absence of lymphocyte activation are activated and focused on the foreign material. As a result of the response, some of the B cells and T cells that were specifically activated give rise to memory cells, which circulate over time and allow the response to a second exposure to be more rapid and more intense, and to last longer.

Immunogens

Strictly speaking, an immunogen is a substance capable of eliciting an immune response, an antigen is a substance capable of reacting specifically with antibody, and a hapten is a small chemical capable of reacting with specific antibody but not able to elicit formation of that antibody. Haptens may become immunogenic when coupled to a "carrier" molecule.

Ability to Elicit an Immune Response

The ability of an immunogen to elicit an immune response depends on a variety of factors. The nature of the prospective immunogen exerts an effect in that it must be foreign to the circulation of the host to which it is exposed and must not have previously induced a state of tolerance in the host. The chemical nature of a substance is important in determining whether it will be immunogenic and this includes its molecular size and complexity. No clear-cut thresholds exist but, in general, the bigger and more complex the better. Usually, different regions of an immunogen react with B cells and T cells. B-cell epitopes of an immunogen (also called antigenic determinants, haptenic groups) are those areas that combine specifically with immunoglobulin (Ig) on the surface of B cells, stimulating these cells to divide, differentiate, and synthesize specific antibody in the presence of signals from T helper cells. T-cell epitopes of an immunogen (carrier groups) are those areas that are retained after denaturation of the protein in the lysosome/fused vacuole, are able to bind to the major histocompatibility complex (MHC) haplotype proteins present in the processing cells, and combine with specific T-cell receptors (TCR). In rare cases the B- and T-cell epitopes are the same. Macromolecular proteins are thought to be potent immunogens because they possess many T-cell epitopes and consequently stimulate numerous T-cell populations to aid in the immune response. Such large antigens usually have more than one B-cell epitope and many T-cell epitopes. Individuals may not produce antibodies to all of the B-cell epitopes or respond to all of the T-cell epitopes present. The B-cell epitopes that do elicit antibody production differ in the amount of antibody produced against them; that is, they differ in *immunopotency*. At the molecular level, an immunoglobulin is specific for B-cell epitopes that are 6 amino acids or 4 sugars in size, whereas T-cell epitopes are 9 to 12 amino acids long for cytotoxic T cells and 15 to 30 amino acids long for T helper cells. Within a given epitope, individual molecules do not contribute equally to the specificity and such variation represents *immunodominance.* Rare antigens can stimulate a B-cell response in mice without the involvement of T cells. It is not clear whether such situations exist in humans. The *animal* being exposed to the immunogen affects the response, as different species may react differently to a given prospective immunogen; for example, dextrans are immunogenic in mice and humans but not in rabbits and guinea pigs. Individuals of the same species show variation in their responses. The *experimental conditions* of exposure, for example, dose, mode of administration, timing of exposure, and physiologic condition of the exposed host, have a broad effect on the response elicited. Adjuvants are substances that can increase the response to an immunogen if administered with it. They may prolong retention of the immunogen, increase its effective size, stimulate the influx of populations of macrophages and/or lymphocytes, or do more than one of these. The *sensitivity* of the method used to detect the presence of an immune response may determine whether or not a response is measured. Although many immunogens cause obvious changes in a suitable host, some require extremely sensitive techniques for detection of their responses, and their immunogenicity cannot be recognized unless such tests are available.

Heterogenetic Antigens

These antigens are present in different, often related, species. The best known is the *Forssman antigen,* which occurs in the red blood cells (RBC) of guinea pigs, horses, cattle, cats, chickens, and some bacteria but not in rats or rabbits. This antigen is a polysaccharide. Humans are usually reported as Forssman antigen negative but some individuals are positive in their gastrointestinal mucosa. Forssman antigen negative individuals can produce gastrointestinal tumors that are positive. The human group A red blood cell antigen is related to the Forssman antigen and will cross react with it.

The Lymphatic System and Inflammation

Lymph is a pale, watery, proteinaceous tissue fluid that flows from the intracellular tissue spaces into lymphatic capillaries and then into a series of larger collecting vessels called lymphatics. During passage from the tissue fluid to the lymphatics it becomes progressively enriched in lymphocytes. The lymphatics carry the lymph through regional lymph nodes, where it is filtered through a cellular network of phagocytic cells that trap antigen that it may carry. The lymphatics ultimately join to form the thoracic

duct, which drains into the left subclavian vein near the heart. Once in the blood, the lymphocytes circulate only for 30 minutes or less before entering some kind of lymphoid tissue.

White blood cells (leukocytes) are of five types. Granulocytes have numerous granules in the cytoplasm and are also called polymorphonuclear leukocytes because the nucleus is irregular, lobed, or segmented. They comprise 60 to 70 percent of blood leukocytes and consist of (1) neutrophils, also called microphages, 55 to 68 percent; (2) basophils, 0.5 percent; and (3) eosinophils, 2 to 5 percent. Agranulocytes consist of: (1) monocytes, 3.5 percent, and (2) lymphocytes, 20 to 30 percent. Macrophages are either fixed (in liver, spleen, bone marrow, lymph nodes, etc.) or wandering, and are derived from monocytes.

All of these cells, plus erythrocytes and platelets, are thought to arise from the pluripotential stem cell during hematopoesis (Fig. 1-2). Stem cells first appear in the yolk sac of the developing embryo and then in the fetal liver. After birth, they are located in the bone marrow, where they persist during adult life; if the bone marrow is destroyed in the adult, stem cells are seen in the spleen and sometimes the liver. Stem cells are self-renewing. Some of their daughter cells remain stem cells; others become more differentiated progenitor cells, programmed to yield progeny that differentiate further into particular types of blood cells. The stem cells are rare and the type of progeny cell to which they give rise is influenced by local conditions in terms of stimulating factors released by neighbor cells. Stimulating factors include the interleukins, colony-stimulating factors for granulocytes and monocytes, and erythropoietin. Inhibitory factors include tumor growth factor (TGF— both alpha and beta). The balance of these in an individual cell's local environment is thought to influence its differentiation. The lymphoid cells differ from the other stem cell progeny in not proliferating without some additional stimulation.

Lymphocyte progenitor cells then leave the site of stem cell reproduction and migrate to the *primary lymphatic*

Fig. 1-2 The hematopoietic system.

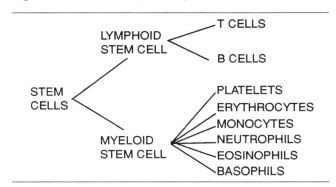

organs, where they undergo proliferation and differentiation independent of any stimulation by antigen, become committed to behave as either B or T cells, and define the specificity of their antigen-binding receptors. Two primary lymphatic organs exist: the thymus, where progenitor cells become T cells, and the B-cell organ equivalent to the avian bursa of Fabricius. In mammals, progenitor lymphocytes probably develop into B cells in the bone marrow, gut-associated lymphoepithelial structures (GALT; e.g., appendix, tonsils), the lymphocyte-infiltrated epithelium that lines mucosal surfaces (MALT), and lymph nodes. The committed lymphocytes leave the primary lymphatic organs and migrate, via the blood, to other *secondary lymphatic structures.* These consist of the spleen, the lymph nodes, and less organized clusters of lymphocytes in many tissues and organs. Here, the lymphocytes reside for a while, leave the blood vessels and enter the tissue, and recirculate via the lymphatics. When they encounter the antigen for which they have a specific affinity, these uncommitted lymphocytes proliferate and further differentiate. The ability of lymphocytes to recirculate from blood to tissues and back through the lymphoid system is unique to these cells and, coupled with their long life span and antigenic specificity, equips them for their central role in the adaptive immune response. The thorough mixing of lymphocytes, particularly in the spleen and lymph nodes, ensures the maximum contact of antigen presenting cells, which have newly encountered antigen, with lymphocytes. The bodywide dissemination of expanded T- and B-cell populations in readiness for a second encounter with the same antigen ensures that memory is available at all sites. Leukocyte entry into tissues is controlled by interaction between the endothelium and adhesion molecules. These latter consist of *selectins* (induced in the endothelial cells by thrombin, histamine, cytokines, etc., and cause neutrophils and other leukocytes to accumulate and roll along the vessel wall), *integrins* (synthesized by leukocytes and strengthen their binding to the epithelium), and recently discovered members of the Ig superfamily molecules. There is a tendency for different types of lymphocytes to "home" to different regions of the lymphoid organs due to either chemotactic factors unique to these regions or some kind of preferential adhesion (specific molecules and their receptors). In general, lymph nodes respond to antigens introduced into the tissues they drain and the spleen to antigens in the blood. The gut, lungs, and external mucous surfaces also have their own less specialized lymphoid organs. Five hundred billion lymphocytes are present in the body. Most leave the blood system through specialized regions called the high endothelial venules (HEV), although in areas of inflammation they can pass through nonspecialized endothelium.

The two fundamentally different classes of lymphocytes, B and T cells, look alike and are differentiated on the basis of cell surface antigens and response to mitogens (compounds that cause mitosis, i.e., cell proliferation). In humans, B cells have immunoglobulin, receptors for the C3 component of complement, and a receptor for Fc regions of immunoglobulins on their surface and respond to pokeweed mitogen. T cells have a receptor for sheep red blood cells on their surface and respond to concanavalin.

In a normal, healthy individual, the majority of lymphocytes seen are small (6–8 μ); they have scanty mitochondria, no endoplasmic reticulum, and little cytoplasm, which forms a slight rim around a dense nucleus. These can be B or T cells and are thought to consist of uncommitted lymphocytes (i.e., those not yet stimulated by exposure to specific antigen) and memory cells. Binding of specific antigen to a small lymphocyte causes it to enlarge (up to 25 μ), proliferate, and further differentiate. Large lymphocytes have more cytoplasm, which is rich in mitochondria and polysomes (protein production), and some B cells have endoplasmic reticulum and a Golgi apparatus (i.e., a secretory system). Some of both B and T large lymphocytes revert to small lymphocytes that circulate over a long time period as *memory cells.* Large T cells can be divided into T helpers, T killers (called cytotoxic T lymphocytes, or CTL), and possibly other types (suppressors?). T helper cells are divided into two subsets according to which cytokines they produce: Th1 are involved in cytotoxic immune responses and secrete interleukin-2 (IL2) and interferon-gamma (INF-gamma); Th2 are involved in antibody-mediated responses and secrete IL4, IL5, and IL10. Most large B cells further differentiate into *plasma cells.* These are even larger (about 2 times), have an eccentric cartwheel-like nucleus, and stain more intensely with basic dyes. They are rarely seen in the peripheral blood and are the most active of all B cells in the synthesis and secretion of immunoglobulins. Leukocytes have been recently differentiated on the basis of surface antigens recognized using monoclonal antibody. These are called *cluster of differentiation* (CD) antigens and over 100 have been defined. Major CD antigens worthy of note at this stage are CD4 on T helper cells and CD8 on CTL T cells. CD3 combines with the T-cell receptor to form the complex involved in antigen recognition.

Natural killer cells have been recognized as lymphocytes that do not have the surface markers associated with B and T cells. They arise in the bone marrow, mature in unknown sites, and are present as mature NK cells in the bone marrow, blood (10–15% of lymphocytes), and spleen (1–2%). Only a few are found in the lymph nodes or thymus. They do not rearrange their Ig or TCR genes, but have CD56 and -16 on their surfaces (these are not specific as both are found on some T cells and other leukocytes). They are able to recognize and kill autologous (self) and allogeneic tumors without requiring an immune response or the recognition of MHC antigens on the target cells. They also can kill, without prior exposure to the antigen, virus-infected cells and so form the first layer of defense before the induction of antibodies and antigen-specific CTL. Because they have CD16 on their surface, they can bind Fc regions of mainly IgG1 and IgG3, and hence attack cells coated with these immunoglobulins—antibody-dependent cellular cytotoxicity (ADCC). Resting NK cells can kill only a few tumors but they can be activated by exposure to cytokines, for example, IL2, to kill virtually all tumors. These lymphokine-activated killer (LAK) cells are almost all NK cells although some T cells are also activated. This is the basis of recent therapy attempts. Note that NK cells appear to require 24 hours to regenerate after killing whereas CTL cells can kill again immediately after a kill.

Cells of the *mononuclear phagocyte system* arise in the bone marrow from stem cells and can mature into varied morphologic forms. They first appear in blood as monocytes, having bean shaped nuclei and finely granular cytoplasm, and then migrate to tissues and mature into macrophages (histiocytes). If activated, which can occur by a variety of stimuli, they can develop into a variety of forms, such as epithelioid cells with abundant cytoplasm multinucleate giant cells from cell fusions, and are given different names according to their location in the body. Macrophages phagocytose foreign material, kill viable bacteria, present some of this material to T cells, and secrete cytokines.

Inflammation

Inflammation is a process initiated in response to injury and is essential for the survival of the host. Because of the nature of the environment and the natural microbial flora of skin and mucous membranes, injury is almost always accompanied by an influx of potentially harmful microorganisms. Inflammation is designed to limit this invasion to the area of injury and prevent spread of microorganisms to the mainstream of the body. Inflammation involves interlocking networks of the complement, clotting, fibrinolysis, and kinin systems and of cellular elements. All these systems are dependent on proteolytic and other enzymatic reactions, which are regulated by activation of inactive precursors by selective proteolysis, positive feedback, stoichiometric inhibition, multistep amplification, and enzymatic degradation of active products. The inflammatory process comprises a series of biochemical and microanatomic changes of the terminal vascular bed and of the connective tissues. These changes are intended to eliminate the injurious agents and to repair the damaged tissue but in some cases the effect can be detrimental to the host. It can be seen as redness (rubor), swelling (tumor), heat (calor), and pain (dolor).

Acute inflammation occurs upon tissue injury. Blood vessels in the injured region become dilated (erythema) so that their permeability is increased and fluid accumulates in the tissue (edema). Initial vasodilation can be due to damage to mast cells by trauma, heat, and ultraviolet (UV) light, resulting in release of vasoactive amines (histamine) and heparin. The Hageman factor (clotting factor XII) is activated with the formation of factor XIa and initiation of the kinin cascade and the coagulation cascade. Clotting of the blood by deposition of fibrin aids in trapping the deleterious agents at the site of injury so that they can be destroyed before spreading to other parts of the body. Kallikrein (chemotactic for leukocytes) and bradykinin are formed. Platelets are also caught up in the clot. Once a clot is produced, the resulting thrombin released causes the conversion of plasminogen to plasmin, which begins digesting the clot. Because of the accumulation of fluid in the area, the local levels of antibody, complement factors, kinins, and opsonins increases and toxins formed are diluted. Platelets, neutrophils, and monocytes release prostaglandins (PG), leukotrienes (LT), and other degradation products, which increase the vascular permeability. PG and LT are derived from metabolism of arachidonic acid, a component of most cell membranes, and are responsible for pain, fever, and attraction (chemotaxis) of polymorphonuclear leukocytes (PMNs) in addition to increasing vascular permeability. Cross-reactive protein (CRP) appears within hours of injury and binds to phosphorylcholine (on the surface of many bacteria), where the complex is able to fix complement. Thus, complement fixation can occur before the formation of antibody with the formation of C3a and C5a, which stimulate mast cells to release amines, and C3b, which sticks to particles and enhances phagocytosis. Physiologic and biochemical changes occur, for example, increased carbon dioxide, decreased oxygen, increased body temperature, and accumulation of organic acids, which may help to deter invading bacteria. Final resolution with tissue repair occurs when macrophages have removed any invading bacteria, fibroblasts appear, and collagen is deposited. The cytokines tumor necrosis factor (TNF) and transforming growth factor β (TGF-beta) are involved in this healing.

Persistence of the deleterious agent following the initial acute inflammatory process can lead to *chronic inflammation,* for example, foreign bodies such as silica or asbestos and urate crystals in gout. In their efforts to remove the agents, the leukocytes release lysosomal enzymes, especially when they die in the area, which cause damage to the surrounding healthy tissue. This situation can lead to chronic immunologic disorders such as rheumatoid arthritis. Chronic inflammation may eventually resolve, especially if the irritant can be removed, or can lead to granulomatous inflammation.

Persistent inflammation can occur that is characterized by the presence of mononuclear cells, that is, lymphocytes, monocytes, plasma cells, macrophages, and epithelioid cells, and is termed *granulomatous inflammation*. Granulomas may form in response to nonantigenic body irritants (nonimmune type) or they may have an immune component. They are especially important in delayed-type hypersensitivity.

Immunologic Inflammation

Inflammation can be induced by injury, trauma, heat, or tissue-damaging chemicals but is also induced by immunologic reactions involving specific recognition of antigen. In cell-mediated immunity (delayed-type hypersensitivity), antigen is processed by an antigen presenting cell (APC) and presented in the context of class II MHC antigen to a Th1 T cell. This results in the activation of the cell with production of mediators (MIF, MAF, INF-gamma, CF, and IL2), causing chemotaxis, vasodilation, fibrin deposition, and granuloma formation. Immune complexes, IgE, and basophils can also participate in inflammatory reactions.

B Cells and the Humoral Immune System

Stem cells programmed to develop into B cells leave the bone marrow (yolk sac and fetal liver before birth) and develop into B cells in a variety of locations equivalent to the avian bursa of Fabricius. They then migrate to secondary lymphatic structures, which provide an optimal microenvironment for antigen processing, cellular interaction, and development of the immune response.

The Spleen

The spleen is a large (200 g in an adult man), capsulated, vascular organ. The splenic artery enters the spleen and divides into arterioles that are surrounded by a sheath of lymphocytes. These are visible macroscopically and called the *white pulp*. In this periarteriole sheath, the T cells surround the arteriole and the B cells mainly lie on top of the T-cell layer and may form follicles. The white pulp is surrounded by a *marginal zone* containing specialized antigen presenting cells and B cells. These arterioles become thinner, lose their sheath, and divide into capillaries that enter into venous sinuses and hence into the splenic vein. The splenic artery and vein are called "travecular" because they are supported by fibrous tissue. These venous sinuses, associated blood vessels, and cords of reticular tissue (Billroth's cords) constitute the macroscopically red

region of the spleen—the *red pulp* (some lymphocytes may be present—T and B cells).

The Lymph Node

The lymph node parenchyma consists of a network of reticular fibers and reticular cells within which motile cells (lymphocytes, plasma cells, and macrophages) are trapped loosely. The node filters out antigen from the incoming lymph. Afferent (incoming) lymph vessels enter around the circumference of the node where they form sinuses. Lymph leaves the node via a vessel at the hilus; blood vessels enter and leave here. Blood and lymph come in close contact.

The node is divided into an outer *cortex* and a *medulla*. The former consists of an external cortex (also called subcapsular cortex), where the lymphoid follicles and their germinal centers are located containing predominantly B cells, and the deep cortex (also called the paracortical, paracortex, or diffuse cortex), which contains the blood vessels and some lymphocytes (mainly T cells). The medulla is less cellular and contains many sinuses with a few macrophages, plasma cells, and T cells. Lymph nodes are found in the groin, the underarm, and the neck and in the mesenteric region. Their HEV (high endothelial venule) for lymphocyte passage is mainly in the paracortex. In the external cortex, lymphocytes cluster together to form darkly staining areas called primary follicles. Some of these primary follicles develop further as a result of antigenic stimulation, to form secondary follicles characterized by a definite structure with a germinal center on their inside. *Secondary follicles* have a polarity when compared to the outer layer (capsule) of the lymph node: Nearest the capsule is a cap of lymphocytes, which comprises those cells in the primary follicle before the germinal center was formed. Below the cap is the *germinal center*, divided into two regions: a zone staining lighter than the cap and containing small lymphocytes (the "light zone") and a zone staining lighter than the cap but darker than the light zone, called the "*dark*" or "*fertile*" *zone*. This dark zone consists of lymphocytes undergoing rapid mitosis, and various phases of development can be seen— plasma cells, large lymphocytes, small lymphocytes— together with some macrophages removing cell debris. Lymphocytes found in follicles are almost always B cells with T cells only rarely identified. However, T cells are necessary for development of the vast majority of germinal centers.

B Cells

Stem cells that are differentiating into B cells are first recognized as pre-B lymphocytes that have μ H chains (with both V and C regions) in their cytoplasm but no Ig on their membrane. They are found in hematopoietic tissue. The next stage is immature B lymphocytes in which L chains (kappa or lambda) are produced to form, with the μ H chains, IgM that is expressed on the cell surface and can react with specific antigen. However, contact with specific antigen (usually self at this stage) does not induce proliferation and development and may cause destruction (induction of tolerance). Migration into the periphery occurs as maturation continues to give mature B cells with both μ and delta H chains being produced and both IgM and IgD appearing as surface receptors. Contact with specific antigen causes proliferation and differentiation to form activated B lymphocytes. Here, most of the synthesized Ig is secreted; some cells produce a different H chain from the initial μ or delta (to form a different Ig class), that is, class switching; some change to an identifiable morphologic type (the plasma cell); and some probably never secrete much Ig but persist as membrane Ig-expressing memory cells. This progressive differentiation of activated B cells requires the influence of cytokines produced mainly by T helper cells (subclass Th2). Memory cells can persist for long periods and actively recirculate between the blood, lymph, and lymphoid organs. Contact with antigen leads to a secondary immune response.

The response of B cells to specific antigen comprises *proliferation* (increase in numbers) and *differentiation* where membrane-bound Ig is secreted and usually changes in terms of its H chain (class switch). The B cell is also a presenter of antigen to T cells and presents antigen at lower concentrations than macrophages. Protein antigens do not induce antibody without the involvement of T (helper) cells; the resting B cell requires two distinct types of signal, the specific antigen plus some soluble product (cytokine) of T helper cells. Lipids and polysaccharides apparently do not require the T-cell involvement (thymus-independent antigens) in mice but the position in humans is not clear. A response to antigen that has never been seen before (a primary response) involves resting B and T cells and takes a certain time course. Exposure to the same antigen at a later date (a secondary response) involves memory B and T cells, which are in greater number than the original inducible resting cells so that the response is faster, reaches a higher level, and lasts longer. With increasing time of the immune response, antibodies produced become of greater affinity (have a stronger binding for the antigens) because of *somatic mutation* and selection of those B cells that produce the higher-affinity Ig. (Some of these going into memory cells will allow the secondary response to occur with a lower level of antigen than needed for a primary response.)

Upon binding to antigen, the surface Ig (which is evenly distributed over the cell surface) forms small groups that migrate to one part of the cell to form a large group that is taken into the B cell (receptor-mediated endocytosis). The cell enlarges, produces more messenger ribonucleic acid (mRNA), more receptors for T-helper cytokines, and more of its class II MHC molecules. Close to the surface IgM and IgD are two other proteins called *Ig-beta* (also called B29) and *IgM-alpha* (also called MB1). When IgM or IgD binds with its specific epitope, it undergoes conformational change that causes IgM-alpha and Ig-beta to activate tyrosine kinase and initiate the antibody production response. Also involved in this first stage of B-cell activation are activation of phospholipase, increase in intracellular calcium ions, activation of protein kinase C, and increase in transcription initiators (c-fos and C-myc).

The antigen is broken down to peptides and these are combined with the class II MHC antigens so that the B cell can now present the antigen to T helper cells. These peptides are not usually the regions of the original protein antigen that combined with the B-cell surface Ig. The T helper cells are presented with peptides in collaboration with class II MHC antigens by both the activated B cells and other accessory cells. Following this presentation, the T helper cells produce cytokines that influence the B cell to carry on with its functions, such as proliferation, secretion of Ig, class switch, and differentiation into plasma cells or memory cells. Other accessory cells, such as macrophages, also produce cytokines that influence the function of the activated B cells.

Immunoglobulins

Immunoglobulins are glycoprotein molecules that can specifically combine with the substances that elicited their formation. However, "natural" antibodies occur at low levels in serum although no known antigenic stimulus has occurred, for example, anti–blood group substances. They are found in serum (20% of total plasma proteins), extravascular fluids, and exocrine secretions, and on the surface of some lymphocytes, for example, saliva, nasal secretions, sweat, milk, colostrum, cerebrospinal fluid (CSF), and ascites fluid. After combination with antigen, they can initiate a series of secondary reactions, such as complement fixation, histamine release, and stimulation of macrophages to phagocytose antigen. Based on electrophoresis, they are classified as gamma globulins and are extremely heterogeneous in terms of specificity. Table 1-1 lists the five classes of immunoglobulins and describes their differentiating characteristics.

The basic unit of structure is a monomer of four peptide chains: two identical light (L) chains (mol. wt. 23,000) and two identical heavy (H) chains (mol. wt. 50,000–70,000). Disulfide bonds (-S-S-) between cysteine residues are found intrachain, that is, joining residues within the same chain, and interchain, that is, joining residues of different

Table 1-1   Properties of Human Immunoglobulins (Ig)

Ig Class	Molecular Weight	Heavy Chain Half-life (days)	% Total Ig	Complement Fixation	Transfer	Location	Function
IgG	150,000	25	80	+	Placenta	Blood—60% Fluids—40% Secretions—0	Major systemic Ig
IgM	900,000	5	6	+ +	None	Blood—90% Fluids—10% Secretions—0	Major early-response Ig
IgA	385,000	6	13	Alternate pathway	Milk	Blood—15% Fluids—low Secretions—85%	Major Ig on mucosal surfaces
IgE	190,000	2	0.002	—	None	Blood—very low Fluids—very low Secretions—100%	Allergic responses
IgD	180,000	3	1	—	None	Blood—low Majority on B cells	Involved in B-cell response

chains (may be H-H, H-L, and L-L). Each chain is composed of a variable (V) and a constant (C) region, so named because many more amino acid differences occur between related chains in the V region than in the C region. Chains are composed of globular regions, about 110 amino acids in length, called *domains* and characterized by an intrachain disulfide bond linking residue 22 (approximate) to residue 88 (approximate). The variable region (V) of the light (L) chain is one domain. The variable region (V) of the heavy (H) chain is one domain. The constant (C) region of the light (L) chain is one domain. The constant (C) region of the heavy (H) chain is three to four domains. The antibody-binding site for specific antigen is formed by three small regions of the V_L and three small regions of the V_H domains coming together in the three-dimensional structure of the folded immunoglobulin to form a cleft or pocket. This area is large enough to bind with four amino acids and six sugars. The hinge region is on the H chain just below the fork between the C_H^1 and the C_H^2 domains (Fig. 1-3) and allows flexibility so that the two binding sites (in the V region) can move in space. Limiting digestion of an immunoglobulin molecule with papain breaks the molecule above the hinge region to yield two Fab fragments and one Fc fragment (Fab is *f*ragment carrying the *a*ntibody *b*inding site and Fc is *f*ragment readily *c*rystallized). Digestion with pepsin yields one F (ab')$_2$ fragment with digestion of the remaining Fc portion, that is, cleavage below the hinge region. Immunoglobulins are sometimes associated with other peptides. J chain is a polypeptide normally found in polymeric forms, and secretory component (SC) is part of the IgA molecule found in secretions. Secondary biologic activities, which occur after Ag/Ab combination, are associated with the Fc fragment region. Immunoglobulins are found in vertebrates only.

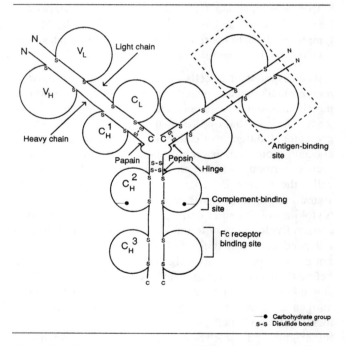

Fig. 1-3 Diagrammatic representation of a human IgG immunoglobulin showing the sites of papain and pepsin digestion.

Classification of Immunoglobulins

The terms "classes" and "subclasses" are used for immunoglobulins and H chains. The terms "types" and "subtypes" are used for L chains. Five classes of immunoglobulin are differentiated based on the H chain present and called IgA (H chain alpha), IgD (H chain delta), IgE (H chain epsilon), IgG (H chain gamma), and IgM (H chain mu). Two types of light (L) chain, called lambda and kappa, are found in all five classes of immunoglobulins, but the two types never occur together naturally in the same individual immunoglobulin molecule; kappa chains show allotypes but no subtypes whereas lambda chains show six or more subtypes with no allotypes. Four subclasses of gamma H chain exist with two subclasses of alpha H chains.

Immunoglobulins as Antigens

Immunoglobulins are large complex protein molecules and act as potent antigens when introduced into a vertebrate circulation in which they are foreign. This property has been used to prepare antisera specific for the different classes of immunoglobulin and for their different regions. Different types of antigens have been recognized. *Isotypes* are present in all members of the same species and are used to divide the immunoglobulins into classes and subclasses of H chains and types and subtypes of L chains. *Allotypes* are present in some but not all members of the same species, for example, blood group antigens. They exhibit a mendelian pattern of inheritance and have been found on gamma H chains (Gm allotypes), alpha-2 H chains (A2m allotypes), and kappa L chains (Inv allotypes). Idiotypes are highly specific determinants that occur on molecules made by a single clone of immunoglobulin-producing cells. The determinant is in, or very close to, the binding site and depends on the 3D structure of the H and L chains in this region. This is the "private" or "unique" idiotype. Inbred mice show private idiotypes plus "shared" or "public" idiotypes found in all antibodies raised against the same antigen.

Pure Immunoglobulins

Exposure of a vertebrate to an antigen results in the production of a large number of different antibodies—different immunoglobulin classes, immunoglobulins specific for different epitopes, and immunoglobulins with different capacities to bind to a given determinant. Detailed knowledge of immunoglobulin structure requires the availability of pure immunoglobulin, and this has been obtained from patients with multiple myeloma and other neoplastic diseases of lymphoid cells in which (usually) a single antibody-producing cell becomes malignant and its progeny secrete a single immunoglobulin into the serum. Such serum proteins (called M proteins, monoclonal proteins, or paraproteins) are easily isolated and purified for study. Bence Jones (B-J) proteins are L chains, usually dimers, that occur in the urine of some of these patients. As a group, patients with multiple myeloma produce only B-J proteins (10%), only whole M proteins (40%), or both M proteins and B-J proteins (50%). Myeloma tumors arise in other animals, for example, MOPC tumors caused by

injection of mineral oil into the peritoneal cavity of inbred strains of mice.

Pure immunoglobulins (monoclonal antibodies) for diagnostic and other work are now prepared using hybridomas. Mice are immunized and their spleen cells fused with mouse tumor cells growing in culture. The resulting hybrid cells are screened for those that produce the specific single immunoglobulin of an original parental spleen cell. These cells produce a pure immunoglobulin in culture and can be grown as tumors in histocompatible mice to produce extraordinary levels of such immunoglobulin, for example, 5 to 15 mg/ml.

Individual Classes of Immunoglobulins

IgG comprises 75 percent of normal serum immunoglobulins, is divided into four subclasses (total IgG = 60–70% IgG1; 14–20% IgG2; 4–8% IgG3; 2–6% IgG4), is the only class able to pass through the placenta (IgG2 is the least able to do so) and therefore is responsible for protection of the newborn, and can fix complement (IgG3 > IgG1 > IgG2) by the classic pathway. IgG_4 cannot use the classic pathway but may mediate in the alternate pathway.

IgA is the predominant immunoglobulin in secretions, comprises 15 percent of serum immunoglobulin, and occurs as a monomer (7S IgA) or polymer to which J chain and secretory component may be attached. It is secreted as a dimer with attached (noncovalently) J chain (10S IgA) and transported through epithelial cells of the basement membrane, which add SC to produce secretory IgA.

IgM comprises 10 percent of normal serum immunoglobulins and occurs as a pentameric polymer made up of five monomer units plus one J chain. It is the predominant early antibody and is very efficient at fixing complement. It is one of the two (with IgD) major immunoglobulins on the surface of B cells.

IgD is at low levels in serum (0.2% of normal serum immunoglobulins) and is present on the surface of B cells.

IgE comprises 0.002 to 0.004 percent of normal serum immunoglobulins, is important in allergy, and is called "reagin." The Fc region of IgE has extremely high affinity for special cell surface receptors on tissue mast cells and basophilic leukocytes. Cross-linking of IgE, bound to these cells, by antigen causes release of powerful vasoactive amines (e.g., histamine).

Genetic Basis of Immunoglobulin Structure

Immunoglobulin chains are specified on the chromosome by fragmented regions of DNA (exons). This information is transcribed into mRNA and translated into protein in a sequence that allows cutting and splitting of both deoxyribonucleic acid (DNA) and RNA. H and L chains are synthesized with an N-terminal piece of about 20 amino acids called a "leader." It is made up predominantly of hydrophobic amino acids and functions to guide the chains to specific receptors on the membrane of the endoplasmic reticulum. The chains then pass into a vesicle where the H and L chains are assembled to form immunoglobulin molecules. The leaders are cleaved off and the mature immunoglobulins are extruded from the cell.

Figure 1-4 shows how light and heavy chains are selected and synthesized.

The first rearrangement involves the heavy-chain locus (found on chromosome 14) and leads to the joining of one D and one J segment with deletion of the intervening DNA (Fig. 1-4). The D segments 5' of the rearranged D and the J segments 3' of the rearranged J are not affected by this recombination. DJ rearrangement may occur prior to commitment of a lymphoid precursor to the B-cell lineage. Following the DJ rearrangement, one of the many V genes is joined to the DJ complex, giving rise to a rearranged VDJ gene. At this stage, all segments 5' of the rearranged D are also deleted. This VDJ recombination occurs only in cells committed to become B lymphocytes and is a critical control point in Ig expression because only the rearranged V gene is subsequently transcribed. The C region genes remain separated from this VDJ complex by an intron (presumably containing the unrearranged J segments), and the primary (nuclear) RNA transcript has the same organization. It is not known whether all the C regions are expressed in the primary transcript. Subsequent processing of the RNA leads to splicing out of the intron between the VDJ complex and the most proximal C region gene, which is C, giving rise to a functional mRNA for the heavy chain. Multiple adenine nucleotides, called poly-A tails, are added to one of several consensus polyadenylation sites located 3' of the CRNA. Genes coding for other C_H classes also have 3' polyadenylation sites, which are utilized when these C regions are expressed. It is thought that cleavage of the primary RNA transcript and splicing are tightly coupled to polyadenylation, since most functional, complete mRNAs have poly-A tails. How these events are coor-

Fig. 1-4 Arrangement of the human genes controlling immunoglobulin structure in their embryonic form.

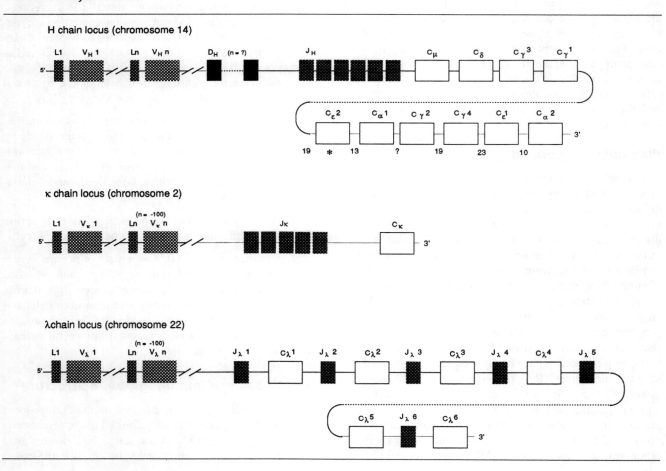

dinately regulated is not known. Translation of the heavy-chain mRNA leads to production of the protein, giving rise to the phenotype of the pre-B lymphocyte.

The next somatic DNA recombination involves a light-chain locus (on chromosome 2 and then on chromosome 22) and follows an essentially similar sequence. One V segment is joined to one J segment, forming a VJ complex, which remains separated from the C region by an intron, and this gives rise to the primary RNA transcript. Splicing of the intron from the primary transcript joins the C gene to the VJ complex, forming an mRNA that is translated to produce the kappa or lambda protein. The light chain assembles with the previously synthesized μ heavy chain in the endoplasmic reticulum to form the complete membrane IgM molecule, which is expressed on the cell surface, and the cell is now the immature B lymphocyte. Rearrangements of Ig genes are the essential first steps in the production of antibodies. In addition, the heavy-chain protein that is synthesized in a developing B cell itself regulates the somatic recombination of Ig genes in two ways. It irreversibly inhibits rearrangements on the other chromosome and stimulates light-chain gene rearrangement. Rearrangements of light-chain genes occur first in the kappa locus. If the kappa rearrangement is productive, giving rise to a kappa protein, subsequent rearrangement of the lambda light chain is blocked. Rearrangement of the lambda locus occurs only if the rearranged kappa genes on both parental chromosomes are unable to code for a functional protein. This explains why an individual B-cell clone can produce only one of the two types of light chains during its life (light-chain isotype exclusion).

The mature B lymphocyte is the functionally responsive stage in B-cell maturation in which membrane-associated μ and delta heavy chains are co-expressed on the surface of each cell in association with kappa and lambda light chains. Both classes of Ig heavy chains have the same V region and, therefore, the same antigen specificity. Simultaneous expression of a single V_H with both C μ and C delta to form the two heavy chains is thought to occur by alternative RNA splicing. A long primary RNA transcript is produced containing the rearranged VDJ complex as well as sequences encoded by C genes. If the introns are spliced out such that the VDJ complex is attached to the C μ RNA, it gives rise to a μ mRNA. If however, the C μ RNA is spliced out as well so that the VDJ complex becomes contiguous with C delta, a delta mRNA is produced. Subsequent translation results in the synthesis of complete μ or delta heavy-chain isotypes.

Additional variation in the V regions is brought about by lack of specificity in the actual base pairs involved at the site of DNA joining and in the accumulation of mutations in the V region during the life of the activated B cell (somatic mutation). Mutations that result in the production of higher-affinity antibody are selected out.

Membrane-Bound and Secretory Ig

The DNA coding for the constant region of the H chain consists of one exon for the C chain plus a small exon coding for a tail piece, one exon coding for a transmembrane piece, and one exon coding for a cystoplasmic piece. If the mRNA is transcribed with all this information, the IgM will be membrane bound. Regulation mechanisms for these alternatives are not understood. Little is known about the other Ig classes.

Class Switching

After antigenic stimulation, mature IgM and IgD producing B cells also undergo class switching allowing their progeny to produce Ig with H chains of different classes. Two mechanisms are involved: orderly deletion of H-chain genes and alternative RNA splicing. The latter takes place early in the differentiation. Class switching at the DNA level is not a random process and is affected by genetic background (individuals and their progeny may have a definite ratio of classes produced), cell milieu (B cells in mucosal regions have a marked tendency to produce IgA), and the secreted cytokines of T helper cells (IL4 for IgE, INF-gamma for IgG2a).

The different immunoglobulin classes are metabolized at different rates and vary from IgE (96% of total is turned over in 1 day) to IgG (6–7% of total is turned over in 1 day; IgG3 is 17%).

Evolution

Immunoglobulins have only been demonstrated in vertebrates. Primitive vertebrates and fish have IgM, amphibians and reptiles have IgM and IgG, IgA appears with birds, IgE with most mammals, and IgD in primates and some other mammals.

Development of the Normal Immune System

The capacity for specific immunologic responses does not develop as an all-or-none phenomenon but rather appears in a stepwise fashion for different antigens. The thymus appears 6 to 7 weeks into embryologic life and by 8 weeks has lymphocytes present with T-cell markers that leave and populate the body. B cells with immunoglobulin on their surface are in the liver at 9.5 weeks and peripheral blood by 11.5 weeks. IgM and IgE appear by 10.5 weeks, and IgG by 12 weeks, all at low levels. IgA is not detected but SC is in the urine. Maternal IgG is significant by 12 weeks. Cord blood usually contains IgM (10% adult level) and a little IgG, IgD, and IgE as well as maternal IgG. In the newborn human, maternal IgG is adequate as opsonin for gram-positive bacteria and viruses but not for gram-negative bacteria (needs IgM). Premature infants have less maternal IgG and are consequently more susceptible to infection, but usually mature at the same rate as full-term babies. IgM shows a rapid rise to adult level by 1 year. Maternal IgG is degraded by 6 to 8 months, and synthesis to adult level occurs by 6 to 7 years. IgA and IgE show a later rise than IgG but reach adult level by 7 years.

Use of Immunoglobulins in the Diagnosis of Disease

Serum levels of the different classes of immunoglobulins are performed in diagnosis of immunodeficiency diseases, specific antibodies are used to diagnose infections (comparison of acute and convalescent sera) or prepared for identification of microorganisms, and immune complexes or autoantibodies are screened in certain disease conditions.

Possible Future Uses for Immunoglobulin

Hybrid antibodies containing two different antigen-binding sites have been used to "home" a chemotherapeutic compound to a specific site in the body. Chimeric immunoglobulins combine specific regions of mouse monoclonal antibodies with human Fc regions to avoid an immune response against them. Antiimmunoglobulins are being tested as vaccines.

Cells Containing Receptors That Bind IgG

Mononuclear phagocytes have a receptor when cytokine activated (called CD64) that binds IgG1 > IgG3 > IgG4 > IgG2. Mononuclear phagocytes, neutrophils, eosinophils, and platelets have a receptor called FcRII (CD32) that binds IgG1 > IgG3 = IgG4 >> IgG2. In both cases, if the cell is phagocytic (all except platelets) the receptors allow the cell to bind to antigen coated with its specific IgG antibody and more easily phagocytose it than if the antigen is not coated. Natural killer cells, neutrophils, eosinophils, and macrophages (but not monocytes) are capable of lysing various target cells, especially if the cell is coated with its specific IgG antibody. This is called antibody-dependent cell-mediated cytotoxicity (ADCC) and occurs because these cells have a receptor called FcIII (CD16) that can bind IgG1 = IgG3, not IgG2 or IgG4.

Transgenic Mice

Linearized DNA of choice (can be manipulated by recombinant DNA techniques) is injected into the pronucleus of recently fertilized mouse eggs, the eggs are transferred to the oviduct of a pseudopregnant female, and development is allowed to continue. Usually, 70 percent of the resulting pups have the injected DNA (called the transgene) at some random site in one of their chromosomes (usually head-to-tail in about 50 copies) and breed true. Such mice have been used to study the effects of genes not normally present, to alter genes controlling development, to alter regulation, and to delete normally present genes.

B-Cell Tumors

Normal cellular genes that code for proteins involved in cell growth and regulation are tightly regulated in terms of their expression. Some of these, called protooncogenes, can cause the cell to become malignant, that is, function as oncogenes, if they are altered by mutation, if they are placed in other regions of the genome by retroviruses (where their regulation is not effective), or if their expression is altered. Because the B-cell DNA is unusually active in terms of its being cut and spliced, it has an unusually high chance of accidentally incorporating pieces of distant genes. In the case of Burkitt's lymphoma the misincorporation is a gene called c-myc. Similar DNA manipulation also occurs in T cells and these are also susceptible to malignancy of the same origin.

T Cells and the Cellular Immune System

The thymus arises from an anlage (the first assembly of cells in an embryo, which constitutes the beginning of a future tissue, organ, or part) of the third and fourth endodermal pharyngeal pouches. This anlage progressively loses its ties with the pharynx, its central lumen disappears, and it migrates to its final position in the upper thorax. The thymic and parathyroid primordia are the same. The thymic anlage is then colonized with stem cells from the yolk sac (early in fetal life), the fetal liver (later in fetal life), and the bone marrow (after birth).

The mature thymus is divided into lobules (small, 0.5–2.0 mm, globular areas) by connective tissue and continuity between lobules is provided by narrow bridges of parenchymal tissue. Thymic parenchymal tissue consists of a network of epithelial cells that delineate spaces in which lymphocytes accumulate. Staining shows that each lobule is divided into two parts. The *cortex* is a darkly staining outer area of the lobule that is very rich in lymphocytes. These lymphocytes are mainly of the small type, and show a high incidence of mitosis, indicating rapid proliferation. Some have already acquired T-cell membrane antigens. There is also evidence that a large number of these lymphocytes die locally. The *medulla* is the central area of the lobule that stains lightly and is much less abundant in lymphocytes. Those present are more mature than the cortical lymphocytes, that is, they contain a higher percentage of large lymphocytes, are able to respond to mitogens, and can induce the graft-versus-host response. Some of the epithelial cells in the medulla form aggregates in which the cells are piled and coiled on and around each other. These structures are called *Hassall's corpuscles or Hassall's bodies*. The function of Hassall's bodies remains obscure, but, because their blood supply resembles that of an endocrine gland, it has been suggested that they secrete something into the circulation that may influence thymocyte development. Blood enters each lobule in an arteriole at the junction between the cortex and the medulla. The arteriole divides to form capillaries, which eventually coalesce to form a venule that passes through the corticomedullary junction. The normal, healthy thymus does not contain lymphoid follicles or germinal centers. However, these are present in some pathologic states, such as lupus erythematosus.

T Cell Development

Pluripotential, hematopoietic stem cells migrate from their region of production, and those programmed to eventually become T cells are entrapped in the cortex of the thymus, where they accumulate. It appears that the immature lymphocytes that reach the thymus are at a stage of developing into either T cells or B cells, and it is the location in which they continue maturation that determines their eventual type. Here they divide rapidly but only a small proportion (about 5%) survive to become mature T cells. Such division does not depend upon the presence of antigen. These immigrant, rapidly dividing cells are called *thymocytes* and the region of rapid division and death is located in the deep area of the cortex. As the thymocytes pass from the deep to the surface area of the cortex, they come under the influence of a hormone, thymosin, produced by the epithelial cells of the thymus, which induces the thymocytes to mature. Cells near the surface of the cortex have acquired the T-cell surface antigens. These semi-immature T cells then pass from the cortex to the medulla, where they complete their maturation and acquire the ability to respond to mitogens and react with foreign cells (graft-vs.-host response). They are now indistinguishable from circulating T cells. Mature T cells leave the thymus by passing through the medullary venule wall. The blood vessels of the cortex appear to be impermeable to molecules large enough to be considered antigenic and hence the thymocytes and partially mature T cells are protected against exposure to antigen. The blood vessels of the medulla, on the other hand, are antigen permeable so that it is possible for medullary T cells to be exposed to antigen before they enter the general circulation. The parenchyma of the thymus is not penetrated by lymph vessels. Cell death in the maturation process appears to be a way of selecting positively for T cells that can react strongly with the MHC antigen of the body and negatively against those that do not bind MHC proteins or that react with peptides from the individual's own body. In some cases, cells that can react with self antigens are turned off but not killed. This is called *anergy*.

Thymic Involution

The thymus is largest at the onset of puberty and decreases in size with continuing age. As elderly individuals can obviously mount an effective immune response, there must be other sites where T cells mature. The T-cell receptor is made up of dimers of four possible proteins, called alpha, beta, gamma, and delta. Young people have T cells maturing in the thymus that have mainly TCRs of alpha/beta dimers; older people with maturation outside the thymus have TCRs with gamma/delta dimers.

T Lymphocytes

On leaving the thymus, the mature T cells circulate throughout the blood and lymph systems. They are the major lymphocyte found in the blood and lymph, and also are found to accumulate in the white matter of the spleen, in the perifollicular (little sac) and deep cortical regions of the lymph nodes, and in the bone marrow. T cells have many different surface antigens, called CD. Some are common to all T cells and some serve to divide the T cells into subsets. Major examples are:

TCR: the antigen receptor
CD2: the receptor for sheep RBC in rosette formation
CD3: forms the antigen receptor complex with TCR
CD4: recognizes class II MHC antigens
CD8: recognizes class I MHC antigens

Most T cells that are CD4 positive but CD8 negative (CD4$^+$/CD8$^-$) are T helper cells. They have been divided into two subsets: Th1, which secrete mainly interleukin-2 and interferon-gamma and are involved in cytotoxic immune responses, and Th2, which secrete mainly IL4, IL5, and IL10 and are involved in antibody responses. Cytotoxic T lymphocytes are CD4 negative and CD8 positive (CD4$^-$/CD8$^+$). These kill target cells and are important in viral infection, acute allograft rejection, and rejection of tumors. The majority express the CD8$^+$ antigen and require class I MHC antigen on the target cell for its recognition. They emerge from the thymus as "pre-CTL" cells that are committed to the CTL lineage, have the CD8$^+$ antigen, and have the TCR for a specific antigen, but have no ability to lyse target cells. First stimulation is by contact with specific antigen in a class I MHC antigen context that makes them susceptible to the action of cytokines produced by activated CD4+ T cells (IL2, IL4, IL6, and INF-gamma). In the presence of these cytokines, they mature into CTL cells that have lytic ability. Maturation and differentiation involve the development of membrane-bound cytoplasmic granules, which contain pore-forming protein (perforin or cytolysin), serine esterases, and protein toxins, and the secretion of cytokines. CTL killing is antigen specific, requires cell contact, does not affect bystander cells, and does not injure the CTLs, which can go on and kill multiple target cells. Cross-linking of TCRs on the CTL by specific antigen causes a trigger mechanism, leading to the delivery of a lethal hit. This consists of the secretion of granules in the area of contact, mainly the pore-forming protein, or of protein toxins that enter the target cell and break down the nuclear DNA (apoptosis).

Suppressor T Cells

These are a group of T cells that were thought to inhibit the immune functions of both T cells and B cells. They seem to be preferentially produced in cases of massive antigen exposure and perhaps are responsible for tolerance. They are of the CD8+ type, are able to react directly with antigen without the presence of MHC antigens, and act by secreting proteins and not the usual cytokines.

T Cell Recognition of Antigen

CD4+ T cells recognize peptides (usually derived from microbes and soluble antigens) bound to class II MHC antigens on the surface of accessory cells. CD8+ T cells recognize peptides derived from endogenously synthesized proteins such as viral proteins, bound to class I MHC antigens on cells that are the target of their lytic action. As only peptides can bind to the MHC antigens, T cells can only respond to protein antigens. B cells respond to proteins, polysaccharides, lipids, small bound chemicals, and perhaps nucleic acids. T cells respond to a linear array of amino acids while B cells respond to a linear array of amino acids or to an epitope in its tertiary structural form.

Accessory Cells

Antigen breakdown products are presented to the T cell by accessory cells. These are called antigen presenting cells. Foreign proteins from outside the accessory cells are taken in and partially broken down (antigen processing). Phagocytic cells take in the foreign material by phagocytosis and degrade it. Additionally, B cells react with foreign antigen through their surface immunoglobulin (which initiates the pathway to antibody production) and take in the foreign material by receptor-mediated endocytosis. The antigens are then degraded to peptides. MHC II molecules, present on the surface of antigen presenting cells (APCs), bind the peptides. The MHC II–peptide complex is then presented to the CD4+ T helper cells, where it is recognized as nonself. There are two levels of selection involved. The MHC II molecules can bind peptides 12 to 30 amino acids in length but not all of the possible peptide breakdown products of a given antigen. Also, the CD4+ cells do not have receptors (TCR) for all of the peptides that will be presented. Thus, the T-cell epitope depends on the type of MHC II and the extent of the TCR repertoire present. A few accessory cells are able to present antigen directly to T cells under normal conditions. However, most accessory cells are induced to produce class II antigens when exposed to interferon-gamma resulting from an immune response so that presentation is enhanced.

Foreign proteins synthesized in accessory cells are also partially degraded but by a different route that combines them with class I MHC antigen. The complex is recognized by CD8+ T cells. Here, the recognized peptides are 8 to 10 amino acids long. Again the actual part of a protein presented and recognized by the CD8+ cells depends on the type of MHC II protein possessed by the individual and the TCR repertoire.

The T-Cell Receptor

The antigen receptor on T cells is usually described as a heterodimer consisting of one alpha chain and one beta chain joined together by disulfide bonds. However, as T cells mature extrathymically with increasing age, a different receptor made up of a delta chain and an epsilon chain is found. Each chain has a variable (V) and a constant (C) region and, as they are not secreted, like the membrane-bound IgM they have a transmembrane piece and a cytoplasmic piece. The TCR chains are derived from complex DNA multiple alleles with DNA and RNA splicing and joining. There are not as many V genes for the TCR chains as there are for the Ig molecules, but the joining of VJ and DJ has much more leeway in the TCR system so that more V proteins can actually be produced. However, there are no somatic mutation changes in the TCR so that once the DNA joins are made the specificity is sealed. The TCR is able to recognize the peptide–MHC antigen complex on the antigen presenting cell and is found on the cell surface in association with the CD3 antigen, which is a complex of five polypeptide chains. Many chains (Ig, TCR, class I MHC, class II MHC, CD2, CD3, CD4, CD8, etc.) have domains with V and C regions. These antigens have been grouped together as the *Ig gene superfamily*.

Binding of TCR and Antigen

In the CD4+ T cell, the CD4 antigen recognizes the self class II MHC protein on the presenting cell, and the TCR (complexed with CD3) recognizes the antigenic peptide bound in the cleft of the MHC II molecule. These comprise the specific part of the reaction. However, if nothing further happens, the T cell goes into *activation-induced cell death* or *clonal anergy* (inability to react to this or other stimulation). For proliferation and differentiation to occur, the T cell requires co-stimulatory signals from the binding of a variety of T-cell and APC molecules. As a result of the specific binding, together with a co-stimulatory signal, the TCR influences CD3 to begin molecular events that result in cytokine secretion, cell proliferation, and so forth. Under normal circumstances, these accessory molecules are present and T cells are co-stimulated. The major effects of antigen binding to CD4$^+$ cells are secretion of cytokines (which act on other cells) and cell proliferation. In the cytotoxic CD8$^+$ T cell, CD8 recognizes the self class I MHC protein on the expressing target cell and TCR, complexed with CD3, recognizes the foreign protein on the MHC I protein. Co-stimulatory signals are again required to provide extra stability in the binding. CD3 is influenced to initiate a cascade of molecular events, which in this case results in killing of the target cell.

Adhesion Molecules

These molecules stabilize and strengthen the T cell and APC binding, and provide accessory signals for T-cell activation. They are also involved in T-cell binding to stroma cells. Major groups that have been recognized include extracellular matrix protein receptors and leukocyte adhesion proteins.

Regulation of the Immune Response

It is obvious that an immune response is turned off after a time but the exact mechanisms involved are not yet clear. Several mechanisms have been proposed. Antigens are removed by the effects of the immune response so that stimulation of the B and T cells ceases. Cells already responding eventually die and the response is diminished with their death. A network may also be built up in which newly synthesized Ig molecules have extensive idiotypic regions (some newly formed by somatic mutation) and the body will respond by making antibodies against these idiotypes and neutralizing them. Positive feedback can arise where Ig binds to unstimulated B cells through the Fc receptor, effectively preventing their binding of antigen. Cytokines that downregulate the immune response may be produced. Suppressor T cells may exist and act to suppress the effects of T helper and B cells.

Cytokines

Cytokines are mediators that function as up and down regulators of immunogenic, inflammatory, and reparative host responses to injury. Lymphocytes produce *lympho-*

kines and monocytes or macrophages produce *monokines*. They differ from hormones in that they are not produced by specialized glands, that they act on cells near their site of production rather than on distant target cells, and that they are not present in serum under normal circumstances. They are peptides or glycoproteins with a molecular weight ranging between 6000 and 60,000 daltons. Examples are:

Interleukin-1: produced mainly by macrophages and influences a vast array of cells. It causes bone marrow cells to increase their production, macrophages to produce other cytokines, T cells to produce lymphokines, B cells to proliferate, and PMNs to increase their metabolic rate. For nonlymphoid tissue it affects adipocytes, chondrocytes, epithelial cells, osteoclasts, brain cells, synovial cells, smooth muscle cells, hepatocytes, aderenal cells, and fibroblasts.

IL-2: produced by T cells and large granular leukocytes. It activates T and NK cells and causes B cells to proliferate.

IL-3: produced by T cells and promotes growth of early hematopoietic cells.

IL-4: produced by T helper cells and is a growth factor for T and B cells. It affects the switch to epsilon H chain in the choice of IgE. It also promotes mast cell growth.

IL-5: produced by T helper cells. It stimulates B cells and eosinophils and promotes the switch to IgA.

IL-6: produced by fibroblasts and others. It affects B cells.

IL-7: produced by stroma cells and is a lymphocytic growth factor for pre-B and pre-T cells.

IL-8: produced by macrophages and others. It is a chemotactic agent for neutrophils and T cells.

G-CSF (granulocyte colony stimulating factor): produced by monocytes and others and generates neutrophils.

M-CSF (macrophage colony stimulating factor): produced by monocytes and others and generates macrophages.

Interferon

Type alpha, produced by leukocytes, and type beta, produced by fibroblasts, have antiviral activities and stimulate macrophages and NK cells. Type gamma is produced by T cells and NK cells and induces membrane antigens such as MHC.

Tumor Necrosis Factors

Type alpha is produced by macrophages and others and type beta by T cells. Both have inflammatory, immunoenhancing, and tumoricidal properties. At low concentration they bind to TNF-R1 on thymocytes and CTLs to cause cell proliferation. At high concentration they bind to TNF-R1, as above, and to TNF-R2 of CTLs to increase their cytotoxicity. They also bind to fibroblasts to increase their proliferation, and to other cells to increase cytokine production.

Transforming Growth Factor

This factor comes from platelets, bone cells, and others and is involved in wound repair.

PMNs have traditionally been limited to roles of phagocytosis and release of preformed enzymes. Recently, they have been shown to synthesize and release cytokines (e.g., IL1, TNF, and IL6) to modulate both B- and T-cell activities.

Complement and the Major Histocompatibility Locus

Complement

Complement is a series of blood proteins that, upon specific activation, acts as an enzyme cascade and functions to effect an acute inflammatory response that concentrates cells of the immune system where they are needed. It results in cell lysis in cases in which activation occurs on cell surfaces. Activation occurs by two methods plus the nonspecific effects of proteolytic enzymes.

The Classic Pathway

This pathway is initiated by antigen binding with specific antibody (Fig. 1-5). Two IgG (IgG4 does not activate) molecules attached adjacently on the antigen or one pentameric IgM molecule bound to the antigen is sufficient to initiate the pathway. As a result of the antigen binding, the Fc portion of the immunoglobulin is changed, probably as a result of an allosteric shift in three-dimensional structure. The new Fc structure is capable of binding C1q, which in its turn changes shape and reacts with a proprotease (C1r) to activate it into a protease. The activated C1r protease partially digests a proesterase C1s to form an esterase. C4 is bound to the complex and is partially digested by the activated C1 to give a piece C4a, which goes into solution, and a piece C4b, which remains bound to the complex. The removal of C4a reveals a binding site on C4b for C2 and the bound C2 is partially digested to C2a by activated C1. When C2a is bound to C4b, it can split factor C3 in two, C3a (called anaphylatoxin) and C3b. The latter may drift off into the serum and be degraded, may be released and bind to cells with specific C3b receptors, may complex with serum factor B to enhance C3b production, or may remain attached to the complex. The complex binds and splits factor C5 to yield C5a, which is released and has anaphylatoxic activity and is chemotactic for leukocytes, and C5b, which remains in the complex and binds with C6

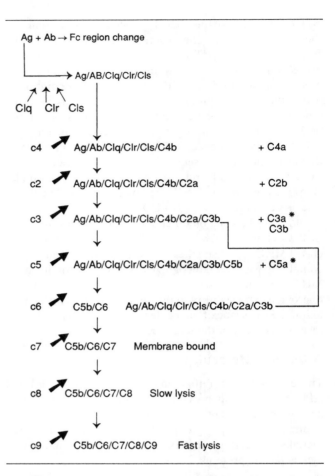

Fig. 1-5 The classic complement pathway. *, products with anaphylatoxic activity.

with the release of C5bC6. The C5bC6 complex binds in solution with C7 and the C5bC6C7 complex has chemotactic properties and can bind to cell membranes. When membrane bound, the C5bC6C7 complex binds C8 and can slowly lyse cell membranes. However, it is the additional binding of C9 that imparts the ability to rapidly lyse cell membranes. The effect of the complete cascade is to lyse cell membranes and to release factors that cause the inflammatory response.

The Antibody-Independent Alternate Pathway

Two serum proteins involved with the alternate pathway have been identified and called factors B and D. Factor B normally forms reversible, short-lived complexes with C3 in the fluid phase of the serum. Factor D can react with these complexes to change factor B to Bb. C3Bb can react with C3 to form C3a and C3b. Under normal circumstances, the C3a and C3b produced are broken down by specific inhibitors. Activators of the alternate pathway, such as yeast cell wall (zymosan), plant polysaccharide (inulin), endotoxin, or aggregates of immunoglobulins, especially IgA and IgG, act by binding the C3b produced to their surfaces, protecting it from breakdown. The protected C3b binds factor B, and the C3bB complex is acted on by factor D to form C3bBb. This protected complex, called S-C3bBb, is an enzyme that can start the complement cascade at the step that converts C5 to C5a and C5b. S-C3bBb has a short half-life. In addition to reacting with C5, the S-C3bBb complex can react with another blood protein, properdin, to form a complex that is much more stable but can still activate the cascade at the C5 step. Cobra venom acts on factor B so that it forms a much more stable complex with C3 and so enhances the alternate pathway.

Nonspecific Activation

Proteases, such as plasmin and thrombin, and bacterial and lysomal enzymes, can enhance the reaction by factor D on the C3B complex to initiate the alternate pathway and can also interact with C1 to start the classic pathway.

Regulation of the Cascade

Specific molecules in the serum have been found that inactivate various products of the cascade. For example, C1INH binds to activated C1 and inhibits esterase activity, beta-1 H interferes with the interaction of C3b and C5, C3bINH combines with beta-1 H to degrade C3b, C6INH inhibits activated C6, and anaphylatoxin inactivator cleaves off the terminal arginine from C3a and C5b to make them less biologically active.

Enhancement

C3b, released in both the classic and alternate pathways, binds to factor B and then reacts with factor D to give C3bBb. C3bBb is an enzyme that can react with C5, as described above, and also with C3 to produce C3b and C3a. As an enzyme, C3bBb can convert many molecules of C3, enhancing C3b formation.

The Breakdown of Factor C3

After the breakdown of C3 to C3a and C3b, the C3b is further degraded by a variety of soluble proteins in the blood. C3b is first degraded to iC3b by factor H or to CR1 and factor I and then to C3c or C3d and C3g. These breakdown products are bound to certain cells by specific receptors, where they have definite biologic effects. Receptor CR1 is found on erythrocytes, phagocytes, B cells, and others, and aids phagocytosis by binding C4b/C3b and iC3b. Receptor CR2 is present on B cells, some T cells, NK cells, ADCC effector cells, and others and has immunoregulatory properties when it binds C3d and C3d/C3g. Receptor CR3 is present on phagocytes and aids ingestion

when it binds iC3b. Receptor C3aR is found on neutrophils, T cells, and others and has immunoregulatory properties when it binds C3a and C4a. It is also present on mast cells and basophils where it is involved in histamine release and on smooth muscle cells where it is involved in contraction. A receptor for C5a is present on mast cells and basophils (histamine release), endothelial cells (increased vascular permeability) and on neutrophils and macrophages (chemotaxis).

Biologic Functions of Complement

Lysis of cells, as the end product of the cascade, opsoninization, and phagocytosis due to products of the cascade on the surface of microorganisms that can bind to specific receptors on phagocytes are biologic functions of complement. Inflammation is caused by the effects of C5a, C3a, and C4a components on mast cells, which stimulate histamine release, and on muscle cells, causing vascular contraction. C5a is a chemoattractant for PMNs.

The Complement Fixation Test

This assay depends upon the fact that when antibody and antigen combine to activate the complement cascade the complement factors are depleted. In certain diseases, so much inflammation occurs as a consequence of antigen, antibody binding, and complement activation that the level of complement factors in the blood drops. This decrease is measured as a means of monitoring the progress of the disease or the effectiveness of therapy, in such diseases as rheumatoid arthritis. Normally, the removal of complement factors is counterbalanced by synthesis so that the level is fairly constant. In an in vitro complement fixation test, an antigen and antibody are allowed to combine and a fixed amount of complement is added so that removal of complement factors can be detected by the lysis of sheep red blood cells by bound anti-sheep RBC serum. Lysis of sheep RBC indicates that complement is not "fixed" and that no reaction occurred between the original antigen and antibody. If the original antigen and antibody combined to activate the complement cascade and remove complement factors, then the sheep RBC are not lysed.

The Kinin Cascade

The kinin cascade is another important mediator-forming system in the blood. It results in the formation of bradykinin, a nonapeptide with potent ability to cause increased vascular permeability, vasodilation, hypotension, pain, contraction of many types of smooth muscle, and activation of phospholipase A2, causing activation of cellular arachidonic acid metabolism. Factors involved are high-molecular-weight kininogen (HMWK), clotting factor XI, prekallikrein, and the Hageman factor (HF). When contact is made with a negatively charged surface such as lipid A in gram-negative cell walls, HF is cleaved and activated. Activated HF enhances cleavage of additional HF and cleaves factor XIa from XI. Factor XIa then activates the coagulation cascade, and cleaves off kallikrein from the prekallikrein-HMWK complex. The kallikrein attacks HMWK to release bradykinin. The latter has a short life and is degraded. These events occur in the inflammatory reaction.

Arachidonic Acid Metabolism

Arachidonic acid is a 20-carbon, 4 double-bond fatty acid liberated from membrane phospholipids by both the sequential action of phospholipase C and diacylglycerol lipase and the direct action of phospholipase A2. Once liberated, it can be metabolized to yield many products that are active in inflammatory responses. Mast cells, found in connective tissue, form prostaglandin D2 (PGD2) by cyclooxygenase reactions. PGD2 causes erythema and wheal-and-flare vasodilatory responses, mediates neutrophil infiltration into skin, and acts as a chemotactic agent for leukocytes. Mast cells found in mucosal areas form leukotrienes (LT) by lypooxygenase activity on arachidonic acid. Four major biologically active compounds are produced: LTB4, LTC4, LTD4, and LTE4. These cause smooth muscle contraction and wheal-and-flare reactions.

The Human Major Histocompatibility Locus

The major histocompatibility locus (MHC) in humans is called the human leukocyte antigens (HLA) region and is present on the short arm of chromosome 6. It is a region of chromosomal DNA that codes for a variety of proteins, which have been divided into three groups.

Class I Antigens

These antigens are recognized because of their involvement in transplant acceptance or rejection and because they are potent immunogens. They are transmembrane proteins of approximately 43,000 daltons with three domains, only two of which have intrachain disulfide linkages. They are coded for by three loci (HLA-A, HLA-B, and HLA-C), of which many allelic forms exist. They are found on the surfaces of all nucleated cells and allelic forms can exist co-dominantly in heterozygous cells. Each class 1 antigen is associated noncovalently with a small polypeptide (12,000 daltons) called beta-2 microglobulin. Testing for class I surface antigens is done by the *microcytotoxity test,* in which mononuclear cells (lymphocytes and monocytes) are separated from a patient's blood and placed in the well of a microtiter plate together with a test antiserum and complement. Cells that have the test antigen bind antibodies, fix complement, and lyse. Lysis is seen by adding eosin, a red dye that can enter and stain lysed cells. Cytotoxic T cells have receptors that recognize class I antigens on a target cell and can kill it when the two cells have identical class I antigens.

Class II Antigens

These antigens are recognized by their ability to stimulate lymphocytes from genetically different individuals in the *mixed lymphocyte reaction* (MLR). Blood leukocytes from one individual are mixed with those of another and the *T cells,* which outnumber the B cells in blood by a factor of 4 to 1, are stimulated by any non-self surface antigens. Proliferation of T cells is measured by uptake of radiolabeled thymidine resulting from replication of DNA. Both populations respond. In most cases, the reaction of the recipient lymphocytes to the donor cells is of major concern and a one-way test can be set up using killed donor cells. Class II antigens are transmembrane heterodimers made up of two polypeptide chains. They are found on B lymphocytes, activated T cells, macrophages, and dendritic and other accessory cells. Three loci control these antigens in humans (HLA-DR, HLA-DQ, and HLA-DP).

Genes, which code for some of the complement factors (C2 and C4) and the properdin factor B, are found between the HLA-A, -B, and -C regions and the HLA-D region. Class II antigens are involved in the presentation of antigen by the accessory cell to the T helper cell.

Some diseases are more prevalent in individuals with a specific HLA antigen. Of note is ankylosing spondylitis; 90 percent of patients with this inflammatory disease of the spine have HLA-B27. However, not all individuals with this gene develop the disease.

Structure/Function Relationships in the MHC Molecules

MHC molecules can be regarded as a partially closed hand. Antigenic peptide may or may not fit into the groove formed by the hand, which thus confers specificity. Amino acids oriented out of the groove react with the TCR of the T cells. Different allotypes of one MHC antigen will not all react with the same peptide so that the actual T-cell epitopes of a given antigen will differ between allotypically different individuals.

Immunologic Tolerance and Immune Regulation

Failure to respond immunologically to an antigen may be due to more than one cause. *Paralysis* occurs in cases in which there is a massive amount of antigen so that the efforts of the immune system are insufficient to remove the invading agent. *Nonresponsiveness* or low response occurs where there is a hereditary absence of cells able to respond to a given antigen. This effect is complex and fine tuned. *Immunologic tolerance* is a state of the immune system that, with respect to one or more specific antigenic determinants, is manifested by an absence or diminished capacity to express either cell-mediated or humoral immunity, or both.

The major property of immunologic tolerance is its specificity, which endows the immune system with two cardinal features, tolerance of self and the ability to recognize and respond to non-self. Such a property allows an effective defense against all foreign antigens whether they be infectious agents, toxins, or tissue antigens in neoplastically transformed cells. Loss of self-tolerance occurs in autoimmune disorders and an understanding of the mechanisms involved is necessary for treatment of these diseases and also in the control of transplant rejection, allergic diseases, and immunotherapy of cancer.

Factors found to be important in the induction of tolerance include *maturity,* since tolerance is easiest to induce during embryonic or neonatal life; *immunogenicity,* since it is much easier to induce tolerance to a weakly immunogenic agent than to a highly immunogenic one; *form,* since a substance injected in its monomeric form often induces tolerance but is immunogenic if allowed to aggregate because macrophages more readily phagocytose the larger form; *dosage,* since tolerance can be induced by opposite extremes of dosage; and *nonmetabolizable substances,* since the continued presence of antigen may induce tolerance.

Differences in the Responses of B and T Cells

Both T and B cells are susceptible to induction of tolerance but T cells become tolerant at lower doses of antigen and remain tolerant for longer periods of time than do B cells.

Mechanisms of Immunologic Tolerance

There are many ways of attaining the identical final result of specific immune unresponsiveness and not all of these mechanisms have been explained.

Unresponsiveness in B Cells

This condition may be due to clonal abortion and receptor blockade. At a very early stage of development, the B cells have only IgM on their surfaces and are deleted if they contact an antigen. This serves as a mechanism for abort-

ing cells that react with self antigens, but would also remove cells capable of binding the foreign antigen if contact were made at this stage. If a large number of receptors on a B cell are engaged by their specific antigen and no cytokine help comes from T cells, then the cell may be suppressed or destroyed by the effect. This is termed clonal deletion.

Unresponsiveness in T Cells

By analogy with the B system, both clonal deletion and clonal abortion have been proposed. In addition to the selective mechanisms involved in both T- and B-cell maturation, with their definition of "self" and "non-self," these lymphocytes are subject to regulation by the soluble factors produced in an immune response, to anti-idiotype antibodies produced in network control mechanisms, and to feedback effects of antibodies. The question of whether or not suppressor T cells are involved in this regulation is still moot.

Hypersensitivity

In some cases, exposure to an antigen can result in an altered state in which re-exposure to that antigen, or a structurally similar substance, elicits responses that are pathologic to the body. This state is called *hypersensitivity.* Hypersensitivity responses can arise *immediately* (from half an hour to 3 hours) and subside within 1 to 15 hours or can be delayed (taking 1–2 days to show up and a few weeks to subside).

Gell and Coombs have classified hypersensitivity as:

Type 1: anaphylactic, atopic, or immediate hypersensitivity diseases in which the IgE immunoglobulins behave abnormally

Type 2: cytotoxic or alloimmunization in which the antigen binds to cells and reaction with antibody results in cell lysis

Type 3: mediated by immune complexes

Type 4: delayed-type hypersensitivity (DTH) reactions

Immediate-type Hypersensitivity

In the discussion of all allergic responses, the immunogen is called the *allergen* or *sensitizer,* immunization is called *sensitization,* and the immunized individual is called *sensitive, hypersensitive,* or *allergic.* Type 1 states of hypersensitivity are caused by reaction of allergen with IgE antibodies (often called reagins) and the reaction is called anaphylaxis or an anaphylactic reaction. *Systemic or generalized anaphylaxis* occurs when the allergen is introduced intravenously into sensitized individuals. The reaction begins within a few minutes and leads to shock (acute peripheral circulatory failure), vascular engorgement, and asphyxia due to bronchial and laryngeal constriction. If death does not result, recovery is complete within an hour. In humans this is a rare event and occurs in sensitized individuals stung by insects (bees, wasps, and hornets) or sensitized individuals injected with horse serum used as antitoxin or penicillin (this drug may also elicit DTH). *Cutaneous anaphylaxis* occurs when the allergen is injected into the skin. In sensitized individuals itching at the site of injection begins almost at once and within minutes a pale irregular wheal (round elevation of the skin) surrounded by a zone of erythema (redness) forms. This is called a *hive* or *uticarium*, and the response is called the *wheal-and-flare reaction*. The reaction is maximum at about 10 minutes, persists for 10 to 20 minutes, and then gradually subsides. It is used clinically to specify a patient's range of allergies. *Passive cutaneous anaphylaxis* occurs when the serum from a sensitized individual is injected, usually after dilution, into the skin of a nonsensitized individual. After a latent period of at least 10 to 20 hours, the allergen, which is injected into the same site, elicits the wheal-and-flare reaction. This is a common technique for study of allergy in laboratory animals, into which the antigen is injected together with a dye (Evans blue) to measure leakage from cutaneous blood vessels. This was called the Prausnitz-Küstner test but is no longer used in humans because of the risk of hepatitis and acquired immunodeficiency syndrome (AIDS). *Atopy* is a form of allergy in which the response is elicited by exposure to a variety of environmental antigens, such as pollen, fungi, animal danders, house dust, or foods. When individuals with atopy ingest or inhale the appropriate allergen, hives or the manifestations of hay fever or asthma promptly develop. The tendency for the development of atopy is hereditary.

Mechanisms of Type 1 Hypersensitivity

In humans these effects are caused by IgE. The allergens not only elicit IgE but also cause the production of IgG and other Ig. This has led to the form of allergy treatment in which a sensitized individual is immunized with small amounts of allergen in the hope of stimulating IgG production. This will act as blocking antibody to remove the allergen before it comes in contact with the IgE. IgE molecules are cytotrophic; that is, they bind specially to *mast cells* and *basophils*, and, as they bind only to human cells, are called homocytotrophic. Mast cells are found throughout the body, especially near blood vessels and nerves, and beneath epithelia. They arise in the bone marrow and mature in the tissues. Most likely, connective tissue mast cells arise independently, whereas mucosal

mast cells require IL3 and IL4 from T cells to mature. Both they and basophils have a receptor for the Fc region of IgE called Fc epsilon R1 (FceR1). There is a much lower affinity receptor for the epsilon chain called FceRII on B cells, macrophages, and eosinophils. IgE binds through its Fc portion to receptors on mast cells and basophils. Allergens bind to their specific IgE to elicit the type 1 reaction. However, an allergen must be multivalent and form a *cross-linking bond* between adjacent IgE molecules. For this reason, univalent haptens can block the reaction but cannot elicit it. Cross-linking results in release of *primary mediators* as soon as it occurs followed by synthesis and release of *secondary mediators*. Primary mediators consist of histamine, which is stored in granules of mast cells and basophils ready for release and has inflammatory effects; *serotonin*, to which humans are refractile; and enzymes, such as aryl sulfatases. Secondary mediators consist of lipid mediators (prostaglandins, arachidonic acid–derived mediators, and platelet activating factor) and cytokines produced by mast cells. *Therapy* is based on reducing mast cell activation with sodium cromolyn; counteracting leukotriene effects by bronchodilators, such as epinephrine and theophylline; and reducing cytokine synthesis with corticosteroids.

Regulation of IgE and Its Role in Immunity

IgE-producing plasma cells are not rare. They are conspicuous in mucosa of the intestinal and respiratory tracts but less obvious in spleen and peripheral lymph nodes. This evidence, together with the very low level of serum IgE and the possible hazardous effects of anaphylaxis, suggests that IgE production must be under very tight control. Immunization conditions that result in allergy involve not only the allergen but include other factors as well. IgE must have some beneficial effect in order to be maintained in humans. A hint of this may come from the fact that high serum IgE levels are found in some helminthic parasitic infections. IgE reactions can stimulate eosinophils that are able to damage this group of parasites. Unfortunately, the validity of this hypothesis can be questioned because most of the IgE is not specific for the parasite.

Cytotoxic or Alloimmunization

This type of immunization results in cell lysis after the cell-bound antigen has reacted with its specific antibody. In the majority of cases, this is a consequence of activation but sometimes it is induced by antibody-dependent cytotoxic cells (ADCC). Examples of type II hypersensitivity are incompatible blood transfusions, hemolytic disease of the newborn, drug-induced hemolytic anemia and thrombocytopenia, Goodpasture's syndrome, and some of the rejection response against organ or skin grafts.

Immune Complex Reactions

In these reactions, complexes deposited at various sites in the body activate the complement cascade and damage tissues in the area of the deposit. *The Arthus reaction* results from circulating antibody reacting with antigen to produce immune complexes at the site of injection, causing inflammation. *Serum sickness* arises from injection of heterologous serum into a previously exposed host resulting in the formation of immune aggregates, which localize in many areas of the body and initiate local inflammation, and the killing of tissue cells in the area. *The Schwartzman reaction* is a skin reaction that is of interest because it resembles the Arthus reaction in appearance although in reality the tissue damage is caused by endotoxin.

Delayed-type Hypersensitivity Reactions

These reactions are modeled by the tuberculin reaction in which inflammation occurs many hours after the cutaneous injection of an extract of *Mycobacterium tuberculosis* in tuberculous guinea pigs but has no effect in normal animals. Similar DTH reactions occur with other infectious agents and such sensitivity has been used to diagnose infections and to screen individuals for previous infections (e.g., mumps, leprosy, brucellosis, psittacosis, lymphogranuloma venereum, mumps, many fungi, some protozoa). The effects are caused by cell-mediated immunity in which the ultimate effector cell is the activated macrophage. It is the primary defense against intracellular bacterial infection and consists of two phases. In the *cognitive phase*, accessory cells present the antigen to CD4$^+$ T cells. These antigen presenting cells may be Langerhans cells of the skin, which carry antigen to the draining lymph node and present it to T cells; macrophages, which when stimulated by bacterial cell wall products secrete IL1, which is chemotactic for T cells; endothelial cells of the postcapillary venules; and B cells. This is followed by the *activation phase*, in which secretion of lymphokines and proliferation occur. Involved are the following:

Interleukin-2

IL2 causes proliferation of antigen-stimulated CD4$^+$ cells and increased synthesis of lymphokines, including itself. It can stimulate bystander T cells to secrete lymphokines.

Interferon-Gamma

INF-gamma causes antigen presenting cells to express their class II MHC antigens for antigen presentation. It is the most potent macrophage-activating cytokine and is the most important mediator in DTH.

TNF and LT

TNF and LT act on venular endothelial cells to augment their ability to bind and activate leukocytes. Under the influence of TNF and other cytokines, the venular endothelial cells perform a variety of functions that contribute to inflammation, including production of vasodilating compounds (prostacyclin); alteration of their surface proteins to adhere sequentially neutrophils, lymphocytes, and monocytes; secretion of cytokines; and shape alteration to forms that favor leakage of both cells and proteins into the tissue spaces. Once leukocytes enter the tissues, they may die in a few days (especially neutrophils), may become activated (especially T cells and monocytes), or may leave through the lymph system. Activation increases the receptor molecules expressed on the cell for matrix molecules (integrins), which are important in the binding of leukocytes to vascular endothelium and extracellular matrices.

Activated Macrophages

Once blood monocytes leave the circulation and enter tissues at sites of DTH reactions, they differentiate into macrophages. This change is called macrophage *activation*. Such activated macrophages kill microorganisms and tumor cells, stimulate acute inflammatory reactions by secreting mediators, are more efficient accessory cells for T cells by increasing their expression of class II MHC molecules, and produce substances (cytokines and growth factors) that modify the local tissue environment with initial tissue destruction and later replacement with connective tissues. If antigen stimulation persists, macrophages become chronically activated and secrete additional cytokines and growth factors that cause the original tissue to be replaced by fibrous tissue. They can undergo morphologic changes and cluster around particulate sources of antigen (e.g., tubercle bacillus) to produce palpable nodules called *granulomas.*

Contact Skin Sensitivity

Allergic contact dermatitis is induced, and its expression elicited, simply by contact of low-molecular-weight chemicals with intact skin and is responsible for common allergic reactions in humans to poison ivy plants, synthetic chemicals, drugs, and cosmetics. The actual immunogens are not the simple chemicals themselves but covalent derivatives that they form with skin proteins. Once established, this form of allergy can persist for years but it tends to wane with time. A patch test to evaluate its persistence can increase sensitivity. The major inflammatory reaction that is elicited resembles the tuberculin reaction and is considered a DTH reaction.

Transfusion and Transplantation Immunity

Transfusion

Erythrocyte alloantigens are responsible for problems with the transfusion of blood. Alloantigens are described below.

The ABO System

This system, which depends on different forms of an RBC surface glycopeptide, separates humans into the blood groups as outlined in Table 1-2. All human RBC, including group O, have an additional antigen called H, which is a variation of the glycoprotein involved in A and B. Normal individuals do not produce anti-H antibodies. However, some individuals, first found in Bombay and hence Bombay-type, do not have the H antigen and therefore produce anti-H antibodies.

The A, B, and H antigens are found on RBC, the surface of many epithelial cells, and most endothelial cells. Eighty percent of people have these antigens also present in secretions (secretors). The property is controlled by a gene called Se, with the nonsecretive form (se) being recessive so that heterozygous individuals, Se/se, are secretors.

The naturally occurring isohemagglutinins are IgM immunoglobulins and what triggers their production is unknown. They may be antibodies produced against the polysaccharides of intestinal bacteria that cross react with the AB antigens. This is supported by the fact that they are not present at birth but appear during the first year of life as the gut becomes colonized.

The Minor Blood Groups

These groups, which are RBC surface antigens distributed allotypically, rarely are involved in transfusion reactions unless the patient has had multiple transfusions in the past. There are no isohemagglutinins. They comprise the MN

Table 1-2 The ABO System

Genotype	Phenotype	%*	Serum Antibodies
AA	A	42	Anti-B (agglutinates AB and B groups)
AO	A		
BB	B	9	Anti-A (agglutinates AB and A groups)
BO	B		
AB	AB	3	No anti-A or anti-B
OO	O	46	Both anti-A and anti-B

*White, North American population.

blood group, the Ss antigens, the Rh antigens, the Kelly group, and the Duffy group. The Rh group causes the syndrome of hemolytic disease of the newborn when an Rh$^-$ mother has an Rh$^+$ fetus (Rh$^+$ from the father) and produces IgG anti-Rh antibodies that pass through the placenta and lyse the fetal RBC. Immunization of the mother with the Rh antigen occurs mainly at parturition, rather than exposure to fetal RBC passing through the placenta. However, the latter occurs in 1 percent of cases during the first pregnancy. Consequently, the disease usually arises during the third or fourth pregnancy. Treatment is to replace the fetal RBC at birth but preventative measures can be undertaken to prevent the mother being exposed to fetal RBC at parturition so that future pregnancies will not be complicated by the Rh antigen. One widely used preparation is called RhoGAM and consists of human anti-Rh antibodies given 72 hours before parturition. The antibodies combine with the fetal Rh antigens so that the mother is not exposed to them.

Transfusion Reactions

These reactions normally occur between the recipient's antibodies and the donor cells. Three types of immune reactions can occur. Hemolytic reactions are the most serious and result mainly from ABO incompatibility caused by clerical or laboratory error. They can also arise from Rh incompatibility or incompatibility in minor blood group antigens if the recipient has been previously exposed. Severe hemolytic reactions occur within minutes of transfusion and consist of diffuse muscle pain, headache, nausea, and sometimes vomiting and fever. A state of shock with renal failure can result. Febrile episodes are usually the result of reactions with minor blood groups that arise from repeated transfusions with blood mismatched for minor groups. Allergic reactions range from mild uticaria to systemic anaphylactic shock.

Cross Matching

Cross matching is performed to prevent transfusion reactions. A minor cross match (not usually performed in the United States or Canada) consists of mixing the donor cells with the recipient serum and observing for agglutination. A major cross match consists of the above along with another test in which the donor cell and recipient serum are mixed, the cells are washed, and anti-immunoglobulin (Coombs' test) is added to detect antibodies associated with donor cells. In cases of extreme emergency, unmatched blood from a universal donor (type O, Rh$^-$) can be used.

Transplantation

Transplantation of cells or organs from one individual to another has become routine in some cases, such as kidneys, and frequent in others, such as heart and lungs. Except for monozygotic twins, cells of individuals from a given species differ in many surface molecules. These molecules are identified as "foreign" in another host.

Relationships Between Donor and Recipient

An autograft is a graft from one area of the body to another in the *same* individual. The graft is recognized as "self" (autochthonous) and no immune responses are involved. *An isograft or syngraft* is from one individual to another who is genetically identical (syngeneic). The two individuals are said to be "histocompatible." *An allograft* is from one individual to another of the same species who is genetically dissimilar, and a *xenograft* is from a donor of a different species.

The implied role of the immune response in graft rejection comes from the observation of *first- and second-set rejections* in which the rejection response to a second identical allograft between two individuals is faster than the rejection of the first graft. The capacity to mount a second-set rejection response can be transferred from one individual to another by transfer of lymphoid cells. The transferred rejection is specific. This is termed adoptive transfer. *Histologic examination* of the site of rejection reveals lymphocytic and mononuclear infiltration appearing like the reaction found in delayed-type hypersensitivity. Specific T cells and circulating antibodies are induced to an allograft or a xenograft. Although antibodies are the major component of RBC rejection in incompatible blood transfusions, they have little role in the rejection of other tissues, and it is the T cells that constitute the major immunologic component responsible for rejection of transplants. T cells recognize specific alloantigens, become activated, and release lymphokines, which recruit inflammatory cells to the site of the reaction.

Clinical Characteristics of Allograft Rejection

Hyperacute rejection occurs within a few minutes to a few hours of transplantation and is the result of preformed antibodies to the graft induced by previous transplantations, transfusions, or pregnancies. Complement is activated and the graft undergoes swelling, interstitial hemorrhage, thrombosis with endothelial injury, and necrosis. The recipient often has fever, leukocytosis, and renal shutdown. Therapy consists of removal of the graft and procedures to keep the patient alive until the response subsides. *Acute rejection* involves recipients not previously exposed to the allograft antigens and is the common type of rejection in individuals for whom the transplanted tissue is a mismatch and who have not been sufficiently immunosuppressed. It usually begins a few days after transplantation and results in rejection in 10 to 14 days. Immunosup-

pressive therapy needs to be increased at the first sign of acute rejection and can reverse the process. The disadvantage of such therapy is that it is nonspecific, and life-threatening complications can occur when nonimmune, rapidly dividing cells are also suppressed. Agents in current use include mitotic inhibitors (e.g., azathioprine); corticosteroids, which are suppressors of the inflammatory reaction and reduce lymphocyte numbers; and cyclosporin. The latter is specific for antigen-activated T cells and has become the mainstay of transplantation therapy despite its nephrotoxicity. *Chronic rejections* occur months to years after the graft has "taken." It is slow and progressive and by the time it is detected the immune injury has taken place so that immunosuppressive therapy is not effective.

Tumor Immunity

Transplantation of tumors between syngeneic animals results in destruction of the tumor and a repeat transplantation to faster tumor elimination. The timing of the rejection indicates the involvement of immunologic mechanisms with memory.

Tumor Antigens

Some antigens on the surfaces of malignant cells may constitute new structures unique to the cancerous cell and absent from normal cells. Other antigens may represent structures that are common to both cell types but "masked" on normal cells and "unmasked" on malignant cells. Still other tumor cell antigens may be present on fetal or embryonic cells but absent on adult cells. These are oncofetal or oncodevelopmental antigens. Such antigens are found on tumors induced by chemical or physical carcinogens, on tumors induced by viral infection, and on spontaneous tumors. Carcinogen-induced tumor antigens exhibit little or no cross-reactivity. Many human tumors are probably induced in this way (e.g., smoke, radiation) and the absence of cross-reactivity makes immune therapy difficult and only possible on an individual tumor basis. Tumors induced by DNA or RNA oncogenic viruses exhibit extensive immunologic cross-reactivity. These antigens are encoded by the virus and referred to as tumor-associated antigens (TAAs). Occasionally, the virus-infected cell undergoes deregulation and expresses oncofetal antigens encoded by the cell. Oncogenic viruses can be classified into groups according to a variety of physical and biologic properties, and within each group, and sometimes between groups, extensive cross-reactivity occurs among the TAAs. Several human cancers show cross-reactivity in the tumor antigens from different patients and this suggests that they may be of viral origin; examples include Burkitt's lymphoma, nasopharyngeal carcinoma, T-cell leukemia, colon carcinoma, and melanoma. Many tumors express on their surfaces, or secrete into the blood, products normally present during embryonic and fetal development that are absent, or at very low levels, in normal adult tissue. They are not immunogenic in the autochthonous host as exposure during development causes tolerance. They are detected using antisera prepared in allogeneic or xenogeneic systems. Examples are the *carcinoembryonic antigen (CEA)*, found predominantly in patients with cancer of the gastrointestinal tract and also sometimes in lung cancer, pancreatic cancer, and breast cancer, and the *alpha fetoprotein*, found in hepatomas and testicular malignancies.

The Immune Response to Tumors

Evidence indicates that both the humoral and cellular immune effector systems play an important role between the tumor and the host. Humoral mechanisms include lysis by antibody and complement, antibody- and complement-mediated opsonization, and antibody-mediated loss of tumor adhesion. Cell-mediated responses comprise cytotoxic T lymphocytes, ADCC, destruction of tumor cells by activated macrophages, and NK cells.

Role of the Immune Response

It has been suggested that the normal immune system keeps malignancies under control. The immune system has been selected for this role during evolution because it allows the identification and destruction of neoplastic cells that arise by somatic mutation and loss of differentiation in animals that are extremely complex and long-lived. This ability to eliminate tumor cells as they arise may be limited by location of the tumor at sites not accessible to the immune system, by tumor cells that change their surface antigens or lose them altogether, or by enhancing or blocking factors. In addition, suppressor cells may be induced as part of the immune response to turn off the reaction, and the tumors may produce a variety of substances, such as prostaglandins, that act to suppress the immune system. In some cases, the tumor increases in size at a rate that is too rapid for the immune system to respond and maintains a size that is too great for the response to be effective.

Immunodiagnosis

Immunodiagnosis is performed to detect antigens specific for tumor cells and to assess the host's response to the tumor. At the moment, immunodiagnosis of cancer does not constitute a reliably accurate method of choice for the early detection of malignancy. It is, however, proving useful clinically in monitoring the progression, or regression, of certain tumors. Monoclonal antibodies are extremely specific for tumor antigens and, when radio-labeled, can be used to visualize both the tumor mass and small metastases using computed tomography (CT).

Tumor Immunoprophylaxis

Immunization against an oncogenic virus would be expected to provide prophylaxis against the virus and against the subsequent induction of tumor by the virus. This has proved to be true in certain cases. For example, chickens can be protected against Marek's disease and cats against feline leukemia and feline sarcoma. However, there are no appropriate immunogens for the protection of humans against spontaneous tumors.

Immunotherapy

Although there have been hopeful results, cancer immunotherapy has not yet proved to be an effective treatment when used alone or in conjunction with surgery, chemotherapy, or radiation. Trials have been performed using specific cancer antigens or agents that nonspecifically enhance the immune system, for example, bacillus Calmette-Guérin (BCG). Lymphokines have been tested and the latest approach is the use of LAK cells. Here, the patient's own lymphocytes (from the circulation or from the tumor) are grown in tissue culture in the presence of IL2 (producing lymphokine-activated killer cells) and are reinjected into the patient. Dramatic results have been recorded with some patients but side effects are serious and the work is still in progress. The use of radioisotopes or toxins attached to tumor-specific monoclonal antibodies is being attempted.

Autoimmunity

Many diseases have been described in which an immune response against some "self" antigen is evoked with pathologic consequences. The nature of these responses is as varied as the immune response itself, with possible involvement of antibody, complement, immune complexes, and cell-mediated immunity. Many animal models have been developed to study these phenomena but almost all involve active immunization with a known antigen. However, the inducing agents for most of the well-recognized, naturally occurring human autoimmune diseases remain unknown. Possible explanations for the cause of these diseases include failure of the deletion of self-reacting T and B cells during their development, re-occurrence of such clones by mutation of nondeleted clones (i.e., the presence of *forbidden clones*), breakdown of control mechanisms that keep self-reactive clones in check, and the occurrence of cross reaction between self antigens and the antigens of invading microbes.

Examples of Autoimmune Diseases

Antibody-Mediated Autoimmune Diseases

Autoimmune Hemolytic Anemia

Patients with this disease present with anemia and evidence of hemolysis, which must be shown not to be the secondary effects of other disease states. The symptoms are due to antibody directed against RBC surface antigens either activating the complement cascade leading to lysis (hemoglobin often appears in the urine in this case) or acting as opsonizers. It is customary to divide the antibodies responsible into warm autoantibodies, which react with the red cells optimally at 37°C, and cold agglutinins. The former are primarily IgG antibodies that arise after overt or subclinical virus infections and react with Rh surface antigens. Because Rh antigens are scarce and complement activation requires the close alignment of two IgG molecules, lysis is rare but phagocytosis is enhanced. The Coombs' test is used to look for these antibodies in the sera of patients suspected of having the disease. Treatment consists of initial administration of steroids with removal of the spleen if these do not eliminate the symptoms after 3 to 4 months. Cold agglutinins attach to the RBC only at temperatures below 37°C and are specific for antigens present on glycophorin, a major constituent of RBC surface. A syndrome similar to autoimmune hemolytic anemia may be induced by drugs, such as penicillin, where the drug binds to RBCs and antibodies against the drug attach to it, activate the complement cascade, and lyse the RBC.

Myasthenia Gravis

In this disease, autoantibody binds to acetylcholine receptors at neuromuscular junctions resulting in severe muscle weakness and eventual death from respiratory failure. There is some link to the thymus as many patients have thymoma and removal of the thymus sometimes leads to regression of the disease. There are molecules on the surfaces of thymocytes that cross react with acetylcholine receptors, but whether these are involved in stimulating the disease is not known.

Immune Complex–Mediated Autoimmune Diseases

Systemic Lupus Erythematosus (SLE)

This disease gets its name from the frequent early symptom of a reddish rash on the cheeks that resembles the wings of a butterfly rather than the face of a wolf. Many organs of the body are attacked with fever, joint pain, and damage to the central nervous system (CNS), the heart, and the kidneys. The origin of the disease is unknown. However, some strains of encapsulated bacteria (e.g., *Klebsiella pneu-*

moniae) induce the formation of antibodies that cross react very strongly with DNA because of the similar phosphorylated backbone of DNA and capsular polysaccharides. A typical feature of patients with SLE is their production of antibody to double-stranded DNA, and the disease is thought to result from the action of these anti-DNA antibodies. Normal breakdown of tissue cells results in release of DNA. The DNA can lodge in a variety of areas of the body and inflammatory events (especially complement activation and cell lysis) can be initiated when anti-DNA antibody binds to it. Alternatively, the antibody and DNA can form soluble circulating complexes that lodge in a variety of sites (this may be seen histologically in some patients and is called "lumpy-bumpy" deposits) where they can activate the complement cascade and cause inflammation. The basement membrane of the kidney is a prime site for lodging of DNA or the complexes with resulting destruction of function (glomerulonephritis).

Rheumatoid Arthritis

Patients with this disease produce an abnormal IgM antibody called rheumatoid factor that is specific for a determinant on the Fc region of the patient's own IgG molecules. Complexes of the IgM and the IgG antibodies are deposited in the synovia of joint fluid where they induce an inflammatory reaction with resulting joint swelling and pain. Breakdown of the attracted neutrophils releases hydrolyzing enzymes that destroy the sliding surfaces needed for joint function. After repeated bouts of inflammation there is replacement of the cartilage by fibrous tissue resulting in immobilization and subsidence of the inflammatory reaction.

T Cell–Mediated Autoimmune Disease

Hashimoto's thyroiditis is a disease of the thyroid, primarily found in middle-aged women, that leads to the formation of a goiter (enlarged thyroid) and destruction of the thyroid gland. The cause of the disease is unknown and the evidence for the involvement of T cells is indirect. There is infiltration of mononuclear cells into the thyroid follicles with their progressive destruction. The gland attempts to regenerate and becomes enlarged. When destruction reaches a level where normal amounts of thyroid hormone cannot be produced, the symptoms of hypothyroidism appear. These include dry skin, puffy face, brittle hair and nails, and a feeling of cold. Because infiltration of mononuclear cells is a characteristic of T cell mediated hypersensitivity reactions and such infiltration occurs here, the disease is thought to involve T cells.

It is possible that *multiple sclerosis* has autoimmune components involving T cells because the lesions (demyelinization of CNS) resemble those of delayed-type hypersensitivity and a similar syndrome can be induced in animals by immunization with myelin.

Deficiency in Complement Components

Some patients with apparent autoimmune diseases are found to be deficient in some complement components.

Disorders of the Immune System

Aberrations of the immune system arise as a result of primary disorders of the cells involved or as the secondary effects of other irregularities. The outcome can be immunodeficiency or, conversely, specific overactivation, usually hypergammaglobulinemia in the latter case. Conditions that produce secondary immunodeficiencies include lymphoreticular malignancies, leprosy, myotonic dystrophy, sarcoidosis, and treatment with x-rays, steroids, and cytotoxic drugs. Secondary gammopathy and abnormal proliferation of immunoglobulin-producing lymphoid cells may be seen in nonlymphoreticular malignancies, rheumatoid disorders, and some chronic infections.

Primary Immunodeficiencies

Primary immunodeficiencies can occur in the B cells, in the T cells, or in both B and T cells. All result in a much increased susceptibility to infections and analysis has clarified the role of the different segments of the immune response in host defense against specific pathogenic agents.

B-Cell Deficiencies

The most dramatic example of B-cell deficiency is *Bruton's agammaglobulinemia,* which is an X-linked birth defect characterized by an absence of circulating B cells. Serum IgG antibody is very low and other gammaglobulin classes cannot be detected. Patients with this disease are usually protected by maternal IgG antibody for the first 6 months of life and then become susceptible to acute, overwhelming pyogenic infections of the sinopulmonary tract including otitis media, bronchitis, pneumonia, and meningitis. Skin infections have also been reported. Causative agents include pneumococci, *Haemophilus influenzae,* streptococci, and gram-negative rods. Response to antibiotic therapy is not prompt and rarely complete. Attempts to replace the deficient immune response involve the administration of commercially available gammaglobulin in anticipation that antibodies to common pathogens will be present. Although patients with this syndrome have survived into the third and fourth decades of life, the prognosis must be guarded. Chronic lung disease and severe mental handicaps may arise from the bacterial infections and some individuals

have developed lymphoma and leukemia. Despite apparently adequate immunoglobulin therapy, several individuals have developed fatal echovirus infections.

Some infants present symptoms that mimic those of Bruton's agammaglobulinemia in the first year or two of life because of a lag in their B-cell development. This syndrome is called *transient hypogammaglobulinemia of infancy.* Treatment requires administration of gamma globulin with monitoring of serum IgA levels, or examination for lymphocytes carrying B-cell markers, to determine whether B-cell development is occurring. Deficient B-cell function appearing at any age, most commonly between the ages of 15 and 35, is characteristic of *acquired hypogammaglobulinemia.* T-cell disorders usually appear at a more advanced age, with a consequent increase in susceptibility to a range of potential pathogens and development of malignancies.

Deficiencies in specific classes and subclasses of immunoglobulins have been described, and individuals with low levels of serum IgA (secretory IgA levels may be normal) appear to be quite common, at 1 per 400 to 600 persons in the population. Patients with this selective IgA deficiency show a higher than normal rate of recurrent sinopulmonary bacterial infections, allergy, gastrointestinal tract diseases, autoimmune diseases, and certain types of malignancies. Gamma globulin therapy cannot be used and blood transfusions may be complicated by the development of anti-IgA antibodies, necessitating the use of packed, washed red blood cells.

T-Cell Deficiencies

An embryonic defect in the development of the third and fourth pharyngeal pouches occurs in *Di George's syndrome* and results in hypoparathyroidism, heart defects, abnormal facies, and production of a small thymus. T cells are much reduced in number and are apparently nonfunctional, although some antibody production may be detected. In cases in which the other defects can be controlled, T-cell immunity has been reconstituted by transplantation of fetal thymus material.

A poorly understood defect of T cells occurs in *chronic mucocutaneous candidiasis,* where cellular immunity to *Candida albicans* is impaired although the response to other antigens appears to be normal. Endocrinopathy involving the parathyroid, adrenal, and stomach glands is involved in this syndrome and is the major cause of death.

Deficiencies of Both B and T Cells

The most clear-cut form of deficiency of both B and T cells occurs in *severe combined immunodeficiency disease* (SCID), where there is a complete absence of both B- and

T-cell functions and consequent susceptibility to infection with a wide variety of bacteria, viruses, fungi, and protozoa. An otherwise rare pathogen, *Pneumocystis carinii,* is a common cause of lethal pneumonia in patients with this syndrome and the pathogen, and has been implicated as the cause of death in patients with AIDS. Reconstitution of the immune system has sometimes been successful using histocompatible bone marrow, fetal liver transplants, and fetal thymus transplants. Recently, attempts to repair the defect at the stem cell level by gene therapy techniques have showed some success. Incompleteness of available tissue-typing methodologies has resulted in death from graft-versus-host disease in some attempted transplantations. Sterile supportive units have been used to maintain some individuals awaiting transplantation material. Variable defects in T-cell and B-cell functions are presented by individuals with *Nezelof's syndrome, Wiskott-Aldrich syndrome, short-limbed dwarfism,* and *ataxia-telangiectasia.* Each case must be evaluated individually and therapy designed accordingly. Thymoma, in which malignant spindle cells replace the thymic parenchyma, has been described as impairing both B- and T-cell functions.

Phagocytic Dysfunction Disease

In addition to extrinsic factors that may affect the function of phagocyte cells, such as lack of antibody, intrinsic defects have been identified that result in impaired activity. In some cases, the specific enzyme deficiency within metabolic pathways necessary for the killing of engulfed bacteria has been identified, for example, lack of glucose 6-phosphate dehydrogenase. Susceptibility resulting from such intrinsic defects varies from mild, recurrent skin infections to severe, overwhelming systemic infection, with both often involving organisms usually considered of low virulence.

Complement Deficiencies

Deficiency in complement is rare and is usually restricted to specific components of the cascade. The evolution and maintenance of the complicated complement cascade argues for its importance in host defense but individuals lacking this system are not always highly susceptible to infection.

Hypergammaglobulinemias

Malignant conditions involving B cells are not rare, probably due to the intense genetic activity involved in the production of immunoglobulin, and usually result in massive production of a single immunoglobulin as the result of the involvement of a single clone. All classes of immunoglobulins are represented in the hypergammaglobulinemias,

with IgM individually recognized in macroglobulinemia. In some cases the complete molecule is not produced and heavy chains are found in the serum. Other cells can be affected as a result of the immune activity; for example, osteoclasts are activated by cytokines to dissolve bone in multiple myeloma.

Acquired Immunodeficiency Syndrome

This disease is discussed in the section on viruses, but is mentioned here because destruction of the T helper cells and loss of immune function occur as a result of infection.

Clinical Evaluation

Some clinical features are associated with specific immunodeficiency disease, such as ataxia-telangiectasia and short-limbed dwarfism, whereas others are indicative of likely immune involvement. Recurrent, chronic infections with incomplete response to treatment, for example, are highly suspicious in terms of an immunodeficiency. Less indicative are skin rashes, chronic diarrhea, growth failure, and hepatosplenomegaly. Often, the infectious agents isolated from disease offer a clue to the specific deficiency involved; for example, sinopulmonary infections with pyogenic organisms suggest lack of a B-cell response.

Evaluation of a suspected immunodeficiency depends upon the immune system function thought to be involved. B-cell function can be determined by quantitation of serum immunoglobulins or specific antibodies, by response to active immunization (using a nonviable vaccine), or by B-cell quantitation. Cell-mediated responses can be measured in skin tests and T cells quantified by a white blood cell count with differentiation. Phagocytic activities can be determined by examining latex particle uptake.

Physiologic and Environmental Influences of the Immune System

The immune system has anatomic and physiologic relationships with other parts of the body and these can influence it.

Psychoneuroimmunology

Endings of primarily sympathetic efferent nerves are found in the thymus, spleen, and lymph nodes, indicating anatomic connections between the nervous system and the immune organs. In addition the connection between the nervous system and the endocrine system (hypothalamus and pituitary glands) forms an indirect link as the endocrine system can influence the immune system. Opportunities for interactions are extensive. Lymphocytes and macrophages have receptors for neurotransmitters (acetylcholine and norepinephrine), endorphins, enkephalins, and some endocrine hormones, including adrenocorticotropic hormone (ACTH), corticosteroids, insulin, prolactin, growth hormone, estradiol, and testosterone. In turn, lymphocytes are capable of producing ACTH and endorphin-like compounds. Neurons in the brain can recognize prostaglandins, interferons, interleukins, and inflammatory mediators such as histamine.

Aging

Older people are more vulnerable to life-threatening infections, cancer, and autoimmune diseases than are young adults, and there is some evidence that this can be associated with a decline in immune responsiveness with age.

Nutrition

Good nutrition is obviously essential for the maintenance of health and only a healthy individual can mount a good immune response. Excess food intake has been possibly implicated as increasing incidence of infections and some cancers.

Environmental Effects

Toxic chemicals in the environment can increase the rates of infectious diseases and cancers. Whether these are causing their effect by initially suppressing the immune system is not clear.

Methods in Immunology

Antigen/Antibody Reactions

The actual binding of an antibody to its specific antigenic determinant (epitope) is the primary reaction. This is difficult to detect and methods usually depend on the secondary phenomena, such as precipitation, agglutination, and complement fixation. These often involve *crosslinking* of antigen molecules by specific antibody and occur because the antibody is divalent (bivalent) and the antigen multivalent. Because the antigen/antibody (Ag/Ab) reaction is so highly specific, it has been used to detect either Ag or Ab, and the methods that have been developed for this detection have been grouped together under the term "serology."

The primary reaction is reversible and the tightness of the binding can be expressed as the association constant (K). Serum antibodies are heterogeneous and when they react the constant is termed K_o, the average association constant. The forces involved are weak noncovalent bonds, including hydrophobic bonds, hydrogen bonds, electro-

static forces, and van der Waal's forces. Because these forces involve low levels of energy, Ag/Ab complexes can be readily dissociated by low or high pH, high salt concentrations, and chaotropic ions that efficiently interfere with the hydrogen bonding of water molecules, for example, cyanates. In cases in which the epitope is a hapten, the reaction has been examined by the hapten-inhibition test, equilibrium dialysis, and fluorescence quenching.

Secondary Reactions

In *agglutination reactions* an antibody reacts with a multivalent insoluble particle to give cross-linking until visible clumps are formed. At high concentrations of antibody, agglutination cannot occur and the test is said to demonstrate a prozone. With erythrocytes, the repulsive zeta potential between cells allows agglutination with IgM but not with IgG. With the latter, anti-human IgG is used in the Coombs' test to agglutinate RBC with bound IgG.

Precipitation Reactions

These reactions take place between antibodies and *soluble* antigens, with lattice formation occurring to give an insoluble precipitate. Excess antigen or excess antibody results in the formation of Ab/Ag complexes but not the formation of lattices large enough to become insoluble. Thus, maximum precipitate formation occurs at a zone of equivalence. For this reason, precipitation reactions can more easily be performed in gels. By allowing the antibody or the antigen, or both, to diffuse into the gel, the diffusion gradient allows for the formation of conditions necessary for the zone of equivalence. Gels can be used in many ways, such as single diffusion in one dimension, double diffusion in one dimension, double diffusion in two dimensions (the Ouchterlony method), or combined with electrophoresis.

Radioimmunoassays

Radioimmunoassays employ isotopically labeled molecules and can measure extremely small amounts of antigen, antibody, or Ag/Ab complexes.

Complement Fixation Tests

These tests use the binding of complement in antigen/antibody combinations as a means of detecting such combinations.

Solid-phase assays bind monolayers of proteins onto the surface of plastic, react these with their specific antibodies, and detect binding using specific anti-Ig immunoglobulins. These anti-Ig immunoglobulins can be labeled with isotope solid-phase radioimmunoassay (SPRIA) or with an enzyme-linked immunosorbent assay (ELISA). Haptens that do not bind to plastic may be bound to paper, for example, the radioallergosorbent (RAST) test for IgE detection. *Inhibition tests* can be variants of practically all immunoassays in which an unknown is compared against a known for its ability to inhibit an immunologic reaction. *Neutralization tests* measure the ability of antisera to prevent the toxic effects of a chemical or the growth of a virus. *Opsonization* depends on the ability of specific antibody to aid macrophages in their engulfing of bacteria. *Fluorescence tests* use antigen or antibody coupled to a compound that fluoresces under UV to determine the location of immunoreactive compounds.

Cell-Mediated Reactions

Cell-mediated reactions involve the blastogenic responses of lymphocytes, rosette formation, the mixed leukocyte reaction, and the detection of lymphokines. Skin tests are used to identify the immune state in terms of allergy or response to previous infection.

Vaccines

Immunity to Microbes

Immunity is mediated by both humoral and cellular reactions, with different types of microbes stimulating distinct lymphocyte responses and effector mechanisms.

The survival of microbes is critically influenced by their ability to evade the immune response and the response elicited may itself cause tissue injury and disease. Extracellular bacteria may produce disease by stimulating inflammation or producing toxins. These bacteria are rapidly killed by phagocytes under normal circumstances, but increased numbers can stimulate the production of antibodies, involving both B and CD4$^+$ T-cell stimulation, which represent the main defense. Immunoglobulin G causes opsonization, IgG and IgM neutralize toxins, and IgG and IgM activate the complement system. Some staphylococcal toxins are the most potent naturally occurring T-cell mitogens known and these can induce vast numbers of CD4$^+$ cells to respond and release large amounts of lymphokines, producing an effect mimicking endotoxic shock. This is the *toxic shock syndrome.* Many bacteria are resistant to digestion when engulfed by phagocytic cells and natural immunity is quite ineffective in their control. Acquired immunity involves the stimulation of CD4$^+$ T cells by the breakdown products of some of these engulfed bacteria. The CD4$^+$ cells then produce cytokines in the DTH reaction that serve to activate the macrophages and enable them to kill the bacteria. Sometimes, however, even

this is not sufficient. Natural immunity to viral infections consists of the production of type 1 interferon and the ability of NK cells to kill virus-infected cells. Specific antibodies are important in the early stages of viral infection. They can neutralize the virus by binding to its surface and preventing entry to the host cell, enhance phagocytosis, and activate the complement cascade, which calls leukocytes to the infected area. Once the infection is established, the primary protective mechanism is that of the CD8$^+$ T cells, which can recognize and lyse virus-infected cells. Little is known concerning the immunity to parasites. Many parasites can alter their surface antigens to evade the specific immune response and this makes the design of possible vaccines difficult.

It can be successfully argued that protection against diseases by immunization (immunoprophylaxis) is the greatest achievement of biomedical science in terms of the saving of human life. If sufficient individuals can be immunized, the population develops "herd immunity" and the transmission is interrupted. The infectious agent will die out unless it has another reservoir. Successful immunization programs require, however, the intelligent implementation of other measures, both hygienic and sanitary, to generally improve the public health so that individuals can mount an immune response to the vaccines.

Immunoprophylaxis may be active, to generate an immune response after exposure to be an antigen, or it may be passive. With active immunity, it is important to generate an immune response with memory before possible exposure to an infectious agent. The usually recommended schedule for vaccination in the United States is:

Diphtheria toxoid, pertussis, tetanus toxoid (DPT), with trivalent oral polio vaccine (TOP) at 2 months, 4 months, 6 months, and 18 months, with a booster before school at 4 to 6 years and as indicated thereafter, although tetanus toxoid with a reduced level of diphtheria toxoid may be recommended at 10 years.

Measles, mumps, and rubella vaccines at 15 months, with boosters at 18 to 24 years and thereafter. Influenza and pneumococcus vaccines are recommended after the age of 65. Selective vaccination of specific groups is recommended against influenza, hepatitis B, pneumococcus, *Haemophilus influenzae, Neisseria meningitidis,* tuberculosis (BCG), rabies, anthrax, and the travelers' diseases of yellow fever, cholera, typhoid fever, and plague.

Basic Mechanisms of Protection

Vaccination is generally intended to serve as a primary stimulus to the immune system so that subsequent exposure to the natural infectious agent will result in a secondary immune response that will be more rapid and of greater magnitude. In addition, a series of vaccinations can be given to maintain ("boost") the response. The newborn is endowed with IgG of maternal origin, which can provide antitoxic, antiviral, and some types of antibacterial protection. The infant at this stage is capable of producing IgM and can respond to toxoids and inactivated or attenuated viruses. Some vaccines (e.g., pertussis) induce a state of tolerance if given too early. After a few months, the maternal IgG has declined and the infant is able to produce IgG and mount a cellular response. Timing of immunizations becomes a question of balancing the need to immunize as soon as possible with the capability of the infant to respond. Individuals over the age of 60 start to mount a reduced primary response, although they can respond effectively to the pneumococcal vaccine, but appear to retain the ability to mount a secondary response to antigens to which they have been previously exposed.

Routine immunization against some infectious agents is simplified if they are of a single antigenic type. Other agents, however, are of several antigenic types, such as poliovirus and pneumococcus, and successful immunization requires exposure to all of the important types. Immunization at the same time with multiple types seems to have no effect on the responses elicited. The usual site for vaccine injection is the arm, especially into the deltoid muscle, and studies have shown that this often gives a better response than injection into the buttocks. Polio vaccine is normally given orally rather than by arm injection.

Hazards

Attenuated organisms used in vaccines may revert to the virulent form or may cause disease in their attenuated state in immunocompromised patients. As a general rule, these vaccines should not be given to pregnant women because of possible damage to the fetus.

Pertussis vaccine occasionally causes serious problems, such as encephalopathy in the infant. It consists of heat-killed *Bordetella pertussis* and, despite the controversy surrounding its use, has continued to be recommended because the complications of whooping cough outweigh the risks of vaccination. Tetanus and diphtheria toxoids may provoke local hypersensitivity reactions. This seems to be especially true of diphtheria toxoid; thus, a smaller dose is used when adolescents and adults are given booster. Preservatives are used in some vaccines and patients can become allergic to these; the medium in which viruses are grown can cause similar effects.

Recent Approaches to Vaccine Production

Synthetic vaccines offer the hope of protection with fewer side effects. Examples of some current approaches are use of synthetic peptides, vectors altered by recombinant DNA technology, and the use of anti-idiotype immunoglobulin.

Passive Immunity

Passive immunity occurs naturally when antibodies pass from the mother to the fetus and to the newborn in the colostrum. Antibodies can be transferred artificially. They are obtained from pooled human blood and are used in possible outbreaks of hepatitis virus; they are sometimes prepared from donors who are selected after a booster dose of specific vaccine. Indications for the use of immune globulins include Rh pregnancy problems, cases of tetanus, chickenpox in leukemics at risk, rabies, and hepatitis B infections. Additional special case indications include botulism, typhus, Rocky Mountain spotted fever, black widow spider bite, coral snake bite, and crotalid snake bite.

Questions

1. The cellular immune response is mediated by:
   A. B cells
   B. T cells
   C. Both B cells and T cells
   D. Endothelial cells
   E. Skin cells
2. The humoral immune response:
   A. Results in the production of antibody by differentiated B cells
   B. Involves T cells only
   C. Requires macrophages to present antigen to B cells
   D. Is part of the natural (or innate) immune system
   E. Occurs in the bursa of Fabricius in mammals
3. T-cell epitopes are those regions of an immunogen that:
   A. Bind specifically to IgM and IgD on the surface of B cells
   B. Bind to Fc receptors on macrophages
   C. Are bound by MHC antigens, presented to T cells and for which specific T-cell receptors are present
   D. Bind to receptors on polymorphonuclear leukocytes and aid in the subsequent opsonization of the immunogen
   E. Do not survive the digestion of the immunogen that occurs following phagocytosis
4. Heterogenetic antigens:
   A. Are found in some members of a given species
   B. May show idiotypic variation
   C. Are specific to macrophages
   D. Are found in unrelated species
   E. Occur on the cell surface of platelets

5. It is true to say that the lymphatic system:
   A. Is the richest source of secretory IgA
   B. Is primarily involved in the innate response to infection
   C. Drains into the left subclavian vein near the heart
   D. Is very rich in platelets
   E. Is a major carrier of adrenal hormones to the brain

6. In humans, the primary lymphatic organs include:
   A. The thymus and the liver
   B. The spleen and the kidney
   C. The bursa-equivalent regions and the thymus
   D. The stomach and the lung
   E. The parathyroid and the thymus

7. Molecules present on the surface of B cells but **not** on T cells include:
   A. A receptor for sheep red blood cells and another for pokeweed mitogen
   B. IgM and IgD plus receptors for the C3 component of complement
   C. A receptor for concanavalin and the TCR receptor
   D. CD4$^+$ and CD8$^+$
   E. A receptor for the Fc fragment of IgA plus CD28

8. It is true to say that natural killer (NK) cells:
   A. Arise in the bone marrow
   B. Rearrange their Ig genes
   C. Express their TCR genes
   D. Require presentation of antigen by macrophages in the context of the MHC complex
   E. Have IgG molecules on their cell surface

9. Macrophages:
   A. First appear in the blood as immature T cells
   B. Mature into plasma cells when activated by contact with T helper cells
   C. Are the major source of specific immunoglobulin
   D. Have both IgM and IgG on their cell surface
   E. None of the above

10. In an acute inflammatory reaction:
    A. Kallikrein and bradykinin are **not** formed
    B. Prostaglandins and leukotrienes are **not** released
    C. Cross-reactive protein appears, binds to bacterial cell walls, and begins the complement cascade
    D. Specific immunoglobulins are formed within hours
    E. The Hageman factor is **not** involved

11. The spleen contains:
    A. Hassall's corpuscles
    B. Regions seen macroscopically as red and white
    C. Bursa of Fabricius cells
    D. Regions derived embryologically from the third pharyngeal pouch
    E. Islet of Langerhans cells

12. A lymph node contains the following anatomic regions:
    A. A cortex and medulla
    B. Low endothelial venules for lymphocyte passage
    C. No primary follicles
    D. No germinal centers
    E. Regions of red and white pulp

13. Immature B lymphocytes:
    A. Have both IgM and IgD on their surface and can react with antigen to produce immunoglobulin
    B. Produce L chains and μ H chains to form surface IgM
    C. Produce only μ H chains intracellularly with no surface Ig
    D. Have not yet begun cutting and splicing of their immunoglobulin genes
    E. Are busy cutting and splicing DNA involved in the structure of the T-cell receptor

14. Activation of mature B cells by contact with their specific antigen results in:
    A. Activation of trypsinase
    B. Decrease in intracellular calcium ions
    C. Activation of tyrosine kinase by IgM-alpha and Ig-beta
    D. Decrease in transcription initiators
    E. Increased production of deoxyribonuclease

15. The actual antigen binding site in an immunoglobulin molecule is formed:
    A. By the hinge region between CH-1 and CH-2
    B. By the first 23 amino acids of the V-H and V-L forming a cleft
    C. In the Fc region of the structure
    D. When three hypervariable regions in both the V-H and V-L domains come together in the three-dimensional structure
    E. By the carbohydrate moiety attached to the H-C3 region

16. The maturation of a B lymphocyte involves:
    A. Cutting and splicing of genes involved in the TCR
    B. Selection and production of the required MHC antigen for contacting the antigen
    C. Rearrangement of the immunoglobulin genes
    D. Production of CD3
    E. Much cell death of lymphocytes migrating through the thymus

17. Bence Jones proteins are produced by:
    A. Some patients with multiple myeloma
    B. The majority of patients with Bruton's agammaglobulinemia
    C. Patients with severe combined immunodeficiency disease
    D. Patients with AIDS
    E. Patients with Wiskott-Aldrich syndrome

18. The T-cell receptor can be made up of a dimer of:
    A. Alpha and delta chains
    B. Beta and delta chains
    C. Gamma and beta chains

D. Alpha and beta chains

E. None of the above

19. Helper T cells:

A. Have CD8 on their cell surface

B. Have IgM on their cell surface

C. Have CD4 on their cell surface

D. Are able to lyse virus-infected cells

E. Have IgD on their cell surface

20. Secretory component is:

A. Synthesized by B cells

B. Attached to secretory IgM

C. Synthesized by epithelial cells

D. Attached to IgG found in saliva

E. Necessary for the passage of IgG through the gut mucosal cells

21. The mucosal immune system includes the:

A. Popliteal lymph nodes

B. Spleen

C. Gut-associated lymphoid tissue

D. Thymus

E. Adrenal glands

22. The most important feature of immunologic tolerance is its:

A. Dependence on the stage of life of the tolerant individual

B. Dependence on dosage

C. Specificity

D. Dependence on the genetic makeup of the individual

E. Dependence on the nature of the tolerated substance (tolerogen)

23. Antigenic cross-reactivity is shown by tumors induced by:

A. Smoking

B. Oncogenic DNA viruses

C. Ultraviolet irradiation

D. Carcinogens

E. Exposure to radioactive isotopes

24. The ability of the immune system to deal with a tumor is influenced by the:

A. Location of the tumor

B. Ability of the tumor to change its surface antigens

C. Ability of the tumor to secrete blocking factors

D. Ability of the tumor to secrete protaglandins

E. Combination of all factors listed in A, B, C, D

25. As compared to a primary response, a typical anamnestic response yields:

A. About the same antibody level but the level persists longer

B. More antibody but the level is slower to develop

C. A much higher antibody level that also persists longer

D. A higher antibody level that, however, declines much more rapidly

E. A lower level of antibody that declines rapidly

The remaining questions are groups of 5. For each numbered item, choose the lettered choice with which it is most closely associated. Each choice may be used once, more than once, or not at all.

Questions 26–30. Select the type of immunoglobulin that is most closely associated with each numbered phrase or statement.

A. IgA

B. IgM

C. Kappa L chains

D. IgE

E. IgG

26. Inv allotypes

27. Able to pass the placenta

28. The first immunoglobulin class produced in an immune response

29. Has SC component when found in secretions

30. Is known as "reagin"

Questions 31–35. Select the surface marker that is most closely associated with each numbered phrase or statement.

A. CD4

B. CD3

C. CD8

D. CD2

E. CD28

31. Recognizes class 1 MHC antigens

32. Recognizes class 2 MHC antigens

33. Forms the antigen receptor complex with TCR

34. Binds to B7 on the antigen presenting cell to provide a co-stimulatory signal

35. The receptor for sheep red blood cells

Questions 36–40. Select from the list of compounds the numbered phrase or statement with which it is most closely associated.

A. C3a

B. C3b

C. Arachidonic acid

D. Class 1 MHC antigens

E. Class 2 MHC antigens

36. Recognized by CD4 on T helper cells

37. Is liberated from membrane phospholipids

38. Recognized by CD8 on cytotoxic T cells

39. Is anaphylatoxic

40. Is broken down into a variety of protein products in the blood

In questions 41–45, classify the diseases listed according to the Gell and Coombs' classification.

A. Class 1

B. Class 2

C. Class 3

D. Class 4
E. Class 5
41. Atopy
42. Allergic contact dermatitis
43. Serum sickness
44. Hemolytic disease of the newborn
45. Cutaneous anaphylaxis

In questions 46–50, for each numbered item choose the lettered choice with which it is most closely associated.
A. The ABO antigens
B. The Rh antigen
C. An allograft
D. A syngraft
E. Isohemagglutinins
46. IgM antibodies
47. Minor blood group antigen(s)
48. Involves genetically different individuals
49. Major blood group antigen(s)
50. Involves genetically identical individuals

In questions 51–55, for each numbered item choose the lettered choice with which it is most closely associated.
A. Antibody-mediated autoimmune disease
B. Immune complex–mediated autoimmune disease
C. T cell–mediated autoimmune disease
D. Complement component deficiency
E. IgE-mediated autoimmune disease
51. Hashimoto's thyroiditis
52. Rheumatoid arthritis
53. Autoimmune hemolytic anemia
54. Myasthenia gravis
55. Systemic lupus erythematosus

In questions 56–60, for each numbered item choose the lettered choice with which it is most closely associated.
A. Deficiency in B cells, T cells normal
B. Deficiency in T cells, B cells normal
C. Deficiency in both B and T cells
D. Deficiency in phagocytic cells
E. Deficiency in complement component(s)
56. Di George's syndrome
57. Transient hypogammaglobulinemia of infancy
58. Bruton's agammaglobulinemia
59. Severe combined immunodeficiency disease
60. Ataxia-telangiectasia

In questions 61–65, for each numbered item choose the lettered choice with which it is most closely associated.
A. Agglutination
B. Precipitation
C. Hapten inhibition
D. ELISA
E. Opsonization

61. Measures the primary reaction between antigen and antibody
62. Involves an insoluble antigen
63. Usually involves a bound antigen, reacted with its antibody, and detected using enzyme-labeled immunoglobulin specific for the antibody
64. Requires the build-up of a lattice of antigen/antibody combinations
65. Measures the effect of antibody binding on the ability of cells to phagocytose

In questions 66–70, for each numbered item choose the lettered choice with which it is most closely associated.
A. Extracts of *Bordetella pertussis*
B. Attenuated poliovirus
C. Pneumococcal polysaccharides
D. Measles, mumps, and rubella
E. Typhoid fever
66. Recommended only in cases of proposed foreign travel
67. A booster is recommended at the age of 18–24
68. Requires representation of three different strains
69. Used as a vaccine despite serious problems with side effects
70. Recommended in individuals over the age of 65

Answers

1. B T cells mediate the cellular immune response and help B cells respond in the humoral response.
2. A The humoral response is the production of antibodies by B cells after their activation and during and after their differentiation into plasma cells.
3. C Immunogen is broken down into peptides in the antigen presenting cells (macrophages and B cells), bound to specific MCH II proteins, transported to the cell's surface, and presented to CD4 + T cells. If specific receptors exist on T cells, the peptides in question are T-cell epitopes. In the case of "foreign" protein synthesized internally, peptides are bound to specific MHC I proteins and presented to CD8 + T cells.
4. D
5. C The lymphatic system collects tissue fluid and returns it to the blood supply when it drains into the left subclavian vein.
6. C In humans, the thymus is the primary lymphatic organ where T cells develop. B cells, which develop in the bursa of Fabricius in birds, mature in various sites of lymphatic tissue thought to be equivalent to the bursa.
7. B Surface IgM and IgD on B cells give them their specificity for the antigen response.

8. A All cells found in the blood arise from stem cells in the bone marrow.

9. E The properties listed are those of B and T cells. Macrophages appear in the blood as monocytes and mature into macrophages in different tissues. The site of the differentiation leads to the different names for the macrophages; for example, Kupffer cells are liver macrophages.

10. C Kallikrein, bradykinin, prostaglandins, and leukotrienes are all released in inflammation, and complement is fixed initially by the C-reactive protein.

11. B

12. A High endothelial venules, germinal centers, and primary follicles are characteristic of normal lymph nodes.

13. B Immature B cells have begun cutting and splicing of their immunoglobulin genes and produce surface-only IgM with both kappa and lambda light chains present.

14. C Tyrosine kinase activation is the result of combination between the antigen and its antibody.

15. D

16. C Cutting and splicing of the immunoglobulin genes are involved in determining the specificity of the Ig produced by an individual cell and in the class switch following activation.

17. A Bence Jones proteins are dimers of light chains formed from the overproduced immunoglobulin in many patients with multiple myeloma.

18. D T-cell receptors are made up of alpha and beta chains when the T cells mature in the thymus and from gamma and delta chains when the T cells mature in nonthymic regions.

19. C Helper T cells have CD4 on their surface, which allows contact with antigen presenting cells through the MHC II antigen.

20. C Secretory component is synthesized by epithelial cells and is attached to IgA molecules before they are released into the lumen of the gut.

21. C Lymphoid tissue associated with the gut forms the mucosal immune system.

22. C All the properties listed are characteristic of tolerance but it is the specificity that is the major quality of immune tolerance.

23. B Oncogenic viruses produce specific surface antigens that allow some cross-reactivity.

24. E

25. C Because of the pool of specific T and B memory cells, the secondary response can be detected sooner, involves production of more antibody, and lasts longer than a primary response.

26. C Kappa light chains have allotypic forms termed *Inv*.

27. E IgG is the only immunoglobulin able to pass through the placenta.

28. B IgM is produced before the class switch and therefore occurs first in an immune response. IgD is found on the surface of mature B cells but is not secreted at a high level.

29. A IgA has secretory component attached when it is found in secretions.

30. D IgE has been termed *reagin* by allergists.

31. C CD8 on T cells (mainly cytotoxic T cells) recognizes MHC class I antigens.

32. A CD4 on T cells (mainly T helper cells) recognizes MHC class II antigens.

33. B

34. E

35. D

36. E

37. C

38. D

39. A C3a is released in the complement cascade and is anaphylatoxic.

40. B C3b is released during the complement cascade and is broken down into a variety of products.

41. A Atopy involves IgE and is class I.

42. D Allergic contact dermatitis involves a tuberculin-type response and is class IV.

43. C Serum sickness involves antigen/antibody complexes and is class III.

44. B The reaction involves antigens forming part of cell surfaces and is class II.

45. A Cutaneous anaphylaxis involves IgE and is class I.

46. E Naturally found isohemagglutinins are IgM immunoglobulins.

47. B A,B, and O are the major blood groups. Other antigens are considered minor.

48. C

49. A

50. D

51. C

52. B

53. A Autoimmune hemolytic anemia is caused by anti-RBC antibodies.

54. A Myasthenia gravis is the result of antibodies against the acetylcholine receptors at neuromuscular junctions.

55. B SLE results from immune complexes formed by anti-DNA antibodies.

56. B Di George's syndrome is a birth deficiency involving the fourth pharyngeal pouch and results in many symptoms including thymus deficiency.

57. A This syndrome involves a retarded development of the humoral immune system.

58. A Bruton's is the original, classic B-cell deficiency.

59. C As the name implies, both B and T cells are deficient.
60. C This syndrome varies with individual patients but both T and B cells are involved.
61. C The ability of a hapten to prevent the binding of bound antigen with its specific antibody occurs at the level of the initial antigen/antibody binding.
62. A Agglutination involves the clumping together of insoluble antigen.
63. D
64. B Precipitation is the continued formation of a lattice between soluble antigen and its antibody until the complex becomes insoluble.
65. E An opsonin increases the ability of phagocytes to engulf bacteria.
66. E Typhoid fever is not a problem requiring vaccination for those staying in the United States.
67. D Booster shots with the measles, mumps, and rubella vaccine are recommended because the original vaccine of 15 to 20 years ago did not result in lifelong immunity and 18 to 20 years of age is the time of exposure to new populations (e.g., college, military training).
68. B Three serologically different strains of polio virus cause poliomyelitis and have to be immunized against.

69. A The whooping cough vaccine results in some cases of neurologic involvement with resulting death, but the chances of this are currently outweighed by the beneficial effects of vaccination.
70. C Pneumonia is caused by a variety of organisms, and many strains of *Streptococcus pneumoniae* can cause the disease. The current vaccine uses strains that cause the majority of the infections.

Suggested Reading

Abbas, A. K., Lichtman, A. H. J., and Pober, J. S. *Cellular and Molecular Immunology* (2nd ed.). Philadelphia: Saunders, 1994.

Kuby, J. *Immunology*. New York: Freeman, 1992.

Roitt, I., Brostoff, J., and Male, D. *Immunology* (3rd ed.). St. Louis: Mosby, 1993.

Stites, D. P., Terr, A. I., and Parslow, T. G. *Basic and Clinical Immunology* (8th ed.). Norwalk, CT: Appleton and Lange, 1994.

General Bacteriology

Joe A. Fralick

Taxonomy and Nomenclature of Bacteria

Taxonomy is the science of biologic classification. It involves *classification, nomenclature,* and the *identification* of organisms. Classification involves the arrangements of organisms into groups or taxa based on similarities or relatedness. Nomenclature is concerned with the assignment of names to taxonomic groups. Identification is concerned with the process of determining that a particular organism belongs to a particular taxon. A major goal of bacterial taxonomy is to aid the bacteriologist in identifying unknown bacteria and to provide the physician with a fast and accurate determination of a pathogen.

Classification

The early description of organisms as either plants or animals is too simplified, and many systematic biologists place organisms into five kingdoms based on three major criteria: (1) cell type (procaryotic or eucaryotic, (2) level of organization (solitary, colonial, unicellular, multicellular), and (3) nutritional type (absorptive, ingestive).

Two fundamentally different types of cells exist: *procaryotic* and *eucaryotic* (Fig. 2-1). Procaryotic (pro, or primitive nucleus) cells have a simpler morphology than eucaryotic cells and lack a nucleus and nuclear membrane as well as intracytoplasmic organelles such as mitochondria. The eucaryotic cell (eu, or true nucleus) has a membrane-bound nucleus and is found in algae, fungi, protozoa, plants, and animals. All bacteria or procaryotic organisms including the *eubacteria* (true bacteria) and *archaebacteria* (ancient bacteria) are placed in the kingdom *Procaryotae* (or *Monera*).

Nomenclature

The basic taxonomic group in microbial taxonomy is the *species*. Species of higher organisms refer to groups of interbreeding or potentially interbreeding populations that are reproductively isolated from other groups. However, a bacterial species is a collection of *strains* that share many stable properties in common and differ significantly from other groups of strains. A strain is a population of organisms that descends from a single parent organism.

Bacteria are named according to the rules established by the International Code of Nomenclature, which uses latinized names with suffixes to indicate *divisions* (-es), *classes* (-aceae), *orders* (-ales), *families* (-aceae), *genera*, and *species*. At present the trend is to place emphasis on the species and genus, with higher taxonomic levels to be indicated only where genetic evidence is adequate. The first word of a bacterial name is the *generic* name (genus) and is capitalized and italicized (e.g., *Escherichia*). The second word of a bacterial name designates the *species*, and is italicized but not capitalized (e.g., *coli*). Often, the genus name is shortened by abbreviating with a single capital letter (e.g., *E. coli*). Common or trivial names, such as streptococcus or pseudomonad, refer to strains that are physiologically or morphologically similar. Such names are neither capitalized nor italicized and sometimes can be confusing, such as when "bacillus" is used to describe any rod-shaped bacteria. However, some trivial names, such as tubercle bacillus and typhoid bacillus, are used in place of *Mycobacterium tuberculosis* and *Salmonella typhi*, respectively, in the medical literature. A list of approved bacterial names was published in 1980 in the *International Journal of Systematics Bacteriology* and new valid names are published periodically in this same journal.

Several criteria are used in assigning bacteria to a previously defined or a new genus and specific epithet. These include phenotypic classifications, which are based on morphologic, physiologic, metabolic, ecological, and genetic characteristics, and phylogenetic classifications, which are based on evolutionary relationships. The latter are determined from comparisons of proteins, nucleic acid-base composition, and nucleic acid homologies.

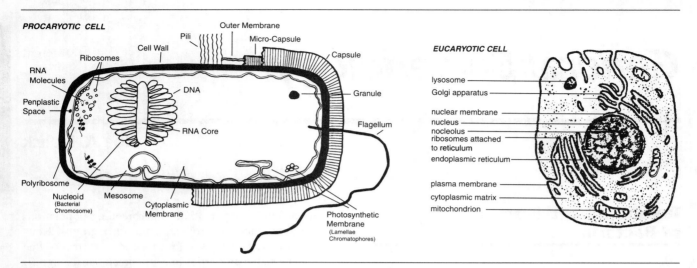

PROCARYOTIC CELL

Outer Membrane
Pili
Micro-Capsule
Cell Wall
Ribosomes
Capsule
RNA
Molecules
DNA
Granule
Penplastic
Space
RNA Core
Flagellum
Polyribosome
Nucleoid
(Bacterial
Chromosome)
Mesosome
Cytoplasmic
Membrane
Photosynthetic
Membrane
(Lamellae
Chromatophores)

EUCARYOTIC CELL

lysosome
Golgi apparatus
nuclear membrane
nucleus
nocleolus
ribosomes attached
to reticulum
endoplasmic reticulum
plasma membrane
cytoplasmic matrix
mitochondrion

Fig. 2-1   Procaryotic versus eucaryotic cell architecture.

Identification

The difficulty of bacterial taxonomy arises from making artificial divisions where no apparent natural species barriers exist, and, despite the uncertainties and problems with the classification in *Bergey's Manual of Systematic Bacteriology*, it is the most widely accepted and used system for the identification of bacteria.

Composition, Organization, and Architecture of the Bacterial Cell

Chemical Composition of the Average Bacterial Cell

Bacterial cells can be harvested by centrifugation and their biomass analyzed by a variety of biochemical techniques. Typically, one finds that approximately 70 percent of the packed cell mass is water, somewhat less than the 90 percent found for cells of higher organisms. Elemental assay of the dry mass of *E. coli* reveals a fairly typical composition of protoplasm that mostly consists of organic compounds. Table 2-1 gives the results of organic analysis of the dry mass of *E. coli* cells growing at 37°C in glucose minimal media.

Some general observations that can be made from analyzing Table 2-1 are as follows:

1. Macromolecules constitute the preponderance (96%) of the dry mass of bacterial cells.
2. Proteins constitute more than one half (55%) of these macromolecules and represent the greatest diversity of different kinds.

3. The ribosomal ribonucleic acid (rRNA) species (23S, 16S, and 5S) are different from eucaryotic rRNA species.
4. While there are many common macromolecules, two are unique to bacteria: *peptidoglycan* and *lipopolysaccharide*.
5. While there are over 1050 different protein species, only 400 different messenger RNA (mRNA) species exist, indicating that many of the proteins are coded in *polycistronic mRNA* molecules (mRNA species that code for more than one gene product).

Variety and Number of Macromolecules

Proteins

We can estimate the number of different proteins and their abundance from analysis of two-dimensional gels that resolve total cell protein (O'Farrell gels). In this technique proteins are separated on the basis of their net charge by means of *isoelectric focusing* in one dimension and on the basis of their apparent size by *sodium dodecyl sulfate (SDS)–polyacrylamide* gel electrophoresis in the second dimension. From such an analysis there are approximately 1050 different polypeptides present in significant amounts (50 or more molecules/ cell) in an *E. coli* cell growing in minimal glucose media at 37°C. This same analytical technique also reveals that the different species of polpeptides may vary in their content over a 10^5-fold range implicating powerful mechanisms for controlling the expression of individual genes.

RNA

The preponderance of RNA (81%) is *rRNA*, comprising three molecular species—*23S, 16S,* and *5S*—present in

Table 2-1 Tabulation of Macromolecule Composition of an Average *Escherichia coli* Cell

Macromolecules	% of Dry Mass	Average Molecular Weight	No. of Molecules/Cell	No. of Different Kinds
Protein	55.0	4.0×10^4	2,360,000	1050
RNA	20.5	1.0×10^6		
23S		1.0×10^6	18,700	1
16S		5.0×10^5	18,700	1
5S		3.9×10^4	18,700	1
tRNA		2.5×10^6	205,000	60
mRNA		1.0×10^6	1,380	400
DNA	3.1	2.5×10^9	2.13	1
Lipid	9.1	705	22,000,000	4
Lipopolysaccharide	3.4	4346	1,200,000	1
Peptidoglycan	2.5	$(904)n$	1	1
Glycogen	2.5	1.0×10^6	4,360	1
Total macromolecules	96.1			
Metabolites, vitamins, precursors, and inorganic ions	3.9			

equimolar amounts (approximately 18,700 copies per cell). *Transfer RNA (tRNA)* makes up most of the remainder of the RNA (15%), of which there are about 200,000 molecules comprised of approximately 60 different species. *Messenger RNA* makes up only 4 percent of the cell's total RNA and represents approximately 400 different species. Messenger RNA of *E. coli* has an average *half-life* of 1.3 minutes; however, not all mRNA species are equally labile and their different half-lives may vary from fractions of a minute to 10 minutes.

DNA

DNA makes up approximately 3 percent of the dry weight of the average *E. coli* cell. The *E. coli chromosome* is known to consist of a circular, covalently closed, double-stranded molecule of approximately four million nucleotide base pairs with a molecular weight of about 2.5×10^9 daltons. Our reference cell has slightly over two complete chromosomes. However, since each daughter chromosome is a copy of the same parental chromosome the cell is genetically *haploid*.

Lipid

The lipid of *E. coli*, excluding lipid A of lipopolysaccharide, is *exclusively phospholipid*. Bacteria do not accumulate neutral fats as reserve materials and their lipids are a functional component of their membranes. Thus, membrane phospholipids comprise 9 percent of the dry weight of the average *E. coli* cell.

Lipopolysaccharide (LPS)

The lipopolysaccharide of *E. coli* is a complex macromolecule. It is composed of three regions: (1) the *lipid A,* (2) the *core oligosaccharide,* and (3) the repeating or *O antigen.* Lipopolysaccharide is found *exclusively* in the *outer leaflet of the outer membrane* and is unique to gram-negative bacteria.

Peptidoglycan

Peptidoglycan is found in all bacteria with the exception of archaebacteria. In gram-positive bacteria, where there are many layers of peptidoglycan, it forms the bulk of the cell envelope. In gram-negative bacteria, such as *E. coli,* where it is only a single layer thick, it still plays an important role in maintaining the structural integrity of the cell.

Bacterial Size and Form
Cell Shape

Bacteria come in a variety of shapes and sizes and can be visualized by dark-field or phase contrast microscopy. These techniques allow the morphology or shape of the bacteria to be determined. Bacteria that possess inflexible cell walls can be classified according to shape as follows:

1. *Cocci:* spherical bacteria
2. *Streptococci:* cocci that are arranged in chains
3. *Staphylococci:* cocci arranged in clusters

4. *Sarcinae:* cocci arranged in packets
5. *Bacilli:* rod-shaped bacteria
6. *Fusiform:* rod-shaped bacteria with tapered ends
7. *Clavate:* club-shaped or bacteria with swollen ends
8. *Cordyneform:* bacteria that exhibit variation in their diameter
9. *Vibrios:* bacillary forms that are bent into the shape of a comma
10. *Spirilla:* bacteria that appear snakelike
11. *Coccobacilli:* bacteria that appear as ovoids or ellipsoids and sometimes occur in pairs
12. *Spirochetes:* bacteria that possess flexible cell envelopes with a "corkscrew" appearance

Bacteria can also show variation in morphology in a pure culture and this is known as *pleomorphism.* Several medically important bacteria are subject to pleomorphism, which underlines the importance of examining fresh, viable cultures.

Cell Size

Bacteria are small, well below the range of what the unaided human eye can see. Typical bacteria are on the order of 1 μm in diameter. It takes approximately 10^{12} bacteria to weigh 1 g and it requires a suspension of 1 to 10 million to be visibly cloudy. It has been estimated that each human carries up to 100 trillion bacteria in the large intestine, which greatly surpasses the total number of the individual's cells.

Being small has its advantages. It allows for very high metabolic rates because the surface-to-volume ratio increases as the size of the cells decreases. Ultimately, biochemical reactions are limited by diffusion, and the smaller the cells, the less limiting it is. Consequently bacteria are capable of high metabolic rates (orders of magnitude higher than those of their eucaryotic cousins).

Bacterial Architecture

Procaryotic Versus Eucaryotic

Bacteria are procaryotes, whereas fungi, protozoa, and *elephants* are *eucaryotes. Procaryotes lack true nuclei* and other internal membrane-bound organelles. They do not carry out endocytosis and are incapable of ingesting particles or liquid droplets. Procaryotes also differ from eucaryotes in important biochemical ways, such as the composition of their ribosomes and lipids. Procaryotes are usually haploid, containing a single (or duplicated) chromosome and extrachromosomal plasmids; eucaryotes are usually diploid or have a diploid phase with multiple chromosomes.

Gram-Positive Versus Gram-Negative

Most bacteria can be subdivided into one of two groups based on their reaction to *Gram's stain.* The major difference between the two groups relates to fundamental differences in the composition and organization of the cell envelope. The cell envelope includes the *cell wall* or *peptidoglycan* layer, which lies just outside the cytoplasmic membrane, and, in the case of gram-negative bacteria, an *outer membrane* (Fig. 2-2). *Gram-positive* bacteria have *thick cell walls* composed of multiple layers (approximately 40) of peptidoglycan, *which are highly cross-linked.* There is no outer membrane. *Gram-negative* bacte-

Fig. 2-2   Gram-positive versus gram-negative cell envelopes. LPS, lipopolysaccharide; LP, lipoprotein.

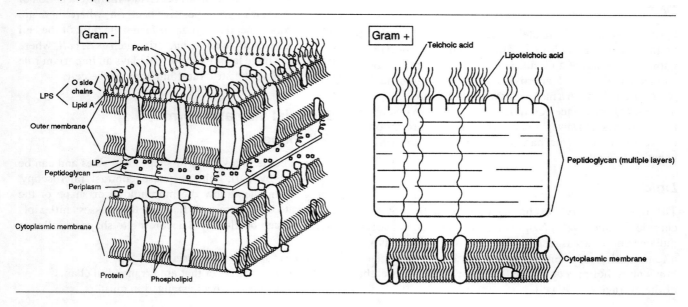

ria have *thin cell walls* of peptidoglycan (often a single layer thick) *with less cross-linking* than gram-positive bacteria and another membrane on the cell surface called the *outer membrane*. Although several explanations have been given for the difference in Gram's stain results, it appears that it is due to the physical nature of the peptidoglycan. If this layer is removed from gram-positive bacteria, they stain as gram-negative. The peptidoglycan is not stained per se but rather acts as a permeability barrier. Both gram-positive and gram-negative bacteria are initially stained by the primary stain crystal violet. The cells are next treated with the mordant ethanolic iodine to promote dye retention. When the gram-positive bacteria are then decolorized with acetone-ethanol, the ethanol is thought to shrink the pore size of the thick, highly cross-linked peptidoglycan and retain the dye-iodine complex. Hence the gram-positive bacteria remain purple. The gram-negative bacteria, on the other hand, have a thin, not as

highly cross-linked, peptidoglycan layer, and the alcohol treatment can extract the purple crystal violet–iodine complex. Hence, gram-negative bacteria must be stained with a counterstain to be seen.

Subcellular Components of Bacteria

Surface Appendages

Both gram-positive and gram-negative bacteria may have proteinaceous surface appendages: *pili* and *flagella* (Table 2-2).

Flagella. Most motile bacteria move by means of flagella, which are long, hollow, whiplike structures made up of polypeptide subunits of *flagellin*. Electron microscopic studies have shown that the bacterial flagellum is composed of three parts: (1) the long whiplike *filament* made up of flagellin; (2) a *basal body,* which is embedded in the

Table 2-2 Summary of the Structural/Functional Relationships of the Subcellular Components of the Bacterial Cell

Structure	Composition	Function
Flagella	Protein (flagellin)	Locomotion
Pili (fimbriae)	Protein (pilin)	Adhesion
Capsule	Polysaccharides	Usually protects from environmental factors
	Polypeptide	Sometimes contributes to virulence
		May prevent phagocytosis
		May be antigenic
		Food reservoir
Cell wall	Peptidoglycan (murein)	Protects from osmotic lysis
		Gives cell rigid structure
		Determines cell shape
Gram-positive	Thick peptidoglycan layer	
	Highly cross-linked	
	Contains teichoic acids	
Gram-negative	Thin peptidoglycan layer	
Outer membrane	Phospholipid, protein, and LPS	Forms hydrophobic barrier
		Unique to gram-negative bacteria
Cytoplasmic membrane	Phospholipid, protein and carbohydrates	Houses many biosynthetic enzymes
		Houses the energy-producing electron transport systems
		Houses many transport systems for sugars, amino acids, etc.
Cytoplasm	Nucleic acids, proteins, and carbohydrates	Primary site for biosynthesis
Bacterial nucleus	DNA (single chromosome)	Genetic storehouse
	No nuclear membrane	
Ribosomes	RNA and proteins	Translational machinery
Inclusions		
Volutin	Polymetaphosphate	Reserve materials
Granulose	Polymers of glucose	
Other	Sulfur, lipids, glycogen	
Endospores	Contain many of the macromolecules of the vegetative cell	Very resistant to environmental factors such as heat, chemicals, and ultraviolet light

cytoplasmic membrane and *acts as a motor* in the turning of the filament in a clockwise or counterclockwise rotation; and (3) the *hook,* which *acts like a universal joint* and links the filament to the basal body. In gram-negative bacteria the basal body has four rings connected to a central rod. The L and P rings associate with the lipopolysaccharide (outer membrane) and peptidoglycan, respectively. The two inner M rings are associated with the cytoplasmic membrane. Gram-positive bacteria have two rings, one associated with the cytoplasmic membrane and one with the peptidoglycan layer.

Bacteria with a single polar flagellum are *monotrichously* flagellated, whereas those with flagella distributed over their surface are *peritrichous. Lophotrichous* bacteria possess a tuft or cluster of flagella confined to one end, and *amphitrichous* bacteria have tufts of flagella at both ends. Being proteinaceous, flagella are antigenic, and are called *H antigens.* Serologic identification of bacterial types via H antigens is useful in identifying various serotypes, especially among *Salmonella* species.

Pili. Pili, or *fimbriae,* are hairlike, hollow-cored appendages that exist on many species of bacteria. Pili are composed of a protein, called *pilin.* Pili often confer adhesive properties to the bacterial cells, enabling them to adhere to various epithelial surfaces, to red blood cells, to surfaces of yeast and fungal cells, and to teeth, as well as to glass. These adhesive properties play an important role in bacterial colonization and thus are sometimes referred to as *colonization factors.* This adhesion is often very specific. For example, the *E. coli* strains that cause traveler's diarrhea adhere through pili to cells of the small intestine where they secrete a toxin that causes the symptoms of the disease. Pili are also essential for gonococci to infect the epithelial cells of the genitourinary tract. A unique pilus called the *sex pilus* or *F pilus* is used for the transfer of deoxyribonucleic acid (DNA) from a donor to a recipient cell during the process of conjugation. Pili, like capsules, can be *antiphagocytic* and may be highly changeable, permitting some organisms to outflank the immune system.

Capsules and Slime Layers

Capsules and slime are located outside the peptidoglycan cell wall and are found in both gram-positive and gram-negative bacteria. If the layer of material is well organized (not easily washed off), it is called a *capsule.* If the material is diffuse (easily washed off), it is called a *slime layer.* In some cases a slime layer is found outside a capsule. Capsules and slime layers are usually composed of *polysaccharides,* but may be constructed of other materials. One important exception is the *polyglutamic acid* capsule of *Bacillus anthracis.* Capsules can be seen with the light microscope when capsule stains are employed. When placed on appropriate media, species that produce large capsules appear mucoid and are referred to as *smooth (S)* colonies, while noncapsular variants of these smooth bacterial cells are called *rough (R)* strains. Capsules are *antiphagocytic,* promote *adherence* to surfaces, *exclude* many hydrophobic antibiotics, *protect against dehydration and bacteriophages, protect against ion and pH fluctuations,* and act as *virulence factors.*

Cell Envelope

Outer Membrane

The outer membrane of gram-negative bacteria is a highly specialized organelle that lies outside the cytoplasmic membrane and the murein/peptidoglycan cell wall and forms the interface between the cell and its environment. In contrast to most biologic membranes, the outer membrane does not allow passage of hydrophobic and amphipathic molecules. It serves primarily as a *selective barrier* that excludes a variety of noxious environmental substances, such as degradative enzymes, antibiotics, and bile salts, while allowing permeation of water-soluble nutrients and ions to the active transport machinery of the cytoplasmic membrane. This specialized function is reflected in its unique composition and molecular architecture. Characteristic components include a limited set of *major outer-membrane proteins* and include in *E. coli* the *porin* family, which form trimeric, transmembrane, nonspecific hydrophilic pores; the *murein lipoprotein,* which covalently anchors the outer membrane to the peptidoglycan cell wall; *OmpA,* which is involved in the integrity of the outer membrane; and a unique major component, *lipopolysaccharide,* which resides exclusively in the outer leaflet of the outer membrane and is essential for the maintenance of the outer-membrane permeability barrier. The size of the outer-membrane pores determines the size of water-soluble solutes that can pass into the cell. In *E. coli,* pores constructed of the porins OmpC and OmpF exclude molecules larger than 700 daltons. The outer membrane also contains approximately 50 other protein species present in much lower copy numbers. Many of these minor outer-membrane proteins have key functions, including specific transport systems (for iron, vitamin B_{12}, maltose, etc.) and enzymatic activities (phospholipase, proteases). In addition, the outer membrane from members of the family Enterobacteriaceae contains a unique polysaccharide, *enterobacterial common antigen.*

Lipopolysaccharide

Probably the most unusual macromolecules of the outer membrane are lipopolysaccharides. These large macromolecules consist of both lipids and carbohydrates, and are composed, chemically, of three regions: (1) the *lipid A,* (2) the *core oligosaccharide,* and (3) the repeating side chain or *O antigen.*

Lipid A is similar in all gram-negative bacteria and consists of two glucosamine disaccharide derivatives with fatty acids esterified to some of its hydroxyl groups. The fatty acids give this region of the macromolecule hydrophobic, lipid-like properties and hence it is this region that is intercalated into the outer leaflet of the outer membrane in place of the usual membrane phospholipids. This portion of LPS also is responsible for the toxicity of LPS (*endotoxin*).

The *core oligosaccharide* can be subdivided into inner and outer segments. The inner core region, which is joined to the lipid A segment, consists of *heptose* and an unusual deoxysugar, *KDO* (3-deoxy-D-mannoctulosonic acid). The outer core, which links with the O antigen, is composed of several sugars. The core oligosaccharide structure is constant within a genus.

The *O antigen* is a short, repeating oligosaccharide polymer that extends from the polysaccharide core. *There is considerable diversity among and within species with respect to the O antigen composition.* Although the O antigen is readily recognized by host antibodies, gram-negative bacteria may rapidly change their O antigen structure thereby outfoxing their host. Also since the O antigen extends from the surface of the cell it may also prevent the antibody from reaching the cell surface. Lipopolysaccharide also serves the cell by providing its surface with a net negative charge, thereby promoting the binding of cations, and resulting in a heavily hydrated and charged surface. This, in turn, prevents access of hydrophobic substances, such as antibiotics, detergents, bile salts, and other surface-active agents, to the membrane and accounts for the relative resistance of gram-negative bacteria to these agents.

Cell Wall

The bacterial cell wall is a *huge macromolecule* made up of *peptidoglycan,* a polymer unique to bacteria. This polymer consists of disaccharide repeating units of *N*-acetylglucosamine in B-1,4 linkage with *N*-acetylmuramic acid and hence is sometimes referred to as the murein cell wall. The disaccharide repeating units are covalently linked to one another through peptide linkage. The *N*-acetylmuramic acid moieties each have a tetrapeptide side chain attached by an ether linkage. This tetrapeptide often consists of alternating D- and L-amino acids, three of which, *D-glutamic acid, D-alanine, and mesodiaminopimelic acid, are not found in proteins.* In some bacteria the mesodiaminopimelic acid is replaced by L-lysine. These tetrapeptide side

chains are cross-linked through a pentapeptide interbridge often consisting of glycine. This polymeric fabric forms a sac the size and shape of the organism. Since the peptidoglycan sacculus of gram-negative bacteria is only one layer thick, the cross-linking can occur only between glycan chains that are in the same plane. Alternatively, the multilayered nature of the gram-positive peptidoglycan also permits the formation of cross-links between glycan chains above and below the plane. Hence, *gram-positive bacteria have more cross-linkages than do gram-negative bacteria.*

The rigid peptidoglycan corset allows bacteria to survive in media of lesser osmotic presure than that of their cytoplasm. In the absence of a cell wall, the membrane bursts and the cells lyse. This can be demonstrated experimentally by removing the peptidoglycan with a hydrolytic enzyme, *lysozyme,* which is present in many human and animal tissue fluids. Treatment with lysozyme causes bacteria to lyse in a low-osmotic-pressure environment. If lysozyme-treated bacteria are kept in an isoosmotic medium, they do not lyse but become spherical. Such cells are called *spheroplasts* (for gram-negative cells) or *protoplasts* (for gram-positive cells). The uniqueness of bacterial peptidoglycan makes it a natural target for antibiotics and some of the most clinically effective antibiotics, the penicillins and cephalosporins, act by inhibiting peptidoglycan biosynthesis.

While the cell wall of gram-positive bacteria consists of a thick, highly cross-linked peptidoglycan layer, it also contains a large amount of *teichoic acids, which are unique to gram-positive bacteria.* Teichoic acids are polymers of glycerol (teichoic acids) or ribitol (ribitol teichoic acids) joined by phosphate groups and carrying one or more amino acids (often D-alanine) or sugar (often glucose) substitutes. Teichoic acids, up to 30 glycerol or ribitol units long, may be connected to the C-6 hydroxyl group of the N-acetylmuramic acid of the peptidoglycan cell wall or to the plasma membrane lipids (in this case called *lipoteichoic* acids). All gram-positive bacteria contain lipoteichoic acids, but they may or may not have the peptidoglycan-linked form. Because teichoic acids are negatively charged they are analogous to the LPS of gram-negative bacteria in that they help give the gram-positive cell surface a negative charge. However, teichoic acids are not endotoxic and have no toxic activity.

Cell Wall–Deficient Bacteria

Some bacteria contain no cell envelope other than the cytoplasmic membrane, which in some instances may contain host-derived sterols. These bacteria belong to the class Mollicutes, which contains several taxonomically distinct genera, some of whose members are highly pleomorphic (e.g., *Mycoplasm.*). The wall-deficient bacteria are distinct from *L forms* or *L-phase variants,* which are derived from both gram-positive and gram-negative bacteria through the clinical use of antibiotics targeted at peptidoglycan biosynthesis.

The Periplasm

The periplasmic space (periplasm) lies between the inner and outer membranes of gram-negative bacteria. Because of its location, this space should not be thought of as a single homogeneous compartment but rather as consisting of several distinct microenvironments created by the two boundary membranes and the peptidoglycan layer. The periplasm harbors *hydrolytic enzymes* involved in breaking down complex molecules into simpler precursors, *detoxifying enzymes*, and *binding proteins*, which are involved in the trafficking of specific nutrients to specific transport systems of the cytoplasmic membrane and are also involved as *chemoreceptors* in chemotaxis. The periplasm also contains *membrane-derived oligosaccharides (MDOs)*, which are synthesized in response to the osmolarity of the environment.

Cytoplasmic Membrane

Beneath the cell wall lies the cytoplasmic membrane, which is vital to the cell. The cytoplasmic membrane is composed of a *phospholipid bilayer* in which *integral* or *intrinsic* membrane proteins are embedded. These proteins mediate membrane functions such as *solute transport* and *energy generation*. Proteins more loosely associated with the membrane are called *peripheral* or *extrinsic* membrane proteins. The major phospholipids found in the cytoplasmic membrane are phosphatidylethanolamines, phosphatidylglycerol, and glycolipids. Ribosomes and the bacterial chromosome are also often found in association with the cytoplasmic membrane. In gram-positive bacteria the cytoplasmic membrane may invaginate into a structure called a *mesosome*, and although this term is technically restricted to gram-positive bacteria, similar structures can be seen in gram-negative bacteria called *intracytoplasmic membranes*. The cytoplasmic membrane may fuse with the outer membrane in gram-negative bacteria at adhesion sites called *Bayer junctions*. It is thought (although not proved) that these junctions are involved in the attachment and DNA injection of bacteriophages, in complement-mediated lysis, and in the translocation of proteins and LPS from the cytosol to the outer membrane.

Cytoplasmic Structures

The Nucleoid

In *E. coli* the genomic DNA is a large circular macromolecule that is compacted more than 1000-fold into a microscopically distinct structure called a *nucleoid* or *nuclear body*. The nucleoid is functionally analogous to the eucaryotic nucleus, but there are intriguing structural differences. For example, *the nucleoid is not surrounded by a membrane*. Moreover, assays that detect superhelical tension in bacterial DNA fail to do so in the DNA of higher cells, and chromatin structure appears to be more labile in bacteria.

Ribosomes and Polysomes

Ribosomes are large *ribonucleoprotein particles* that are responsible for translation of the genetic code. Their molecular architecture is complex. The *70S bacterial ribosome* is 38 percent protein and 62 percent RNA and dissociates into *30S and 50S subunits*. The 50S subunit contains both 23S and 5S RNA and 32 different proteins. The 30S subunit contains 16S RNA and 21 different proteins. Polysomes are chains of 70S ribosomes attached to messenger RNA. Ribosome numbers vary according to growth requirements. Under rapid growth there are more ribosomes per cell than under slow growth conditions.

Cytoplasmic Inclusions

Many bacteria store polymers of glucose (glycogen) as membrane-enclosed or nonmembrane-enclosed *glycogen granules* (inclusions). Most bacteria accumulate glycogen without an enclosed membrane. *Glycogen is the major storage material of enteric bacteria* and is produced in the cell when there is an excess of carbon and limitation of nitrogen, sulfur, or phosphorous or the pH is low. When the limiting nutrient becomes available the glycogen is broken down into glucose and shunted into the glycolytic pathway. Inorganic polyphosphate accumulates during the exponential phase of growth as *polyphosphate granules* and decreases as phosphate becomes limiting. The phosphate granules are not surrounded by membranes and are synthesized in the cell by the enzyme polyphosphate kinase. Other names for these phosphate granules include *volutin* and *metachromatic* granules. They are found in the diphtheria bacillus, *Corynebacterium diphtheriae;* in the plague bacillus, *Yersinia pestis;* in mycobacteria; and in others. *Poly-beta-hydroxybutyrate (PHB) granules* represent a lipid storage component of some *Bacillus* and *Pseudomonas* species. They are surrounded by a membrane and accumulate in sporulating cells of *Clostridium botulinum* during the stationary phase.

Endospores

Some gram-positive bacteria can form dormant, resistant structures called *endospores*, including the medically important genera, *Clostridium* and *Bacillus*. When compared with their vegetative counterparts, *endospores are found to be extraordinarily resistant to heat, dehydration, ultraviolet light, and organic solvents*, treatments often used in disinfecting procedures. Because spore-forming pathogens such as *Clostridium botulinum, tetani, and perfringens*, and *B. anthracis*, are responsible for botulism, tetanus, gas gangrene, and anthrax, respectively, and because the sporulation process provides a number of important antibiotics, such as bacitracins, gramicidins, and tyrocidines, the spore is of considerable interest in medicine.

Bacterial Nutrition, Growth, and Energy Metabolism

Bacterial Nutrition

Nutritional Classifications

Bacteria can be classified by their relationships to *temperature* and *oxygen*, and by their *sources of carbon* and *energy*. Bacteria can be divided into two large groups with regard to their nutritional requirements. In one group are the bacteria that subsist on carbon dioxide and minerals, called *lithotrophs*, that use either light energy (*photolithotrophs*) or chemical energy (*chemolithotrophs*). The other group includes all the organisms that need preformed organic components for their carbon source, *organotrophs* (*chemoorganotrophs* and *photoorganotrophs*). All medically important pathogenic microorganisms are chemoorganotrophs, but within this group they have many gradations of nutritional needs. Some, like *E. coli*, are satisfied with glucose as a carbon source and have additional requirements for various inorganic materials and ions. Other pathogenic bacteria are unable to make one or more essential metabolites such as vitamins, amino acids, purines, and pyrimidines. These must be supplied as *growth factors* by the host. Bacteria that have complex nutritional requirements are called *fastidious*. Many pathogenic bacteria are fastidious.

Bacteria can also be classified according to their range of responses to oxygen. For example, bacteria such as the *Pseudomonas* that require oxygen are called *obligate aerobes* while those, such as *Salmonella*, that are capable of growth in the presence of oxygen by respiration or in the absence of oxygen by fermentative metabolism are called *facultative anaerobes*. Bacteria, such as *Bacteroides*, that are killed or inhibited by oxygen are the *obligate anaerobes*. Some bacteria, such as *Streptococcus*, can tolerate an oxygen atmosphere but are incapable of utilizing oxygen in respiration. They are called *aerotolerant* or *aerotolerant anaerobes*. Additionally, there are bacteria that can grow in oxygen-containing atmospheres, but cannot tolerate the normal levels of oxygen present in air (21%). These bacteria are called *microaerophilic* or *capnophilic*.

Bacteria also have an optimum temperature for growth and can be classified accordingly. *Psychrophiles* are bacteria with an optimum growth temperature ranging between *10°C* and *20°C*. Included in this group are *Pseudomonas fluorescens* and many marine bacteria. *Thermophiles*, on the other hand, grow at an optimum temperature of *50°C to 60°C*, and include bacteria from hot springs such as *Bacillus stearothermophilus*. *Mesophiles* have an optimum growth temperature between *20°C* and *40°C* and include most pathogenic bacteria. As might be expected, a reduction in temperature slows down growth and often extends the viability of a culture. In fact, freezing a culture suspended in 20% glycerol is an excellent way to preserve microorganisms. In contrast, an elevation of growth temperatures above the optimum usually reduces viability. Temperatures exceeding 50°C are lethal for most pathogenic bacteria.

Uptake of Nutrients

Bacteria take up mainly small substrates from the medium but rarely macromolecules or phosphate esters. Gram-negative and gram-positive bacteria secrete *extracellular* enzymes across their cytoplasmic membranes that hydrolyze macromolecules. The resulting breakdown products (peptides, oligosaccharides, nucleosides, phosphate, etc.) can then be transported across the cytoplasmic membrane. The cytoplasmic membrane contains specific carrier proteins called *permeases* that facilitate the entry of most metabolites into the cell. The relative abundance of carbohydrates and proteins in the environment is reflected in the affinities of the specific transport systems for these nutrients. For example, the Michaelis constant (K_m) for the transport of carbohydrates is approximately 10^{-4}, but for amino acids it is much more sensitive, varying between 10^{-6} and 10^{-8}. *The three main types of nutrient transport are:*

1. *Facilitated diffusion*, in which transport takes place *without energy expenditure*. This mechanism does not concentrate compounds in the inside of the cell relative to the outside. Uptake is driven by intracellular utilization of the compound and the process involves a stereospecific *carrier* or *binding* protein. An example of a compound that is transported by facilitated diffusion is *glycerol*. The concentration of free glycerol inside the cell is lowered by its phosphorylation to glycerol 3-phosphate during glycolysis, and more glycerol is then taken up to equilibrate with the outside glycerol concentration.

2. *Group translocation*, sometimes called *phosphorylation-linked* transport, is involved in the transport of certain sugars. Substances transported by this mechanism *are*

chemically altered in the process. For example glucose binds to a stereospecific carrier protein (enzyme-2), which then interacts with a cytoplasmic membrane protein called Hpr-P, to yield glucose 6-phosphate. *Energy is required* for the substrate phosphorylation by the phosphotransferase system.

3. *Active transport* differs from group translocation in that *energy is utilized* to drive the accumulation of a substrate, which remains unaltered, *against a concentration gradient*. It also uses stereospecific binding proteins. Active transport is involved in the uptake of various sugars and amino acids. An example is the uptake of lactose, which is concentrated unchanged inside the cell. The cell's *proton motive force* (PMF) is used to drive this process.

Uptake of Iron

Iron is not available in its free form in the blood and many tissues because it is bound to proteins such as transferrin or ceruloplasmin; nevertheless, it is essential for the growth of bacteria. Many bacteria that inhabit the human body have developed ingenious mechanisms to obtain iron. They often excrete chelating compounds known as *siderophores* that *bind iron* with great avidity. Each organism can take up its own particular form of complexed iron. However, in the competition for iron, many bacteria have evolved multiple siderophores as uptake systems, in an effort to gain an edge on other organisms that inhabit the same environment. Some of these siderophores can efficiently extract iron from transferrin.

Bacterial Chemotaxis

Some bacteria recognize nutrients (attractants) and swim toward them and swim away from repellents. This movement toward attractants and away from repellents is called *chemotaxis* and the movement is accomplished by the action of flagella. Flagella spin around from their point of attachment at the cell surface. *Each flagellum has a counterclockwise helical pitch.* When the bacteria contain flagella rotating counterclockwise, bundles form and the bacteria swim in a straight line. However, when flagella rotate clockwise the bacteria tumble in a random fashion. *The two types of motion, swimming in a relatively straight line and tumbling randomly, account for chemotaxis.* In the absence of attractants or repellents, bacteria alternate indifferently between swimming and tumbling. However, when an attractant is present, swimming up a concentration gradient dominates over tumbling. On the other hand, when a repellent is present, swimming down a concentration gradient is dominant over tumbling. The net result is movement toward attractants and away from repellents. Little is known about the involvement of chemotaxis in pathogenesis, but it would not be surprising if it were involved in guiding the bacteria to a cellular target or away from host defenses.

The components of the sensory system that recognize the chemical and detect the changes in concentration are called *chemoreceptors*. These receptors are not of a single protein class. Some are periplasmic proteins that function in the transport of sugars while others are tightly bound to the cytoplasmic membrane and are found concentrated at the poles of the cells. They are often components of transport systems. Hence, *transport and chemotaxis are very closely related*.

Bacterial Growth

When bacteria find themselves in a suitable environment, they grow (multiply) by *binary fission* and double their population size over a period of time called the *mean generation time*, or *doubling time*. For example, *E. coli* growing in a rich nutrient broth at 37°C with good aeration requires about 20 minutes to double its number. Growth will continue until the population reaches a certain density determined by available nutrients or toxic waste products. Until this condition occurs, the bacteria grow in an unhindered manner and are physiologically alike. This condition is called *balanced growth*, since *all cell constituents increase proportionally over the same period of time*. The cell number increases exponentially with time and the bacterial culture in balanced growth is said to be in its *exponential or logarithmic (log) phase* of growth. The explosiveness of exponential growth suggests that a small number of bacteria may initiate a serious infection. For example, bacteria that cause acute meningitis in a child, such as the meningococcus, grow so rapidly in the patient that the physician may need to intervene immediately to avoid a fatal outcome. On the other hand not all pathogens multiply rapidly. Tubercle bacilli divide every 24 hours so that even under optimal conditions the disease they cause is chronic and takes considerable time for manifestation.

If balanced growth went unchecked, a single bacterium dividing twice an hour (doubling time of 30 minutes) would produce a mass equivalent to that of the earth in just 2 days! Obviously that doesn't happen. Instead, when a bacterial culture reaches a certain cell density, either required nutrients are exhausted or metabolites accumulate to toxic levels. A carbon source, a required inorganic compound, or essential amino acid or vitamin may be depleted. For aerobic bacteria, crowding leads to the depletion of oxygen since it is poorly soluble in water. Toxic metabolites, such as hydrogen peroxide, or acids formed by fermentation that are incompatible with growth may accumulate. Factors actually responsible for the slowdown of growth depend on the sensitivity of the strain of bacteria and on the composition of the culture medium (environment). The stage of the culture where active growth is interrupted is known as the *stationary phase*. Bacteria can cause damage to their host even when they are not multiplying. For example, the production of toxins often occurs or is accelerated when bacteria enter the stationary phase. During this phase, some streptococci secrete enzymes that lyse red blood cells and produce proteases that degrade hemoglobin thus supplying them with amino acids and iron. Cessation of growth in other bacteria may lead to sporulation resulting in the production of metabolically inert spores that are extraordinarily resistant to chemical and physical insults. During sporulation the mother cell is lysed, releasing the spore and often large amounts of toxins (e.g., in tetanus, gas gangrene infections).

Eventually, the cells of the stationary culture begin to die and the culture enters the *death* or *decline phase*. This decline in viable cell number is exponential and is the inverse of the log phase. The rate of exponential decline may vary dramatically from species to species.

When cells from a stationary phase culture are transferred into a nutritious environment, the organisms initially must adapt and show a *lag* in cell division for a short period of time. This adaptation period is termed the *lag phase* of growth and its duration is dependent on the strain and the nutritional status of the new environment.

Measurement of Growth

Increases in cell numbers can be measured microscopically, electronically, or by cell mass determination.

Cell Mass

Bacteria can be weighed by *wet weight* or *dry weight* methods. Wet weights are imprecise and seldom employed. There are two general techniques employed for determining cell mass by the dry weight method. With the first, the cells are harvested by centrifugation and washed several times with distilled water. The sample is then dried in an infrared oven at 100°C or *in vacuum* at 80°C. A more common technique is the *turbidimetric method*. Various photoelectric devices, such as the *spectrophotometer,* are employed to measure the optical density or light-scattering properties of a culture, which during exponential growth are proportional to the bacterial density and are commonly plotted as a log function. All of these methods measure the total bacterial mass without regard to the number of living or dead bacteria.

Cell Number

The *Petroff-Hauser* counter is a device similar to a hemocytometer in which a glass slide has calibrated areas etched into it. Because the volume that fills the etched areas is known, the number of bacteria per unit volume can be determined microscopically. The *Coulter counter* or *electronic particle counter* measures the number as well as the size of the particles in a suspension passing through an orifice through which an electric current flows. As the particle passes through the orifice it displaces its volume of electrolyte and is measured electronically. These methods also do not determine the viability of the bacterial cells being enumerated.

Viable Count

To determine the number of live (viable) cells in a suspension, the bacteria are diluted and spread over the surface of an agar plate, which is then incubated. Cells deposited on the agar surface give rise to visible colonies that are counted. The number of cells multiplied by the dilution factor will give the total viable count.

Bacterial Metabolism
Heterotrophic Metabolism

In bacteria, like all living cells, nutrients are converted into substances that are used for *the production of energy* and/or *the production of new carbon skeletons* needed to synthesize other vital cell materials. Medically important bacteria use organic compounds and chemical energy to achieve these goals (*chemoorganotrophs*). These processes are collectively called *metabolism*. When metabolic process involves the breakdown of a nutrient, with the subsequent production of energy, it is called *catabolism*. When the metabolic process involves the biosynthesis of cell material, it is called *anabolism*. *Neither process exists independently in the cell, but both are closely linked* and regulated so that the cell does not waste energy or produce unnecessary cell components.

Energy Production

Energy is produced in the cell by oxidation/reduction reactions. This energy is trapped in the phosphate bond of *adenosine triphosphate (ATP),* often called the *energy currency* of the cell. The phosphate bond energy can be harnessed by heterotrophic cells by two different processes: *substrate phosphorylation* and *oxidative phosphorylation.* Both processes involve *oxidation,* with the subsequent release of *electrons* and *hydrogen*. Substrate phosphorylation takes place most often in the cell during an anaerobic process called *fermentation,* which can be defined as an oxidation process involving the combustion of an organic substrate in the absence of oxygen. The release of electrons and hydrogen results in the reduction of an organic molecule. Oxidative phosphorylation occurs during a process called *respiration*. Respiration may be defined as a process involving the combustion of a substrate with the subsequent release of electrons and hydrogen resulting in the reduction of an inorganic molecule, usually oxygen.

Fermentation Pathways

Fermentation is an anaerobic process that involves the oxidation of organic substrates. For the majority of bacterial species, the most easily oxidized substrates are carbohydrates. In bacteria, as in other living cells, the *Embden-Meyerhof-Parnas (EMP)* pathway is the principal route for carbohydrate catabolism. When the carbohydrate is a hexose and the product is pyruvate, the process is called *glycolysis*. In glycolysis the electron donor (glucose) is oxidized, and the electrons and hydrogen ions that are released are transported by *nicotinamide adenine dinucleotide (NAD)* to the final electron acceptor, which is pyruvate. Energy is conserved during this oxidation or dehydrogenation process and trapped within certain intermediates in the EMP pathway. This energy is associated with the phosphate group of two intermediates: on carbon 1 of 1,3-diphosphoglyceric acid and on carbon 2 of phosphoenolpyruvate. The high-energy phosphate groups within these two molecules are donated to adenosine diphosphate (ADP), resulting in the formation of ATP. Other monosaccharides are capable of entering the EMP pathway (e.g., mannose, fructose, and galactose). These sugars are converted to glucose 6-phosphate or related sugar phosphates in a series of reactions. Hence, the catabolism of glucose to pyruvate via glycolysis can be represented by the following equation:

$$\text{Glucose} + 2\text{ADP} + 2\text{P}_i + 2\text{NAD}^+ \longrightarrow$$
$$2 \text{ pyruvate} + 2\text{ATP} + 2\text{NADH} + 2\text{H}^+$$

Since fermentation is an incomplete oxidation process, a number of end products can accumulate in the cell. For some bacteria such as the streptococci and lactobacilli the fermentation of glucose results primarily in the formation of lactic acid. This reaction serves to regenerate NAD, which can be utilized during glycolysis. In the process, lactic acid accumulates in the cell. Species that produce lactic acid as the principal end product of fermentation are called *homolactic* or, because they produce a single end product, *homofermentative bacteria*. Species that produce equivalent amounts of other end products, in addition to lactic acid, are called *heterolactic* or *heterofermentative bacteria*. Although the end products of fermentation are diverse, they are the result of only a few chemical bond rearrangements, carboxylations, decarboxylations, and NADH-mediated reductions of pyruvate. *Many of these products are useful in the identification of bacteria* in the clinical laboratory. For example, acetonin helps differentiate certain species within the family Enterobacteriaceae. In addi-

tion, speciation of numerous anaerobic bacteria is based upon gas chromatographic profiles of fatty acids such as acetic, butyric, and propionic acid produced during fermentation.

Glucose can be catabolized by pathways other than the EMP pathway. The *Enter-Doudoroff (ED)* pathway, for example, is used for glucose dissimulation by *Pseudomonas* and other obligatory aerobic bacteria. In this series of reactions, pyruvate and D-glyceraldehyde 3-phosphate are produced. Pyruvate is further oxidized to ethanol while the D-glyceraldehyde 3-phosphate is shunted into the EMP pathway. Since only one ATP molecule per molecule of glucose is produced in this pathway, it is only half as efficient as the EMP pathway in energy production. Another major pathway for glucose utilization is the *hexose monophosphate (HMP) shunt,* sometimes called the *pentose phosphate shunt,* where the conversion of 6-phosphogluconate to pentose phosphate permits the five-carbon sugars to enter the pathway. It is thought that most microorganisms utilize both the EDP and HMP simultaneously because these pathways have different functions. *The HMP shunt generates its reducing equivalents as NADH and H$^+$,* which is used for biosynthetic reductions such as fatty acid biosynthesis, *whereas the NADH and H$^+$ generated by the EMP pathway is usually coupled to energy metabolism.*

Amino Acid Fermentation

Many anaerobic bacteria and some facultative anaerobes can ferment amino acids. Most of these species belong to the genus *Clostridium* or are anaerobic cocci. The fermentation of amino acid results in the formation of products that are similar to those produced during glucose fermentation, such as CO_2, pyruvate, acetate, butyrate, and propionate.

Respiration and Energy Production

Fermentation reactions extract energy from organic substrates by substrate phosphorylation but substantial chemical energy remains in the reduced end products of fermentation. This energy can be retrieved by the complete oxidation of the fermentation products to CO_2 and H_2O. This is the mission of *respiration*. In respiration the final electron acceptor is an inorganic molecule. When the inorganic molecule is oxygen, the process is called *aerobic respiration*. When the inorganic molecule is something other than oxygen, the process is termed *anaerobic respiration*.

Aerobic Respiration

Obligate aerobes or facultative anaerobes derive more energy from metabolism in the presence of oxygen than do anaerobic bacteria in the absence of oxygen. In aerobic respiration the EMP pathway can be utilized; however, other pathways play a more important role (e.g., hexose monophosphate shunt). During aerobic respiration the pyruvate that is produced can be further oxidized to CO_2 and water. This oxidation occurs during a process called the *tricarboxylic acid (TCA) cycle* or *Krebs cycle*. Before entering the TCA cycle, pyruvate is decarboxylated to acetyl coenzyme A (acetyl-CoA). During one complete turn of the cycle, the acetyl-CoA is oxidized to CO_2, three molecules of NADH + H$^+$, and one molecule of flavin adenine dinucleotide (FAD) + H$^+$.

The reducing equivalents and electrons generated during glycolysis and the TCA cycle are then presented to the electron transport system (ETS) located in the cytoplasmic membrane. The ETS consists of a series of stable components (flavoproteins, quinones, cytochromes) that are aligned in a sequence of progressively higher oxidation-reduction potentials. Electrons are passed from the more electronegative to the less electronegative components of the system. The final component of the system is cytochrome oxidase, which catalyzes the reduction of molecular oxygen to water. There are three sites in the ETS in which the oxidation produces sufficient energy to extrude a pair of *protons* (2H$^+$) from the cell. This establishes a *proton motive force* or *electrochemical gradient* across the cytoplasmic membrane as a result of the unequal distribution of charges. The cytoplasmic membrane is impermeable to protons. The extruded protons can return to the cytosol via a specific channel in the *membrane ATPase*. The energy drop during this process provides sufficient energy to generate ATP. The mechanisms that account for this process were derived from the *chemiosmotic hypothesis* formulated in 1961 by the British biochemist *Peter Mitchell*. The proton motive force may drive the transport of molecules across membranes and also account for the rotation of bacterial flagella.

Anaerobic Respiration

Respiration occurs in the absence of oxygen in facultative anaerobes. In this case the terminal electron acceptors may be *nitrate, fumarate, sulfate,* or *carbonate*. The pathways for transfer of electrons in anaerobic respiration are similar to those for aerobic respiration except that cytochrome oxidase is supplanted by other enzymes such as nitrate reductase. This enzyme is induced in the absence of oxygen or in the presence of nitrate, or both, and is repressed in the presence of oxygen. Addition of nitrate or fumarate to an anaerobic culture often results in a greater growth yield. However, when these compounds serve as electron acceptors the energy does not approximate that obtained when the culture is grown with oxygen as the final electron acceptor. For example, phosphorylation coupled to fumarate produces approximately one mole of ATP per mole of

fumarate reduced while the reduction of one molecule of nitrate yields two molecules of ATP. In aerobic respiration, by comparison, approximately three ATP molecules are produced for each election pair passing through the ETS.

Biosynthesis

The assembly of precursors into macromolecules requires that the subunit be energetically activated by being coupled to a substituent group containing an energy-rich bond. This bond is usually derived from the energy currency of the cell, ATP, produced during catabolism. Thus catabolic pathways and anabolic pathways are usually coupled through ATP utilizing reactions. However, catabolic pathways provide more than simply the energy to synthesize the new organic molecules needed for the growth. They also provide the carbon skeletons for the synthesis of many precursors of the cell. For instance, amino acid skeletons are derived from acetyl-CoA and from intermediates of the TCA cycle, glycolysis, and the pentose phosphate pathway. Alanine, aspartate, and glutamate are synthesized by transamination, directly from pyruvate, oxaloacetate, and alpha-ketoglutarate, respectively. The TCA cycle is also an important source of precursors for pyrimidine biosynthesis and because of the heavy demand on its intermediates, the cell has evolved reactions that replenish them. A pathway that serves to replace cycle intermediates is called an *anaplerotic* pathway. For example, using either pyruvate or phosphenolpyruvate as an acceptor molecule, CO_2 fixation forms the TCA cycle intermediate oxaloacetate. The *glyoxalate shunt*, which is actually a modified tricarboxylic acid (TCA) cycle, replenishes TCA cycle intermediates and functions as an important anaplerotic pathway. This shunt is also directly involved in the catabolism of fatty acids.

From this discussion it becomes obvious that many catabolic and anabolic pathways share common intermediates, and it would be inaccurate to refer to the EMP pathway or TCA cycle as being wholly catabolic. Pathways involved in both catabolism and biosynthesis are called *amphibolic* pathways, a term that reflects their dual role.

Questions

1. The basic taxonomic group in microbial taxonomy is the:
   A. Kingdom
   B. Class
   C. Family
   D. Genera
   E. Species
2. Phylogenic classifications are based on:
   A. Morphologic characteristics
   B. Physiologic characteristics

C. Evolutionary characteristics

D. Biochemical characteristics

E. None of the above

3. Comparison of the number of different protein species versus the number of different mRNA species in an *E. coli* cell indicates:

A. That a single gene product can be translated from more than one mRNA

B. That some of the mRNA molecules are polycistronic

C. That mRNA is composed of nucleic acid

D. That all mRNA molecules must be polycistronic

E. None of the above

4. Fusiform bacteria are:

A. Spherical in shape

B. Club-shaped

C. Rod-shaped with tapered ends

D. Rod-shaped and arranged in clusters

E. None of the above

5. The number of different species of proteins in a bacterial cell can be estimated from:

A. Amino acid analysis of total cellular protein

B. The number of different mRNA species in the cell

C. Two-dimensional gel electrophoresis analysis

D. One-dimensional gel electrophoresis

E. None of the above

6. Peptidoglycan:

A. Contains fatty acids

B. Contains D- and L-amino acids

C. Defines the periplasmic space

D. Is found only in gram-negative bacteria

E. None of the above

7. Lipopolysaccharide:

A. Contains amino acids

B. Contains fatty acids

C. Is specific to gram-positive bacteria

D. Is a component of the cytoplasmic membrane

E. All of the above

8. Bacteria that have flagella distributed over their surface are called:

A. Monotrichous

B. Peritrichous

C. Amphitrichous

D. Lophotrichous

E. None of the above

9. H antigens are associated with which of the following structures?

A. Capsules

B. Slime layers

C. Flagella

D. Pili

E. Fimbriae

10. The bacterial outer membrane:

A. Is found only in gram-positive bacteria

B. Acts as a diffusion barrier to hydrophobic antibiotics

C. Contains teichoic acids

D. Is involved in active transport of sugars

E. None of the above

11. The periplasm contains:

A. Ribosomes

B. A nucleoid

C. Hydrolytic enzymes

D. Inclusion bodies

E. None of the above

12. Spheroplasts:

A. Have a thick peptidoglycan layer

B. Require an isoosmotic medium for survival

C. Are made from gram-positive cells

D. Are missing their cytoplasmic membrane

E. None of the above

13. Endospores:

A. Are resistant to various disinfectant treatments

B. Have a unique peptidoglycan structure

C. Are the result of cellular differentiation

D. Are medically relevant

E. All of the above

14. A bacterial pathogen that grows maximally at body temperature is classified as a:

A. Thermophile

B. Psychrophile

C. Capnophile

D. Mesophile

E. Lithophile

15. Bacteria that can subsist on CO_2 but cannot tolerate oxygen are called:

A. Chemoorganotropic, facultative anaerobes

B. Chemolithotropic, obligate anaerobes

C. Organolithotropic, obligate anaerobes

D. Chemolithotropic, aerotolerant anaerobes

E. None of the above

16. Facilitated diffusion involves:

A. Uptake of a nutrient against a concentration gradient

B. A chemical modification of the nutrient being transported

C. Utilization of energy

D. A stereospecific carrier protein

E. None of the above

17. Bacterial chemotaxis involves:

A. Lipopolysaccharide sensors

B. Swimming and tumbling

C. Pili

D. Gram-positive bacteria only

E. None of the above

18. Siderophores:

A. May be important to a pathogenic bacteria

B. Are found only in gram-positive bacteria

C. Are required for chemotaxis
D. Are porin proteins found in the outer membrane
E. All of the above

19. Balanced growth:
    A. Defines a situation in which all macromolecule synthesis is increasing at the same rate
    B. Occurs in the stationary phase of growth
    C. Is linear in nature
    D. Occurs in the lag phase of growth
    E. None of the above

20. Bacterial cell mass can be determined with a:
    A. Coulter counter
    B. Petroff-Hauser counter
    C. Spectrophotometer
    D. Colony counter
    E. None of the above

21. Sporulation is most likely to occur during the _____ phase of growth.
    A. Log
    B. Lag
    C. Stationary
    D. Death
    E. Exponential

22. Fermentation:
    A. Occurs in the Embden-Meyerhof-Parnas (EMP) pathway
    B. Is an aerobic process
    C. Is very efficient in producing energy
    D. Is another word for aerobic respiration
    E. None of the above

23. Fermentation reactions extract energy by:
    A. Oxidative phosphorylation
    B. Substrate phosphorylation
    C. Cytochrome oxidase
    D. Proton motive force
    E. None of the above

24. Anaerobic respiration:
    A. Involves cytochrome oxidase
    B. Involves an obligate anaerobe
    C. Does not involve a proton motive force
    D. Does not involve an electron transport system
    E. None of the above

25. Amphibolic pathways:
    A. Replenish intermediate pools
    B. Are involved in both catabolism and anabolism
    C. Are active only under anaerobic conditions
    D. Are active only under aerobic conditions
    E. None of the above

26. Catabolism and biosynthesis are coupled through:
    A. The TCA cycle
    B. ATP utilizing reactions
    C. Anaerobic respiration
    D. Glycolysis
    E. None of the above

Answers

1. E The basic taxonomic group in microbial taxonomy is the species or a collection of strains that share common properties and differ significantly from other groups of strains.
2. C
3. B The fact that there are fewer mRNAs than proteins (see Table 2-1) implies that some of the mRNAs must code for more than a single polypeptide (protein) and hence are called polycistronic.
4. C
5. C The number of different protein species and their relative abundance can be estimated from the analysis of two-dimensional gels that resolve total cell protein based on their charge (isoelectric focusing) and size (SDS-polyacrylamide gel electrophoresis).
6. B The bacterial cell wall is made up of a rigid polymer called peptidoglycan, which defines the cell's shape. This macromolecule contains disaccharide repeating units of N-acetylglucosamine and N-acetylmuramic acid, which are covalently linked by a tetrapeptide that contains both D- and L-amino acids.
7. B The lipid A portion of LPS is an endotoxin and contains fatty acids.
8. B
9. C
10. B The LPS in the outer leaflet of the outer membrane forms a diffusion barrier to hydrophobic antibiotics.
11. C The periplasm contains hydrolytic enzymes involved in breaking down complex molecules into simpler precursors as well as membrane-derived oligosaccharides that are synthesized in response to the environmental osmolarity.
12. B
13. E
14. D Bacteria that grow between 20°C and 40°C are called mesophiles. Body temperature is 37°C.
15. B Bacteria that use chemical energy (CO_2) but cannot tolerate oxygen are called chemolithotropic obligate anaerobes.
16. D Facilitated diffusion refers to uptake of nutrients without the expenditure of energy but involves a stereospecific carrier protein.
17. B
18. A Iron is not available in its free form in the blood and tissues because it is bound by proteins such as transferrin. Bacteria need iron for growth and they excrete chelating compounds (siderophores) that bind iron with great avidity. Some siderophores can efficiently extract iron from transferrin, thus making them virulence factors.

19. **A**

20. **C** The Coulter counter and Petroff-Hauser counter count cell numbers, not cell mass. The colony counter counts viable cells, not cell mass. The spectrophotometer measures light scattering, which is dependent on cell mass.

21. **C**

22. **A** Fermentation is an anaerobic process that involves the oxidation of organic substrates and uses the Embden-Meyerhof-Parnas (EMP) pathway as its principal route. It is not as efficient as aerobic respiration in extracting energy from substrates.

23. **B** Fermentation is an oxidative process involving the combustion of an organic substrate in the absence of oxygen (i.e., substrate phosphorylation).

24. **E** Anaerobic respiration occurs in the absence of oxygen in facultative anaerobes. It involves electron transport pathways similar to those used in aerobic respiration, except that cytochrome oxidase is supplanted by other electron acceptors. The mechanism by which it generates ATP is identical to that of aerobic respiration (via a proton motive force).

25. **B**

26. **B**

Microbial Genetics

Joe A. Fralick

DNA

Hail to thee O molecule
And mighty nucleotide
Wherein our destinies
Indelibly reside.

Omnipotent, ubiquitous
In phylogenetic span
Each pleiomorphic fantasy
Evolves within thy plan.

Thy codons are a poetry
As writ by greatest pen
In base sequential mysteries
Which chromatins defend.

Two sugar phosphate helices
Pyrimidines between
With purines neatly organized
Enumerate each gene.

Thy messages are manifold
Their syntax proteinaceous
Their grammar stereotaxic and
Their grip on life tenacious.

Unwind, uptake and replicate
Until mitotic knell
Transcribe, translate, communi-
cate!
So cell may nurture cell.

And so, with simple gratitude
I wish to close this poem:
Be it ever so humble
There's no place like genome.

Anonymous

DNA: The Molecular Basis of Genetics

Historical Perspectives

The genetic information of all known living cells resides within their deoxyribonucleic acid (DNA). However, the importance of this macromolecule has not always been recognized. From cytologic, genetic, and chemical studies, it was known early in this century that genes were somehow associated with chromosomes and that chromosomes contained DNA and protein. However, until the 1950s it was widely believed that DNA was a repeating polymer of a single type of tetranucleotide unit and that only proteins were of sufficient complexity and size to accommodate the vast amount of genetic information required of the cell's hereditary makeup. The first important evidence that DNA was the genetic material of cells came in 1944, when Avery, MacLeod, and McCarty chemically fractionated Griffith's transforming principle and unequivocally established that its active ingredient was DNA. However, this view was slow to catch on.

In 1950 experiments by Ephrussi-Taylor and by Hotchkiss showed that one cell-free extract may contain several different transforming activities and that transformation can be explained in terms of recombination between the genetic material of the recipient cell and the DNA of the transforming principle. In 1952 Hershey and Chase demonstrated that during the infection of the bacterium, *Escherichia coli*, by bacteriophage T2 only the phage DNA entered the bacterial cell and directed the synthesis of the resulting progeny phage. These studies along with Chargaff's demonstration that DNA could have variable composition, an obvious requirement of hereditary material, did away with the tetranucleotide hypothesis, and the idea that DNA was the genetic material came of age.

DNA Structure

Primary Structure

The nucleic acids DNA and ribonucleic acid (RNA) are polymers of nucleotides. In both DNA and RNA there are generally four types of nucleotides, which are distinguished by their bases: adenine, guanine, cytosine, and uracil in RNA and adenine, guanine, cytosine, and thymine in DNA. Hence, one major distinction in these two nucleic acids is that RNA contains uracil whereas DNA contains thymine. Exceptions to this rule are the presence of thymine in transfer RNA and uracil in the DNAs of certain phages as well as transiently in most replicating DNAs. Ribonucleic acid also contains a variety of other bases.

Another major distinction between RNA and DNA is their sugar-phosphate backbones: RNA contains only ribose; DNA contains only 2-deoxyribose. These nucleotides are linked together as long, unbranched polymers formed by $3',5'$-phosphodiester bridges between the $5'$-phosphate of one nucleotide and the $3'$-hydroxyl of the sugar of the next (i.e., P-5′ sugar-3′-phosphate-5′sugar-3′-phosphate-) and are referred to as polynucleotide chains.

Secondary Structure

The actual molecular architecture of double-stranded DNA was proposed by Watson and Crick in 1953, after they analyzed the results of x-ray diffraction data obtained on purified fibers of DNA by Franklin and Wilkins. Their model had the DNA molecule consisting of two helically intertwined, antiparallel polynucleotide chains held together laterally by hydrogen bonds between complementary pairs of purine and pyrimidine residues on opposite chains. The sugar-phosphate backbones form a right-handed helix with a periodicity of approximately 10.6 base pairs. This model illustrates the classic B-structure of DNA, which has since been shown to be the predominant form of DNA.

An important concept that came out of this model was that of *complementarity,* which was determined by the steric relations of the bases. The complementary base pairs allowed are adenine (A) with thymine (T) and guanine (G) with cytosine (C). Modified bases can also enter into base-pair formation provided they can form hydrogen bonds with another base. Since A always pairs with T, and G with C, the overall content of A in DNA must be equal to T, and the content of G must equal C. Thus the base ratio of double-stranded DNA is $(A + T)/(G + C)$. The base ratios of DNAs from different organisms may vary widely. However, more important, the actual sequence of bases also varies enormously from one organism to another.

The Watson-Crick model suggested that the only specific aspect of DNA that could distinguish one DNA molecule from another was the nucleotide sequence of the four possible purine-pyrimidine base pairs and that the genetic information must, therefore, reside in the code of these sequences.

The double-helix model also suggested a means by which DNA could replicate itself. For if the two complementary polynucleotide chains were to separate and each parental chain were to act as a template for the de novo synthesis of a complementary daughter chain, a pair of DNA molecules would be generated, each half-new, half-old, whose specific purine-pyrimidine base-pair sequence would be identical to that of the parent molecule (i.e., semiconservative replication). This prediction was later confirmed by Meselson and Stahl's density transfer experiment.

A minor form of duplex DNA that may have physiologic significance is the so-called *Z-DNA,* named after its zigzagging sugar-phosphate backbone. This DNA is characterized by a left-handed helix and alternating sugar-base conformation. Cellular proteins have been isolated that recognize this form of DNA, but their physiologic functions remain unknown.

DNA Molecules and Chromosomes

DNA molecules from different organisms and viruses vary greatly in size, structure, and number. Not all naturally occurring DNA is found as a double-stranded helix. The DNAs of certain small bacterial, plant, and animal viruses occur naturally as single-stranded DNAs. However, even these DNAs must go through a transient double-stranded form during their replication. In eucaryotic cells, DNA is found in a number of molecules, but only one molecule is present per chromosome.

The Bacterial Chromosome

The DNA of the bacterial cell is contained in a central region of the cytoplasm, called the nuclear region or *nucleoid* to distinguish it from the membrane-bound nucleus of eucaryotic cells. Both genetic and autoradiographic studies have shown the *Escherichia coli* chromosome to be a circular structure containing about 4 million base pairs and having a circumference of approximately 1 mm or about 1000 times the width of the cell that houses it. How this huge macromolecule is packaged in situ remains to be resolved. However, much of the compaction required is achieved by high-order structure involving the coiling of the axis of the double helix upon itself. This is called *supercoiled* or *superhelical* DNA. Studies by Pettijohn and Worcel have revealed some of the complexity of its organization. After gentle lysis of the *E. coli* cell, the DNA molecule can be isolated in a highly folded and supercoiled state (approximately 70–130 supercoiled domains) complexed with RNA and protein. This structure is often referred to as the *folded chromosome* or nucleoid. Bacterial cells may contain more than one nucleoid, depending on the cells' growth rate and size. Each nucleoid is assumed to be a single replicating or resting chromosome. Bacteria behave genetically as haploid organisms, and therefore each of the nucleoids of a single cell must contain the same haploid genetic sequences. The implications of nucleoid structure on the expression and replication of the bacterial chromosome remain to be fully understood.

Chromosome Replication in Bacteria

The *E. coli* chromosome replicates as a unit in a sequential and semiconservative manner. The duplication of this replicon is initiated at a unique site, the replicative origin (*ori*C), from which replication subsequently proceeds by polynucleotide-chain elongation in two directions simultaneously (clockwise and counterclockwise) to a fixed terminus (*ter*C). This complex process involves a variety of proteins, an active RNA-synthesizing system, and a functional membrane and can be separated into three physiologically distinct stages: (1) initiation, (2) polynucleotide-chain elongation, and (3) termination and segregation of the newly replicated chromosome (Fig. 3-1).

Initiation

The replication of all known double-stranded DNA molecules is initiated at a unique genetic site often referred to as the replicative origin (*ori*). Bacterial plasmids and viruses use a variety of mechanisms to initiate DNA synthesis. However, one feature common to the initiation of all bacteria and phage systems examined is the need for an RNA primer synthesized by a DNA-dependent RNA polymerase. Other proteins (enzymes) are also needed. In *E. coli*, the site of initiation (*oriC*) maps near the *ilv* operon at minute 84 on the genetic map, and with the development of an in vitro replication system, which specifically uses an *oriC*-containing template (minichromosomes), much has been learned about initiation. Many of the replication proteins of *E. coli,* characterized by Arthur Kornberg and collegues, are required for in vitro initiation and include: DNA polymerase III holoenzyme, single-stranded DNA-binding proteins, DNA gyrase, primase, RNA polymerase, the histone-like protein HU, and the *dna*A, *dna*B, and *dna*C proteins. Initiation occurs through a series of steps involving the formation of a priming complex and an alteration in the conformation of the *oriC* DNA structure.

Most models that attempt to explain how bacterial cells regulate chromosome replication assume that control is exerted at the level of initiation rather than at the level of polynucleotide-chain elongation. This view is supported by experimental observations that the rate of DNA polymerization remains relatively constant over a wide range of doubling times while the frequency of initiation increases with increasing growth rates.

Polynucleotide-Chain Elongation

Once initiated, DNA replication proceeds by polynucleotide-chain elongation in either a uni- or bidirectional fashion to the replication terminus. The bidirectional mode appears to be common and is the manner in which the *E. coli* chromosome is replicated. Replication proceeds by the addition of nucleotides in the 5′ and 3′ direction. One strand of the DNA molecule appears to elongate rapidly, copying the template of opposite polarity in a continuous manner. The other strand is synthesized discontinuously as small "*Okazaki*" pieces (a few thousand nucleotides long in procaryotes), named after their discoverer, Reiji Okazaki. These small pieces of DNA are joined together by polynucleotide ligase. This mode of DNA replication has been termed *semidiscontinuous*. The continuously synthesized strand is referred to as the *leading strand*, while the discontinuously replicated strand is called the *lagging strand*. The Okazaki pieces are initiated by a short RNA primer, which is later enzymatically removed and the resulting gap repaired.

Fig. 3-1 DNA synthesis at the replicative forks. ssb proteins, single-stranded binding proteins.

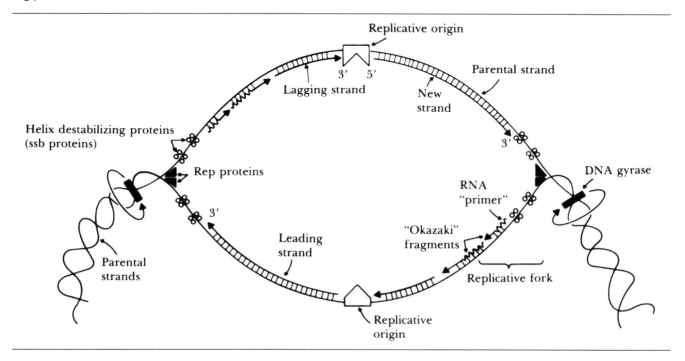

Enzymology

The enzymology of DNA replication is complex and has been extensively studied using in vitro systems reconstituted from purified *E. coli* proteins and a variety of phage and plasmid DNA templates. The following are known to be involved in the replicative process.

DNA Polymerases

Three distinct DNA polymerases (I, II, and III) have been isolated from *E. coli*. All three polymerases synthesize DNA in the 5' to 3' direction and require a primer polynucleotide with a free 3'-hydroxyl end. In all systems thus far examined, the primer has been RNA. All three polymerases also have a 3' and 5' exonuclease activity, which is thought to provide an editing function by which they can remove incorrectly incorporated nucleotides.

DNA polymerase I has an added exonuclease activity; it is able to remove nucleotides in the 5' to 3' direction, which is active on either double-stranded DNA or a DNA-RNA hybrid molecule. It is this latter activity of polymerase I that allows it to remove the RNA primer and replace it with DNA (the process of removing nucleotides from the 5' end of a nick while replacing them by elongating the 3' end is termed nick translation). Nick translation is also essential for DNA repair.

The biologic role of *DNA polymerase II* is not known.

DNA polymerase III is the most complex of the three polymerases, being associated with other proteins to form the pol III holoenzyme. This complex enzyme has the greatest turnover number (rate of elongation) and is the essential DNA-replicating enzyme of *E. coli*.

Polynucleotide Ligases

When the complete 1000-nucleotide Okazaki segment on the lagging strand is polymerized, it is joined to the growing progeny DNA chain by the enzyme DNA ligase. The *E. coli* DNA ligase restores a phosphodiester bond between a 3'-hydroxyl and a 5'-phosphate nick in a double-stranded DNA molecule. This enzyme is essential to DNA replication, DNA repair synthesis, and DNA recombination in *E. coli*.

Helicases

The DNA polymerase III holoenzyme cannot unwind the DNA helix in order to advance during replication. This activity is accomplished by enzymes called helicases. The best-characterized helicase is the *E. coli rep* gene product. The rep protein utilizes the hydrolysis of adenosine triphosphate (ATP) to separate the DNA strands of the double helix at the replicative fork.

Helix Destabilizing Proteins

Helix destabilizing proteins bind to single-stranded DNA and prevent locally denatured DNA from reannealing. In *E. coli,* the destabilizing protein is called the *single-stranded binding protein* (ssb protein), which is essential for replication. This protein is a tetramer that binds single-stranded DNA just behind the rep protein and just ahead of the DNA polymerase III holoenzyme, being displaced by the polymerase as the replication fork advances. Some replication systems employ a single protein that performs the functions of both the helicase and the destabilizing protein. One such example is the gene-32 protein of bacteriophage T4.

Topoisomerases

One of the problems of replicating a closed circular heteroduplex is a topologic one. The unwinding problem that would arise during the replication of a closed circular DNA molecule is formidable. The cell deals with this problem with enzymes that can produce topologic changes in DNA, called topoisomerases or DNA gyrases. The first such enzyme discovered was the omega protein of *E. coli*. This enzyme relaxes negatively supercoiled DNA by breaking and rejoining the DNA backbone, and it has been renamed *eco DNA topoisomerase II*. Recently this enzyme has also been implicated in the initiation of chromosome replication in *E. coli* and may be involved in the separation of newly replicated chromosomes.

Termination of Chromosome Replication

The completion of a round of DNA replication (termination) to yield two daughter chromosomes is an obvious prerequisite for chromosome segregation and subsequent cell division.

In *E. coli*, termination of replication occurs at a genetically specific site named *ter*C. This site is located approximately 180 degrees from the replicative origin in a genetically silent region of the chromosome. The *ter* sequence and its specific binding protein have been characterized in *E. coli*. Two *ter* sequences of approximately 20 base pairs are oriented in such a fashion that when bound by a *ter*-binding protein, termination utilization substance (Tus), one blocks the replicative fork moving clockwise while the other blocks counterclockwise movement.

The termination of a double-stranded circular DNA molecule poses a topologic problem that requires an enzyme for its solution. When a double-stranded DNA molecule is replicated in a semiconservative fashion, the resulting circular daughter molecules (chromosomes) are linked together, preventing their subsequent segregation. Theoretically, these DNA rings could be unlinked by a DNA gyrase (topoisomerases); however, whether this enzyme is actually employed in this unlinking process is not known.

Following the termination of DNA replication, the resulting chromosomes must eventually be segregated into daughter cells. This process is obviously linked to cell division, but the means by which it is accomplished is obscure. An early model, proposed by Jacob, Brenner, and Cuzin in 1963, suggested that the replicating chromosomes were anchored to an envelope between these attachment sites. Although this model is aesthetically pleasing, studies aimed at examining this hypothesis have been contradictory.

DNA Replication Machinery

The replication of the bacterial chromosome is complex, involving the participation of a large number of replication proteins. Both physiologic and genetic studies have supported models in which this macromolecule is replicated by the assemblage of replication proteins into a so-called replication apparatus, or replisome, which is somehow activated at the beginning (initiation) and destroyed or inactivated at the end (termination) of each replication cycle. The existence of such a replication complex could explain how the cell regulates the stoichiometry (chromosome copy number) and timing of chromosome duplication by controlling its number, its rate of assembly, and the timing of its activation.

Mobile Genetic Elements

The concept that chromosomes are static structures that pass unchanged from generation to generation has been abandoned in favor of a more dynamic view. Genetic analysis of chromosome organization has revealed DNA rearrangements that have been brought about by *mobile genetic elements*. These genetic elements are characterized by their ability to insert as discrete DNA segments at more-or-less random locations in the genome. These transposable elements are found as natural constituents of procaryote chromosomes, plasmids and bacteriophage genomes. The two major classes of transposable elements are *insertion elements* and *transposons*.

Insertion Elements

Insertion sequences (IS) are discrete genetic entities that are able to insert into new sites on the same or a different replicon. Insertion elements *are not autonomous replicons*. They compose the simplest class of mobile genetic elements and usually contain a single gene that codes for an enzyme, *transposase,* which is essential for the *transposition* of the IS element. Most IS sequences have similar structure and contain approximately 1000 base pairs of

duplex DNA. A variety of different IS elements are found in bacterial genomes and plasmids, some of which may be found as multiple copies in a single replicon. One consequence of IS sequences is that they provide portable regions of homology that *may bring about DNA rearrangements*. This occurs through the general homology-dependent recombination system (*rec*A system in *E. coli*) and may include *deletions, duplications, translocations,* and *fusions* of replicons. The transposition of IS elements may also inactivate genes (by inserting into them or providing transcriptional/translational termination sequences) or cause the activation of inactive genes by providing functional promoters.

Transposition involves the replication of only the IS element and its insertion into the target DNA. It is independent of the general, homology-dependent recombination system and involves little specificity for the DNA sequences into which they can be integrated. The termini of IS elements contain *inverted repeats* of approximately 10 to 40 base pairs. These repeats are unique to each IS element and provide a site of recognition for the transposase. Hence, a given IS element can only induce the transposition of IS elements that have the same end sequence (i.e., belong to the same IS family). The transposition of IS elements also results in the duplication of a small number of base pairs of the target sequence, apparently as a result of specific staggered cutting and ligation, and the replication process. Transposition of IS sequences usually involves the movement of the IS element out of the donor DNA and its insertion into the target DNA, which may or may not be the same replicon.

Transposons

A second class of mobile genetic elements closely related to IS elements and very important to medicine are *transposons*. Transposons may carry a wide variety of genes; however, most important to medicine are those involved in antibiotic resistance. Essentially every antibiotic used today may be rendered ineffective by one or more antibiotic-resistant genes, which in turn may be carried by a transposon. Some transposons carry multiple antibiotic-resistant genes.

There are basically two types of transposons. The simplest involve the auxiliary gene(s) flanked by two copies of an IS element. Transposition occurs through the reversal of the IS elements at the ends of this transposon. An example is the Cm^r transposon, Tn9, which carries only the structural gene for CM^r between two IS1 elements. A second, more complicated type of transposon does not utilize IS elements at its ends per se and is exemplified by the beta-lactamase Tn3 transposon. This transposon does not have flanking IS elements. Rather, it contains two genes with products involved in transposition: transposase and resolvase. The transposition of this transposon (and its relatives) is complicated and involves its duplication, leaving a copy at its original insertion site and a new copy at a new insertion site.

A recently discovered class of transposons in *Streptococcus* confers antibiotic resistance and provides its host with the ability to transfer these transposons via conjugation. These transposons induce conjugation between two cells, allowing for the transposition of the transposon from the donor DNA to that of the recipient. The transfer of other donor chromosomal genes has not been demonstrated and the precise mechanism of this transfer is not understood. It is believed, however, that these *conjugative transposons* play a major role in antibiotic resistance in *Streptococcus*.

Bacterial Plasmids

In addition to its chromosome, the bacterial cell may also harbor one or more extrachromosomal genetic elements capable of autonomous replication, called *plasmids*. While these genetic components may confer important characteristics on their bacterial host, they are not, under most conditions, essential to cell viability. However, plasmids play an important role in both the antibiotic resistance and the virulence of many pathogens.

Molecular Nature

Most plasmids are double-stranded circular DNA molecules that range in size from 5 to 140 megadaltons, corresponding to approximately 7 to 200 genes, respectively.

Plasmids are *replicons* in the sense that they can replicate autonomously from the bacterial chromosome, although they are heavily dependent on their host's replicative machinery. Some plasmids may also integrate into the bacterial chromosome and thus be replicated passively.

Autonomously replicating plasmids are usually segregated with the bacterial chromosomes during cell division. However, when two different plasmids are present in the same cell, unequal segregation at cell division may occur, resulting in two different cell populations, each harboring only one type of plasmid. If this occurs, the plasmids are said to be *incompatible*. If both plasmid species are maintained, they are said to be *compatible*. Compatibility is a frequently used criterion to classify plasmids and there are approximately 25 different compatibility groups in plasmids found in Enterobacteriaceae.

The number of plasmid copies per cell is regulated by the plasmid itself and is referred to as *copy number*. Plasmids are classified according to their copy number; low-copy-number (1–2/cell) plasmids are called *stringent* plasmids, and high-copy-number (10–100/cell) plasmids are called *relaxed* plasmids.

Functions

Plasmids code for a variety of so-called nonessential functions yet confer important characteristics on the host bacterium. They are therefore often classified according to the properties they confer on their hosts. These include drug resistance (*R factors*), the ability to transfer their own and other DNA by conjugation (*conjugative plasmids* such as the F plasmid), the ability to produce antibacterial proteins (*bacteriocin* or *colicin plasmids*), the ability to produce toxins (*toxigenic plasmids*), and the ability to utilize or degrade specific metabolites (e.g., F-lac plasmid). Plasmids are also called *virulence plasmids* if they carry genes that provide pathogenic properties to their host, for example, the production of toxins and enterotoxins or proteins that enable the bacteria to colonize tissue or adherence proteins. Plasmids that do not have identifiable properties are called *cryptic plasmids*.

Conjugative Plasmids of Gram-Negative Bacteria

Conjugative plasmids are among the largest plasmids and code for the genes whose products are required for their conjugative transfer (see section entitled Mutation and Variation in Bacteria for a discussion of conjugation). The genes, which code for the DNA transfer machinery, reside in an operon termed *tra* for transfer (the *tra* operon of the F plasmid contains more than 13 genes). This operon is under the control of *fertility inhibition (fin)* genes, whose gene product acts as a repressor. (For a discussion of genetic repression, see section entitled The Organization and Expression of Genetic Material: Transcription, Translation, and Regulation.) Normally the *tra* operon is repressed, and therefore only a few of the cells carrying a conjugative plasmid can transfer it. An exception to this rule is the F plasmid, whose *tra* operon is derepressed, and nearly 100 percent of the cells carrying the F plasmid can transfer it.

Conjugative plasmids are not normally transferred to other cells carrying the same plasmid. This is due to a regulatory phenomenon called *entry exclusion* in which pair formation (association of donor and recipient bacteria by conjugative pili) and DNA transfer (process of conjugative transfer of single-stranded DNA) are blocked. Conjugative plasmids can also bring about the conjugative transfer of chromosomal genes. This process is termed *chromosomal mobilization* and in the case of the F plasmid requires its integration into the host chromosome (see section entitled Mutation and Variation in Bacteria).

Conjugative Plasmids of Gram-Positive Bacteria

Unlike gram-negative bacteria, relatively few gram-positive bacteria are known to carry conjugative plasmids. However, conjugative plasmids have been found in *Bacillus, Streptomyces, Streptococcus,* and *Clostridium* strains. Conjugation in gram-positive bacteria is quite different from that of gram-negative bacteria (see section on conjugation in Mutation and Variation in Bacteria).

Bacteriocinogenic Plasmids

Bacteriocinogenic plasmids produce bactericidal substances known as *bacteriocins* or *colicins.* Bacteriocins differ from antibiotics in that they are proteins that act exclusively on the same or closely related species of bacteria. Bacteria that produce them are resistant or immune to their action. This immunity has been shown in some cases to be the result of immune proteins that bind to the bacteriocin and inactivate it. There are a variety of different bacteriocins, and each is highly specific with regard to the means by which it kills the cell. Like bacteriophages, the bacteriocins bind to specific receptors located on the outer surface of the bacterial envelope. The sites of action of these bactericidal proteins include the cytoplasmic membrane (i.e., inhibition of oxidative phosphorylation), the ribosome (i.e., inhibition of protein synthesis), and the enzymes involved in RNA and DNA synthesis, as well as the DNA itself (i.e., DNA degradation).

Drug-Resistance Plasmids

In Gram-Negative Bacteria

Resistance to antibiotics and other chemotherapeutic agents has been found to exist in a variety of microorganisms. In fact, individual strains now often show resistance to several antibiotics simultaneously. Such multiple-drug resistance is specified by extrachromosomal elements called *drug-resistance factors,* or *R factors.* R factors are usually self-transmissible (i.e., conjugative plasmids).

R factors were discovered in the 1950s during an outbreak of bacillary dysentery in Japan. They were first found in a strain of *Shigella flexneri* that was resistant to chloramphenicol, streptomycin, tetracycline, and the sulfonamides. Multiple resistance to these antibiotics was transferable to sensitive strains of *Shigella,* as well as to strains of *Escherichia, Klebsiella, Proteus, Salmonella,* and other enteric bacilli. Epidemiologic studies have shown a worldwide increase in the number of resistant organisms since the advent of antibiotic therapy and the use of antibiotics in animal feeds.

Although resistance to a wide variety of antibiotics has been found, a single R factor specifying simultaneous resistance to all antibiotics has not been reported. Multiple resistance to combinations of three, four, or five antibiotics is common, and among the most frequently encountered drug-resistance patterns are resistance markers to ampicillin, streptomycin, tetracycline, and the sulfonamides.

Genetic studies have revealed that R factors can be divided into two distinct functional groups: the *resistance transfer factor (RTF)* and the resistance determinant (*r determinant*). The RTF is thought to be similar to an F factor in function, since it is responsible for the replication and distribution of the plasmid during cell division and for plasmid transfer by conjugation. The r determinant, on the other hand, contains the genes that specify antibiotic resistance. It has recently been shown that most of the drug-resistant genes are carried by highly mobile transposons, genetic elements that are capable of transposing themselves (hopping) from one DNA molecule to another or from one location to another on the same DNA molecule. *Thus, multiple drug-resistant determinants are actually a collection of transposons, each carrying a particular antibiotic resistance gene.* The RTF and r determinants may exist independently or be associated as a composite RTF-r determinant plasmid. The stability of such a complex varies for each R factor and may be stably associated with an RTF in *E. coli* but may dissociate when transferred to salmonellae. Antibiotic-sensitive strains containing an RTF have been found in nature, as have r determinant–carrying cells that contain no RTF. The DNA boundaries between the r determinant and RTF elements in composite molecules have been shown to contain insertion sequences (IS elements) that account for their ability to associate and dissociate (i.e., IS elements promote crossover).

The medical significance of R plasmids is obvious. The selection for R plasmids by antibiotic therapy and the transfer of these plasmids in an infectious fashion between a variety of different bacterial species provide a constant and continuing threat to the effectiveness of treatment of bacterial disease with antibiotics. The distribution of R factors is worldwide, and the degree and number of different drug-resistant factors are on the increase. Furthermore, R factors are not only found in Enterobacteriaceae but are also in such pathogens as the anaerobic *Bacteroides* and *Neisseria* species. For example, a strain of *Neisseria gonorrhoeae* has been found that harbors an R factor that confers resistance to penicillin, the antibiotic most often used to combat this pathogen. From hybridization studies, it has been concluded that this R factor came from the enterobacterial R-factor pool. A similar plasmid has been found in *Haemophilus influenzae,* one of the causative agents of meningitis. These observations serve to illustrate an important danger, the ability of R factors to cross the genus barrier and be transferred from common inhabitants of humans (i.e., *E. coli*) to transient pathogenic strains. Trans-

Microbial Genetics

ferable drug resistance is probably not a new phenomenon, and its noticeable emergence in recent years is likely the result of indiscriminant and widespread use of antibiotics both in medicine and agriculture.

In Gram-Positive Bacteria

Small drug-resistant plasmids are also found in gram-positive bacteria. These plasmids are not usually called R factors. The best known are the plasmids associated with penicillinase production, which are called penicillinase plasmids. Penicillinase plasmids may also control resistance to erythromycin or to certain metal ions, such as mercury, cadmium, lead, and bismuth. Plasmid-mediated resistance of the staphylococci to tetracycline, chloramphenicol, and kanamycin has also been reported. Unlike most R factors, penicillinase plasmids are not transferred by conjugation. However, their transduction has been reported.

Plasmid-specific antibiotic resistance has also been observed in other types of gram-positive bacteria. For example, various streptococci strains have been found to contain plasmids conferring resistance to erythromycin, clindamycin, chloramphenicol, streptomycin, kanamycin, sulfonamides, and tetracycline. Thus far no streptococci plasmids have been found that produce beta lactamases (beta lactams are the antibiotics of choice in the treatment of streptococcal diseases); however, as with R factors in gram-negative bacteria, it may be only a matter of time before they emerge. Unlike the penicillinase plasmids, some of the streptococci plasmids are transferable by conjugation.

Virulence Plasmids

In the past 15 years, there has been compelling evidence that members of the genus *E. coli* found in the gut of humans and domestic animals are responsible for a significant proportion of diarrheal diseases. These include infantile diarrhea, cholera-like disease in adults, traveler's diarrhea, and colibacillosis in young domestic animals. These diarrheal diseases are elicited by two distinct mechanisms: the invasion of the intestinal mucosa by the bacteria, causing an acute inflammatory response, and the production of enterotoxins, which stimulates the secretion of water and electrolytes. Plasmids have been implicated in both mechanisms. For instance, some pathogenic *E. coli* produce an enterotoxin; possess a common surface antigen, K88, an adhesive surface protein that allows the bacterium to adhere to epithelial cells; and produce an alpha hemolysin. K88 antigen, enterotoxin, and alpha-hemolysin production are all governed by transmissible plasmids, designated as *K88, Ent,* and *Hly,* respectively. Furthermore, it has been demonstrated that the transfer of

K88 and Ent plasmids to normal resident *E. coli* strains converts them to pathogenic strains capable of eliciting diarrheal disease in pigs. Obviously, this is but one example of the involvement of plasmids in pathogenesis, the extent of which remains to be completely understood.

Bacteriophages

Bacteriophages (viruses/phage) are infectious agents that replicate as obligate intracellular parasites in bacteria. Their life cycle includes an extracellar phase in which they are metabolically inert and an infectious phase in which they utilize their host to multiply. These viruses, or *virions,* are very small and can only be visualized by electron microscopy.

Phage Morphology

Bacteriophages contain protein and DNA or RNA as major components. A few phages contain lipid and are sensitive to organic solvents, such as chloroform. The genome of the phage is usually comprised of a single molecule of single- or double-stranded, linear or circular, DNA or single-stranded linear RNA. The protein forms the *phage coat* or *capsid,* which protects the phage genome. Phages differ in their physical structure from species to species but generally fall into one of three basic shapes: (1) *icosahedral tailless,* (2) *icosahedral heads with tail,* and (3) *filamentous* (Fig. 3-2).

Phage Production

The events that lead to the production of new bacterial phages are the following:

Adsorption

Infection of bacteria is initiated by the *adsorption* of phage to specific *receptors* on the surface of the bacterium. These receptors may be protein, such as the porin proteins of the outer membrane of gram-negative bacteria, or lipid in nature, such as lipopolysaccharides (LPS) of the outer membrane of gram-negative bacteria, or a combination of both. Lipopolysaccharides, teichoic acids, flagella, and pili can serve as receptors. Different species of phage often use different surface receptors and the same phage species can mutate to use more than one receptor (*host-range mutant*).

Penetration

Adsorption is followed by the passage of the phage DNA or RNA into the cell. Some phages, such as the tailed phage, use an injection mechanism to accomplish this. For example in the tailed T-even phage the tail tube is inserted

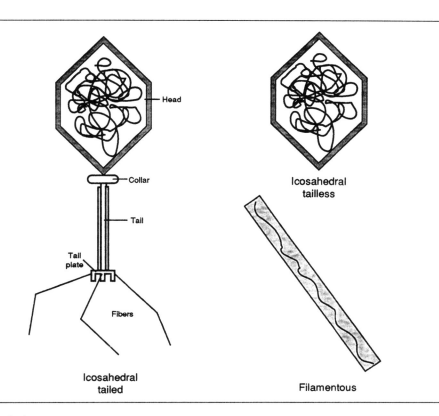

Fig. 3-2 Structures of phages.

through the bacterial cell wall and the phage DNA, contained in the phage head, is extruded through this tube, directly into the host cell. With some tailless phages the nucleic acid is temporally sensitive to nuclease attack, suggesting that it is released and exposed before entering the cell.

Phage Replication

Once inside the bacterial cell the phage may replicate itself many times over and eventually lyse its host. The means by which this is accomplished varies for different phages. However, following most infections the bacterial host loses its ability to replicate and/or transcribe its DNA. The phage RNA or DNA is then replicated to produce many copies of its genome and phage-specific proteins are synthesized within the bacterium. The phage nucleic acid is synthesized by either phage-specific DNA and RNA polymerases or by the addition of specificity elements to modify bacterial polymerases. In either case, many of the host's replication proteins are involved. The initial-phage messenger RNA (mRNA) is usually synthesized by the bacterial DNA-dependent RNA polymerase. This phage mRNA usually codes for a phage RNA polymerase or proteins that modify the host RNA polymerase to recognize *phage promoter sequences*. Another strategy involves

the phage head proteins that are injected along with phage DNA. These modify the bacterial RNA polymerase to recognize viral promoters so that virus genes, instead of bacterial genes, are transcribed.

Phage mRNA synthesis is regulated and its protein products usually synthesized sequentially as needed (i.e., *early mRNA* encodes for the phage-specific enzymes early in the infection and *late mRNA* encodes for the capsid proteins later). The early mRNA directs the synthesis of protein factors and enzymes that allow the phage to take over the metabolism of its host. For example, some early virus-specific enzymes degrade host DNA halting host gene expression and providing precursors for phage DNA replication.

Ribonucleic acid phages must encode their own replication enzymes because the bacterial hosts do not contain enzymes that can replicate RNA. The single-stranded RNA also serves as mRNA. One of the first gene products synthesized from RNA phage is *RNA replicase,* which is an RNA-dependent RNA polymerase. This enzyme copies the original RNA (plus-strand) and produces a double-stranded intermediate called the *replicative form (RF).* The RF is then used to synthesize thousands of copies of plus-strands of phage RNA, some of which are used to make more double-stranded replicative forms and some of which are used as mRNA to make phage proteins. Eventually, the plus-strands of phage RNA are packaged into a maturing virion.

Single-stranded DNA phages replicate their genomes using a similar strategy. They use host DNA polymerase to produce double-stranded (RF) forms before either transcription or replication occurs. The RF form then directs the synthesis of additional RF and single-stranded copies of the phage DNA.

Phage Assembly

The assembly of phages usually requires three types of proteins: (1) *structural proteins,* which are found in the mature phage particle; (2) *assembly proteins,* which often have catalytic activities and which help assemble the phage (e.g., packaging of the nucleic acids in the phage heads or assembly by modification of tail protein components), and (3) *release proteins,* involved in the emancipation of mature phage from the cell (e.g., lysozyme). The suspension of the newly released phage is called a *lysate.*

Virulent and Temperate Phages

Bacterial viruses can be classified into two major groups, *virulent* or *temperate,* depending on their reproductive cycle. Virulent phages have only a single alternative, to lyse the host cell (*lytic cycle*). Temperate phages, on the other hand, can either lyse the host cell, resulting in the production of many progeny phages, or replicate their genome along with the host cell, resulting in a clone of infected cells that may continue dividing for many generations (*lysogenic cycle*). The replicating phage genome, called a *prophage,* may persist either integrated into the bacterial chromosome (usually at a unique genetic locus), such as the prophage of lambda, or as an autonomously replicating plasmid, such as the generalized transducing P1 phage of *E. coli.* Each of these infected bacterial cells carrying a prophage can, under the appropriate conditions, produce infective viruses. This relationship between the temperate phage and its bacterial host is called *lysogeny,* and the bacteria that carry these prophages are called *lysogens.* The *induction* of a lysogen is the process by which the prophage propagates infective viruses and eventually lyses its host (i.e., enters the lytic cycle) (Fig. 3-3).

The process by which a temperate phage, carrying nonessential genes that are expressed, changes the host's phenotype is called *lysogenic conversion.* Some of these changes are of medical importance and result in alterations in the pathogenic properties of the lysogen. For example the gene coding for the diphtheria toxin in *Cornybacterium diphtheriae* resides in the temperate phage B. The production of the erythrogenic toxin in *Streptococcus pyogenes*

Fig. 3-3 Lysogenization and prophage induction.

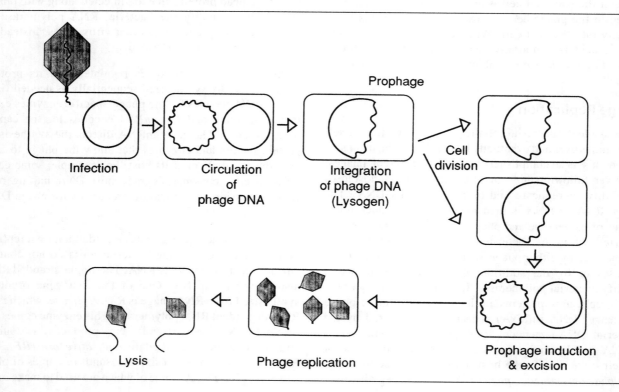

Infection — Circulation of phage DNA — Integration of phage DNA (Lysogen) — Prophage — Cell division — Prophage induction & excision — Phage replication — Lysis

and the O-antigen specificity (LPS structure) in *Salmonella* are also controlled by temperate-phage genes during lysogeny.

The Organization and Expression of Genetic Material: Transcription, Translation, and Regulation

In the 1940s, Beadle and Tatum employed the fungus *Neurospora crassa* to investigate gene activity. They found that specific mutations directly affected specific enzymatic activity. To account for these results, they proposed the one-gene, one-enzyme theory. Since that time, we have found that many enzymes are composed of more than one polypeptide and that mutations in more than one gene can affect the activity of such enzymes. Therefore, the one-gene, one-enzyme theory has been modified to a one-gene,

one-polypeptide relationship. Recently it has been found that in some genomes the same nucleotide region may code for more than one polypeptide. Hence, the concept of gene has come to refer to a very specific DNA nucleotide sequence, faithfully *transcribed* into the ribonucleotide sequence of an mRNA molecule, which in turn may be (for structural genes) *translated* into the amino acid sequence of a polypeptide chain, which then folds spontaneously, under the correct physiologic conditions, to achieve the three-dimensional conformation characteristic of the native protein (Fig. 3-4). The other transcrips (transfer RNA and ribosomal RNA) are not translated but rather are incorporated directly into the cell's biochemical machinery.

Transcription

The first step in gene expression involves transcribing the genetic information into a usable code. Chemically, transcription is the enzymatic polymerization of RNA using one of the two DNA strands (the *sense strand*) as a template.

Fig. 3-4 The transfer of genetic information from DNA to protein.

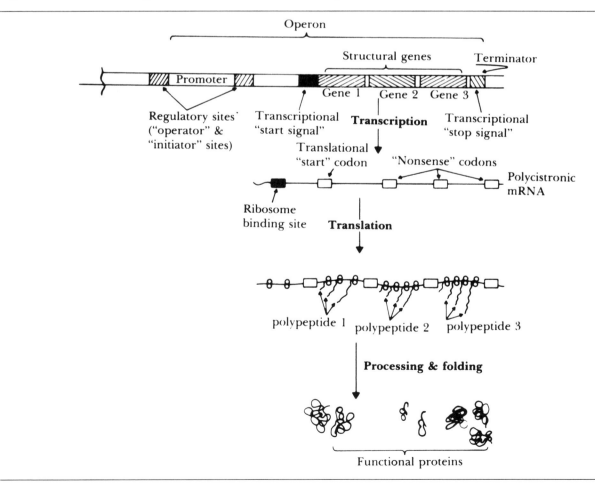

The clearest view of the events involved in this process comes from studies with the bacterium *Escherichia coli,* and we will use this system often as our model (Fig. 3-5).

The Transcriptional Unit

The transcriptional unit is a stretch of DNA nucleotides bordered on one end by a start sequence, or *promoter,* and at the other end by a stop sequence, or *terminator.* The RNA polymerase initiates RNA synthesis at the promoter, using the *sense strand* of DNA to synthesize its complement, and then terminates RNA-chain elongation and disengages from the DNA at the terminator. Each transcriptional unit contains at least one gene and, in procaryotes, often two or more.

Fig. 3-5 Transcription in *E. coli.*

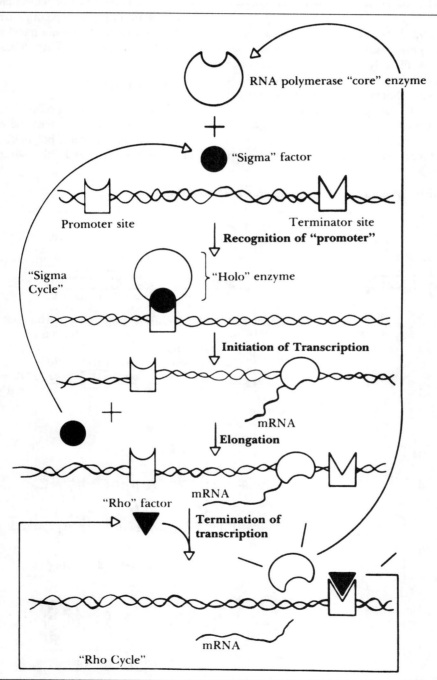

The Promoter Site

The promoter site contains genetic sequences that are organized spatially along the DNA and are responsible for *RNA polymerase recognition* and eventually the initiation of RNA synthesis. Different promoters are used more or less frequently as start signals for transcription, and the degree to which they are used depends largely on the ability of the RNA polymerase holoenzyme to recognize them (i.e., upon sigma recognition).

The Terminator Site

The terminator site is located at the end of the transcriptional unit and is a DNA sequence that *causes the RNA polymerase core enzyme to stop RNA-chain elongation and to disengage from the DNA template.* The completed RNA transcript is released during this process. There are two types of termination sites: those that require a termination protein called *rho* and those that do not. The mode of action of rho is not yet completely understood.

RNA-Synthesizing Machinery

RNA-synthesizing machinery of *E. coli* is the DNA-dependent RNA polymerase. This enzyme is made up of five noncovalently joined polypeptides: one beta subunit, one beta' subunit, two identical alpha subunits, and a sigma subunit. The beta, beta', and two alpha subunits form the *core enzyme* that is responsible for RNA synthesis per se (i.e., RNA-chain elongation). The *sigma factor* is loosely associated with the core enzyme to form the *holoenzyme* and is involved in recognizing the promoter sequence.

Ribonucleic acid synthesis, like DNA synthesis, can be divided into three physiologically distinct stages: (1) initiation, (2) polynucleotide-chain elongation, and (3) termination.

Transcription Initiation

Transcription initiation is a complex, multistep process involving (1) locating the promoter site, (2) opening the DNA double helix and melting in of the RNA polymerase holoenzyme, (3) binding of ATP or guanosine triphosphate (GTP) in the polymerase initiation site, and (4) catalysis of the first and subsequent phosphodiester bonds. After the initiation of RNA synthesis has begun, there is no further requirement for the RNA polymerase to recognize initiation sites, and the sigma factor dissociates from the holoenzyme and recycles with free core enzymes to initiate the synthesis of another RNA molecule.

RNA-Chain Elongation

RNA-chain elongation involves only the core RNA polymerase. During the process, the two DNA strands separate in the region where transcription is occurring, and the next nucleotide to be added to the growing chain is identified by its ability to form a base pair with the next nucleotide in the DNA template. When the correct ribonucleoside-5'-triphosphate is identified, it is enzymatically joined to the nascent RNA chain by RNA polymerase. The RNA chain grows in the 5' to 3' direction. After a particular region of DNA has been transcribed, the melted DNA strands reanneal with each other, and the RNA strand no longer remains hydrogen bonded to that region of DNA. *RNA synthesis can be likened to a bubble traveling down the double-stranded DNA molecule.*

Transcription Products

Transcription products include three different types of RNA molecules, all of which play a role in the translation of genetic information from DNA to protein. These are *mRNA, transfer RNA (tRNA),* and *ribosomal RNA (rRNA).*

Messenger RNAs contain the nucleotide sequence that directly specifies the amino acid sequence of polypeptides. They vary greatly in size, from several hundred to several thousand nucleotides long, and contain only the usual four RNA bases: *adenine* (A), *guanine* (G), *cytosine* (C), and *uracil* (U). DNA segments corresponding to one polypeptide chain plus the start and stop genetic signals are called a *cistron,* and the corresponding mRNA is referred to as *cistronic mRNA.* If the mRNA encodes for a single polypeptide, it is called *monocistronic mRNA.* If the mRNA encodes for more than a single polypeptide, it is called *polycistronic mRNA.*

In addition to start and stop signals for translation, there are other nucleotide sequences in mRNA that act as important signals to the cell's translational machinery. For instance, the start signal for translation often lies well downstream from the 5' end of the RNA transcript. This nontranslated sequence is referred to as the *leader* and it may contain regulatory signals, such as attenuators, that may lead to premature termination of transcription. Untranslated nucleotide sequences are also found at the 3' end of the mRNA and sometimes between cistronic sequences in polycistronic RNA. These sequences are called *spacers,* and their function remains to be determined, although they are believed to be regulatory in nature.

Another important regulatory aspect of mRNA is its short lifetime. Procaryotic mRNA is usually degraded after a relatively short period of time, *the half-life of a typical procaryotic mRNA being a few minutes.* This feature has an important regulatory consequence: If a particular protein is no longer needed, a cell need only turn off transcription of the corresponding gene to turn off the synthesis of its product. This mRNA degradation proceeds from the 5' end by an *RNA exonuclease.*

Transfer RNAs are the smallest of the RNA molecules transcribed and range from 70 to approximately 100 nucleotides long. The structure of tRNA is conserved in nature. Each tRNA molecule can be arranged in a characteristic cloverleaf structure through hydrogen bonding between both normal and modified bases. These RNA molecules are long-lived and contain unusual nucleotides including ribothymidine, dihydrouridine, inosine, and pseudouridine.

The tRNA molecules are involved in decoding the genetic message found in the mRNA by directing the appropriate amino acid to its corresponding codon in the mRNA. There is one or more (usually three or more) specific tRNA species for each of the 20 amino acids found in proteins. Each tRNA molecule has a region called the *anticodon*, which resides in one of the precise base pairings between tRNA and mRNA. The anticodon consists of three bases complementary to the triplet code expressed in the mRNA (*codons*). Each tRNA also contains a 3'-terminal sequence to which one of the 20 amino acids is covalently attached (by a specific aminoacyl-tRNA synthetase). The association between amino acid and tRNA is specific. Only the amino acid specified for by its anticodon can be attached to a given tRNA species. Transfer RNA molecules with covalently attached amino acids are referred to as *charged tRNAs*.

Ribosomal RNAs are components of ribosomes, the cell's protein-synthesizing machine. This RNA is also long-lived and composes the most abundant class of cellular RNA, representing from 60 to 80 percent of the cell's total RNA. However, regardless of its abundance, its function is not completely understood. It is usually thought to play some structural role in ribosome assembly and function.

All ribosomes of a given species of organism have an identical set of rRNAs. Ribosomes of procaryotes contain one copy of three different rRNA species, designated at *23S, 16S,* and *5S* after their sedimentation coefficients. Ribosomes from eucaryotes, on the other hand, contain four different species: 28S, 18S, 5.8S, and 5S RNAs.

Processing of RNA

Processing of RNA refers to the digestion and chemical modification of the primary transcription products (RNA). Transcription products are almost always larger than the final functional form of the RNA. Hence, these transcription products must be digested to some extent by nucleases. Furthermore, since only the four ribonucleoside-5'-triphosphates can be incorporated into RNA during transcription, the primary product of transcription must also be modified to produce the methylated and other chemically altered nucleotides found in RNA. For example, the 28S,

18S, and 5.8S rRNAs found in eucaryotic ribosomes are derived from the same transcript (i.e., are processed by endonucleases). After they are cleaved to the appropriate size, the 28S and 18S rRNA are then methylated at the appropriate sites along the RNA chains.

Similar processing occurs in the maturation of tRNA species. In the case of *E. coli* tyrosine tRNA, the primary transcript is 41 nucleotides longer at the 5' end and 2 nucleotides longer at the 3' end than its final form. After endonucleolytic cleavage of the primary transcript, this tRNA is chemically modified and folded to yield the mature tyrosine tRNA.

Processing of mRNA is less well understood and does not appear to occur in procaryotes. Processing of eucaryotic mRNA is complex. Although the *mRNAs of eucaryotes are monocistronic,* the portion that is used as the template for protein synthesis is usually about one tenth the size of the primary transcript. Obviously it must be processed. During this processing, intervening sequences called *exons* are cut out and rejoined into the final message. It is also known that many eucaryotic mRNA molecules are relatively long-lived (in comparison to procaryotic mRNA), and this may be due to modifications at the ends of these molecules, especially at the 5' end, where a cap consisting of a 7-methylguanosine group is found. The 3' end of most eucaryotic mRNA is modified by a string (up to 200) of adenine moieties (poly A) before the splicing of the exons occurs. The significance of this modification is not understood, although it has been implicated in the stability of mRNA.

Translation

Once the genetic information has been coded into the messenger RNA molecule, the stage is set for the final step in gene expression: the translation of that code into protein. This protein requires a change in the chemical nature of the genetic code and some very sophisticated translational machinery.

The Genetic Code

The genetic code is a collection of base sequences called codons that correspond to each of the 20 amino acids found in proteins and to the start and stop signals of translation. Each *codon* consists of three adjacent ribonucleotides. Since there are four different bases from which these triplets can be made, 4^4, or 64, different permutations or code words are possible. This suggests an excess coding capacity and, in fact, it turns out that the code is highly redundant or *degenerate,* with some amino acids having as many as 6 different codons. This degeneracy is thought to minimize the deleterious effects of mutation. Sixty-one of the 64 possible codons code for specific amino acids and are thus called *sense codons*. The remaining 3 codons do not code for an amino acid and are referred to as *non-sense codons*. These non-sense codons signal for the termination of translation and have been given specific names: *amber codon* (UAG), *ocher codon* (UAA), and *opal codon* (UGA). The start or initiation codons are also *sense codons*. The most commonly used is AUG, which codes for methionine, although in a few instances GUG (which codes for valine) is used. These codons, therefore, have dual roles, since depending on the adjacent nucleotide sequence, they specify either for the insertion of the indicated amino acid or for the initiation of a polypeptide chain with a modified amino acid, N-formylmethionine (fMet). In eucaryotes, unmodified methionine is used at the beginning of polypeptide-chain formation. The initiation codon also determines the reading frame of the mRNA. The mRNA is read as non-overlapping contiguous codons in a colinear fashion (i.e., the linear order of codons corresponds to the linear order of amino acids).

Until recently, the genetic code was considered to be universal, and with but one known exception it is. In 1979, the genetic code of mitochondria was found to be different. The most striking codon differences lie in those involved in the initiation and termination of transcription (in mitochondria, UGA codes for tryptophan, not termination, and AUA for methionine and initiation, not isoleucine).

Another recent surprise has been the finding of *overlapping genes*. It has been shown that in the single-stranded DNA phage of *E. coli*, 0X174, translation occurs in several reading frames from three mRNA molecules. In fact, five different 0X174 proteins obtain some or all of their primary structure from shared base sequences. Similar findings have been found in the animal virus SV40.

Ribosomes

Ribosomes are the cell's protein-synthesizing machinery. It is on these intracellular particles that the genetic code is decoded. They are composed of three different RNA molecules and some 55 different proteins. This macromolecular complex contains the enzymes required for forming a peptide bond and the recognition sites for mRNA and charged tRNAs.

The complete procaryotic ribosome has a sedimentation coefficient of 70S and can be further divided into two major components, a small 30S and a large 50S subunit. The large subunit has 34 different ribosomal proteins and two different rRNAs (a 23S rRNA and a 5S rRNA) present in one copy per ribosome. The small subunit contains 21 different ribosomal proteins and only one rRNA molecule (16S rRNA).

The 30S ribosomal subunit contains the binding site for the mRNA molecule, and it is here, therefore, that the codon-anticodon recognition must take place.

The 50S ribosomal subunit contains portions of the binding sites for the tRNA molecules and various enzymes involved in polypeptide-chain elongation.

The Translation Mechanism

The translation mechanism is complex, involving the multicomponent ribosome, the genetic message (mRNA), some 40 to 60 tRNAs and their corresponding aminoacyl-tRNA synthetases, and a variety of cytoplasmic protein factors involved in the different stages of translation.

The direction of polypeptide-chain elongation is the same as RNA-chain elongation: The ribosome binds to the 5' end of mRNA, which encodes the protein's *N-terminal*, and proceeds in a processive fashion through the sequential addition of amino acid moieties toward the 3' end of the mRNA, which encodes the protein's carboxy-terminal (*C-terminal*) end. This asymmetric process is completed with the translation of the C-terminal residue and release of the polypeptide from the polysome. As with other polymerization processes (DNA and RNA synthesis), translation can be described in terms of three main stages: (1) polypeptide-chain initiation, (2) polypeptide-chain elongation, and (3) polypeptide-chain termination.

Initiation

Initiation of protein synthesis begins with the incorporation of methionine into the N-terminal of the polypeptide chain. This methionine residue is derived from a special species of methionyl-tRNA, called fMet-tRNA (fMet), which is exclusively used in the initiation of protein synthesis. In procaryotic organisms (but not eucaryotic), the initiating methionine moiety contains an N-formyl group that is donated to the methionine from N-formyltetrahydrofolic acid after it has been incorporated into the fMet-tRNA.

The steps in initiation take place on the 30S ribosomal subunit called the *30S initiation complex*, which includes the mRNA, fMet-tRNA, and 30S ribosomal subunit. The association between the mRNA and the ribosome involves a specific association between the 3' end of the 16S rRNA of the 30S ribosomal subunit and the initiation region of the mRNA called the *Shine-Dalgarno sequence*, after its discoverers. This specific association ensures the recognition of the initiation codon.

In addition to fMet-tRNA, mRNA, and the 30S ribosomal subunit, the initiation of polypeptide synthesis requires specific cytosol proteins called the *initiation factors: IF-1, IF-2, and IF-3*. The IF-3 is involved in the binding of the mRNA to the 30S ribosomal subunit. The IF-1 and IF-2 are involved in the attachment of N-formylmethionyl-tRNA to the mRNA-30S ribosome complex. Guanosine triphosphate is hydrolyzed during this process. The initiation factors are recycled (as are the ribosomal subunits). Only after the attachment of fMet-tRNA to the mRNA-30S ribosomal subunit does the 50S subunit join this complex to form the 70S initiation complex.

Chain Elongation

The 70S ribosome has two sites that bind tRNA. One is designated the *A site* (peptidyl-tRNA site). The A site accepts the aminoacyl-tRNA, while at the same time, the *P site* is occupied by a molecule of tRNA to which is attached a partially completed peptide chain or the fMet-tRNA. At either site, the anticodon of the tRNA is positioned to pair with its corresponding codon of the mRNA molecule. Therefore, charged tRNAs enter the ribosomal complex through the A site while the growing chain is carried in the P site.

The charged tRNAs complementary to the exposed mRNA codon enter the A site with the help of two accessory proteins designated as *elongation factors: EF-Tu* and *EF-Ts*. They enter as a charged tRNA-EF-Tu-GTP complex. The binding of the EF-Tu to the charged tRNA requires a free N-terminal. The release of the EF-Tu-GTP from the charged tRNA requires the hydrolysis of the GTP molecule, resulting in an EF-Tu-GDP complex. EF-Tu-GTP is regenerated by an EF-Tu-EF-Ts intermediate.

In the 70S initiation complex, the fMet-tRNA is bound in the P site, and the aminoacyl-tRNA-EF-Tu corresponding to the second codon in the mRNA is brought into the A site. The EF-Tu-GDP is then released, and a peptide bond is formed between fMet and the second amino acid. The initiator tRNA then becomes disassociated from the ribosome and is recycled for future initiation events. The dipeptide, now associated to a tRNA in the A site, is then translocated from the A site to the P site, and the ribosome is moved one codon down the mRNA in the 3′ direction, in preparation for the second cycle of chain elongation. This translocation process requires the participation of a third accessory protein, EU-G, and the hydrolysis of a second GTP molecule. Further elongation of the peptide chain occurs by repetition of the cycle (i.e., binding of aa-tRNA to the A site, peptide-bond formation and translocation). Each peptide bond formed requires the expenditure (hydrolysis) of two GTP molecules.

Polypeptide-chain elongation is very rapid, polymerizing at a rate of 15 to 20 amino acids per second per ribosome. More than one ribosome can translate the same mRNA at any given time, thereby increasing the efficiency of translation. Each ribosome must bind and begin transla-

tion at the initiator codon on the mRNA. The resulting *polyribosome* or *polysome* is an mRNA, containing a row of ribosomes engaged in protein synthesis in varying stages of completion. The translation of large polycistronic mRNAs (in procaryotes) can produce polysomes containing up to 20 or more ribosomes active in polypeptide synthesis.

Termination

Termination occurs when a termination codon is encountered in the A site of the 70S ribosome. Terminator codons are not read by tRNA molecules (with the exception of mutated suppressor tRNAs), but rather by one of two protein *release factors: RF-1 and RF-2*. RF-1 and RF-2 are codon specific, since the former recognizes the codons UAA and UAG and the latter UAA and UGA. Each release factor forms an activated complex with GTP, and it is this complex that binds to the termination codon and brings about the hydrolysis of the bond linking the polypeptide to tRNA in the P site and thus releases the polypeptide from the ribosome. The 70S ribosome then dissociates into its 30S and 50S subunits, which are recycled for further use in translation.

Posttranslational Processing

Protein synthesis is not the final stage of gene expression. Polypeptide folding and subunit association are obviously important for protein function. Furthermore, polypeptides are often processed or modified to produce the mature functional protein. Such modifications include

1. *Removal of the formyl group of fMet at the NH2-terminal amino acid of procaryotic peptides.* This may be accomplished with the enzyme *deformylase*, which removes the formyl group, leaving methionine as the NH-2 terminal amino acid.
2. *Removal of one or more of the NH2-terminal amino acids.* This is catalyzed by the hydrolytic enzyme called *aminopeptidase*.
3. *Cleavage of polypeptides at specific internal sites.* For example, many proteolytic enzymes are synthesized as inactive precursors called *zymogens*, which must be cleaved to produce their active form (e.g., pepsin is formed by cleavage of pepsinogen).
4. *Chemical modification of component amino acids.* For example, the carbohydrate groups in glycoproteins are added onto asparagine, serine, or threonine residues following the synthesis of the polypeptide backbone. In collagen, a large fraction of the prolines and lysines are hydroxylated.
5. *Oxidation of the sulfhydryl groups in two cysteines to form a disulfide bond.* This is a common occurrence and often plays an important role in producing the final conformation of the functional form of the protein.

The Genetic Organization of the Bacterial Chromosome

As previously pointed out, the bacterial chromosome is a closed ring of double-stranded DNA with a molecular weight of about 2 billion daltons. Within the cell this macromolecule exists in a folded, supercoiled state, complexed with RNA, protein, and the cellular membrane. It is the nucleotide sequence of this DNA macromolecule that serves as a repository for all the essential genetic information of the bacterial cell. In this respect, the bacterial genome is identical to that of all other cellular organisms. However, there are many differences in the architecture and gene arrangements between procaryotic and eucaryotic chromosomes.

Gene Arrangement

Bacterial genes that are functionally related are often linked together in transcriptional units called *operons.* For example, in *E. coli,* of the 1000+ known genes, 260 are located in a total of 75 different operons. This is not the case for eucaryotes, where such transcriptional units remain to be demonstrated.

Gene Structure

Gene structure also differs in procaryotic and eucaryotic cells. In eucaryotic, many of the genes contain *introns,* which are noncoding, intervening sequences that must be excised before translation. No such corollary has been found in bacteria.

Regulation

In the human body, every living cell contains the same set of genes, yet in different cell types different genes are expressed. How? Understanding the mechanisms by which gene expression is regulated is the key to understanding such important phenomena as differentiation and development. In higher organisms, deviation from the normal control of gene expression occurs only in rare instances and has been implicated in such pathologic conditions as carcinogenesis, teratogenesis, and certain immunodeficiency syndromes.

Bacteria, *E. coli* in particular, have served as model systems for the study of control or regulatory systems at the cellular and molecular level. The growth of bacteria is seldom complicated by the supracellular controls that buffer the cells of many eucaryotic organisms from the environment. In fact, the mechanisms by which a bacterium's growth rate, composition, and metabolism relate to the environment are relatively visible, and it is therefore not surprising that the existence of a variety of bacterial

cellular regulatory mechanisms has been known and studied for some time. Some of these mechanisms provide control over intermediary metabolism or the synthesis of the many precursors of the macromolecular components of the cell, while other control mechanisms regulate the formation of these macromolecules per se.

The concept that intermediary metabolism is regulated comes from many observations. For instance, regardless of the growth rate, the relative rates of the formation of precursor molecules (e.g., amino acids, nucleotides) match their rates of polymerization into macromolecules. Furthermore, when certain precursors (end products of specific biosynthetic pathways) such as amino acids become available in the growth medium, their endogenous biosynthesis stops immediately, as does the synthesis of the enzymes involved in their production, while the enzymes in certain catabolic pathways are synthesized only if the substrate of that pathway is present. The mechanisms by which these and many other metabolic controls are effected can be divided into two broad categories: One pertains to the regulation of the catalytic activity of key enzymes in metabolism and the other to the regulation of the synthesis of the enzymes themselves.

Both of these mechanisms are mediated by low-molecular-weight compounds called *effectors,* which are formed by the cell as *intermediary metabolites* or enter from the environment. Both mechanisms also involve the operation of a special class of *allosteric proteins* that undergo a conformational change when bound by effectors. In other words, allosteric proteins are the mediators of metabolic change that is monitored by the concentrations of the cell's metabolites or effectors.

Control of Enzyme Activity

The control over enzymatic activity seems to be responsible for the moment-to-moment control over intermediary metabolism. During this regulatory event a metabolite binds to an allosteric enzyme causing it to gain (activation) or lose (inhibition) in catalytic activity (i.e., changes its K_m or V_{max}). Activators and inhibitors are therefore intermediates of metabolism and act as effectors. The process of inhibition by an effector is sometimes referred to as *feedback inhibition.* Feedback inhibition serves to maintain relatively constant internal concentrations of metabolites in the face of changing demands for them and their availability in the medium.

Two generalizations can be made about feedback inhibition of biosynthetic pathways: (1) Usually only the first enzyme of a biosynthetic pathway is regulated. The teleology is obvious; inhibition of a later enzyme in the pathway would cause wasteful accumulations of intermediates of that pathway. (2) The end products of the pathway being regulated act as effectors or feedback inhibitors. This way a cell can monitor and modulate the flow through the various pathways, depending on the concentration of the end products of those pathways.

The flow through catabolic or energy-producing pathways is also regulated at the enzyme level. However, the generalization that the end product inhibits the first enzyme in the pathway is not applicable. Key regulatory enzymes usually are positioned internal to the pathways. In addition to various by-products of metabolism, the end products of catabolism, ATP and reduced pyrimidine nucleotides ($NADH_2$ and $NADPH_2$), as well as their precursors, nicotinamide adenine dinucleotide (NAD), nicotinamide adenine dinucleotide phosphate (NADP), adenosine monophosphate (AMP), and adenosine diphosphate (ADP), also play an important role in the regulation of these pathways.

Control of Enzyme Synthesis

While the regulation of enzymatic activity seems responsible for the immediate moment-to-moment response to metabolic changes, the mechanisms controlling the synthesis of enzymes, *induction* and *repression,* appear less responsive and come into play as the cell attempts to adjust to changes in its environment. For example, the synthesis of the enzymes involved in the utilization of many diverse carbon sources is induced by the presence of these carbon sources, while the enzymes involved in biosynthetic pathways are usually repressed by the presence of their end products.

Specifying for the amino acid sequences of proteins (structural genes) is not the only function of DNA. As previously mentioned, there are also regions of DNA that serve as signals for the initiation of RNA synthesis (promoters) and for the termination of RNA synthesis (terminators) and there are genes that get transcribed but not translated (rRNA and tRNA). There are also genes whose end products are involved in regulating the frequency with which neighboring structural genes are transcribed into mRNA. These regulatory genes provide the cell with a means of controlling the intracellular concentrations of specific structural gene products. Not all structural genes are regulated by regulatory gene products. In fact, the majority are not. Those structural genes that are not regulated are termed *constitutive,* and the proteins they code for are present within the cell in relatively constant amounts regardless of changes in metabolism. However, the relative amounts of different constitutive gene products are different. This is thought to be due to differences in the strengths of their respective promoters (i.e., the strength of the interactions between the promoter site and the RNA polymerase), lifetimes of mRNAs, and efficiency of translation (i.e., ribosomal binding).

The cell's strategies for regulating gene expression include regulating the efficiency by which RNA polymerase initiates transcription of specific genes and the efficiency with which RNA polymerase terminates transcription of specific genes.

Transcriptional Regulation

Those structural genes whose transcription frequency can be regulated have often been found to be clustered into functional transcriptional units called operons. Operons are multigenic clusters of adjacent structural genes that control related functions and that are transcribed as a unit. Operons are regulated at the level of transcription.

Regulatory Elements

Elements that participate in the control of operon expression are those that either generate or recognize the regulatory signal and include the *promoter,* the *operator* and *initiator* sites, and *regulatory proteins* and their effectors.

The Promoter.   As previously pointed out, it is at the promoter site that RNA polymerase binds to the DNA molecule and initiates transcription. The polycistronic nature of operon mRNA is a reflection of the fact that each operon has but one primary promoter. It is at this site that the majority of transcriptional regulation occurs.

The Operator and Initiator Sites   The frequency with which an operon is transcribed depends not only on the affinity of its promoter for RNA polymerase but also on the degree to which the regulatory regions restrict or promote this association. The regulatory regions are of two types. One of these, the *operator site,* is recognized by a regulatory gene product called a *repressor* whose function is to inhibit the initiation of transcription. The other regulatory site is called an *initiator site,* and it is modulated by a different type of regulatory protein called an *activator* whose function is to enhance transcription of its operon. Therefore, the actual mechanism by which control is exerted at these regulatory sites is by influencing the efficiency of mRNA initiation at the promoter. These regulatory sites usually overlap the promoter region.

The Regulatory Proteins and Their Effectors.   The regulatory proteins that recognize the operators are known as repressors. Specific repressors, in their active state, bind to their respective operator site and prevent (repress) the transcription of the corresponding operon. On the other hand, in their active state, the activators bind to specific initiator sites and increase (activate) transcription of their respective operon. In both cases, these proteins are allosteric in nature, so that the configuration that allows for interaction with the operator or initiator is influenced by ligands (effectors). In other words, the effectors determine the functional state of the operon.

Induction and Repression

Induction and repression refer to the functional state of the operon. When an operon goes from an inactive state to an active state, it is said to be induced and is called an inducible operon. On the other hand, when an operon goes from an active state to an inactive state, it is said to be repressed and is called a repressible operon. In general, operons whose gene products are involved in catabolic pathways are inducible and provide the bacterium with the ability to adapt to changes in the availability of metabolic substrates in its environment. The effectors for such regulatory systems are usually the substrates for such pathways. In contrast, repressible systems are generally biosynthetic and provide the bacterium with the capacity to use preferentially metabolic products that become available in its environment.

Positive and Negative Control Mechanisms

Induction and repression refer to the final outcome of regulation. However, the molecular mechanisms by which this outcome is brought about may be due to either positive or negative control mechanisms. Positive control refers to the action of the regulatory protein in its active state—to turn off transcription. However, it should be recognized that, theoretically, operons can be induced or repressed by either positive or negative regulatory proteins simply by altering their active state. In other words, an inducible operon could be induced either by inactivating an active repressor protein or activating an inactive activator protein by an effector ligand (inducer). Using the same logic, a repressible operon could be repressed by either activating an inactive repressor or inactivating an active activator protein by an effector ligand. In the case of negative control, the effector is sometimes called a corepressor. In practice, positive and negative control systems can be distinguished by the response of the operon when no regulator protein is present (i.e., in regulatory mutants). For genes under positive control, expression is possible only when an active activator gene is present, whereas genes under negative control function unless they are switched off by interaction with an active repressor protein.

Regulons

Not all bacterial genes that are controlled as a unit are clustered in an operon. In some cases, they are scattered around the bacterial chromosome and are collectively called a regulon. A regulon, therefore, can be described as a group of genes controlling physiologically related func-tions that are regulated together by the same regulatory protein but that are not grouped together in an operon (i.e., have more than one promoter site). This implies a common regulatory site that is repeated on all of the genes or operons that compose the regulon.

Autoregulation

The classic Jacob-Monod model of regulation of gene expression had an implicit requirement for a regulatory gene whose product had no other function except to control the expression of structural genes. However, today we have recognized that exceptions to that rule exist. Products of structural genes have been recognized to participate in the regulation of the expression of the operon in which they reside. This regulatory system is often referred to as *autoregulation,* or autogenous regulation. In some cases, this protein is the multimeric allosteric enzyme that catalyzes the first step of a metabolic pathway, bringing together two important mechanisms for controlling the biosynthesis of metabolites in bacterial cells, repression and feedback inhibition.

Other Regulatory Mechanisms
Transcription Termination

Gene expression may be regulated not only by alterations in the frequency with which RNA polymerase successfully initiates transcription at specific genetic (promoter) sites, but also by alterations in the efficiency with which the polymerase terminates transcription at specific genetic (terminator) sites. It has been shown that transcription punctuation signals exist not only at the ends of operons but also within them. The presence within operons of signals that terminate transcription and the means of regulating the activity of these terminators (i.e., rho and anti-rho factors) reveal a new dimension of gene control.

Polarity

Polarity, or transcription termination within operons, can be theoretically explained through the use of rho-dependent terminators within the intercistronic regions of operons and by controlling the frequency of activation of such terminators.

Attenuation

Attenuation is a mechanism for regulating operons based on premature termination of transcription of mRNA. Messenger RNAs have a leader sequence of variable length between the transcriptional origin and the beginning of the coding region for the first structural gene. In attenuation, this leader sequence contains several complementary sequences that can take on different secondary structures,

Microbial Genetics

one of which can act as a signal for the abortion of transcription at the attenuator site located downstream within the leader sequence. The other structure is not recognized as a terminator signal. The cell regulates which structure the leader sequence will assume through the translation of a short segment of the leader sequence. Attenuators have been found in several operons involved in amino acid biosynthesis (e.g., the tryptophan, histidine, threonine, and isoleucine-valine operons in *E. coli*).

Translational Control

Theoretically, gene expression could be regulated at translation. Regulation is influenced, for example, by the stability of the mRNA molecule, the frequency at which specific portions of the polycistronic messages are translated, or the availability of the various components of the translational machinery, such as specific tRNAs or their synthetases or initiation factors. Examples for such regulatory systems have been documented in *E. coli* and some of its phages.

Several well-documented examples of *translational regulation involve the regulation of the ribosome-binding site*, preventing translation. One such example involves the translation of polycistronic mRNA coding for ribosomal proteins. Ribosomal proteins bind to ribosomal RNA during the assembly and maturation of the ribosomal subunits. The genes for these proteins reside in ribosomal protein operons and thus their translation results in polycistronic mRNAs. One of the proteins encoded by each of the ribosomal protein operons also can recognize the ribosome binding site of its corresponding polycistronic mRNA and inhibits its translation. This occurs because its rRNA-binding site is similar to that of the ribosome-binding site for the polycistronic mRNA. This rRNA-binding protein will bind rRNA in preference to the ribosome-binding site of its mRNA. Hence when the rRNA for this protein is available its polycistronic mRNA will be translated. However, when the rRNA becomes limiting, the rRNA-binding protein will bind the ribosome-binding site of the polycistronic mRNA and the translation of all ribosomal proteins of that operon will be inhibited.

A second mechanism of regulating the binding of ribosomes to mRNA involves regulation by *antisense RNA*. An example can be found in the regulation of the porin protein OmpF of *E. coli*. The two major porins, *omp*F and *omp*C, are coordinately regulated so that the total amount of protein in the outer membrane remains relatively constant (i.e., when *omp*F is upregulated, *omp*C is downregulated and vice versa). This inverse regulation is partially accomplished by an antisense RNA, termed *mic*F, which is complementary to the 5′ end of the *omp*F mRNA, including its initiation or ribosome-binding site. The transcription of *mic*F RNA correlates with the transcription of *omp*C (they may share a common regulatory DNA region), and hence when *omp*C transcription is induced, *mic*F is also induced, which effectively represses the translation of *omp*F. Antisense RNA regulation has been found in other regulatory systems including genes in transposons and plasmids. Theoretically, the product of any procaryotic or eucaryotic gene could be controlled by antisense RNA, and the potential of this regulatory mechanism for providing antiviral and gene therapy is enormous.

Epigenetic Control Mechanisms

Epigenetic control mechanisms alter the structure of the structural gene product. The folding of the newly synthesized protein and its association with other subunits, leading to a specific three-dimensional conformation, is usually required for the realization of this specific catalytic or other function. Obviously, this folding process and the processes of subunit aggregation and disaggregation may be subject to control mechanisms. Examples of such epigenetic regulation are known in both procaryotes and eucaryotes.

Coordinate Regulation

Thus far we have discussed regulatory mechanisms involving the control of individual operons or regulons. However, there are a number of systems in bacteria for regulating the expression of several different operons at the same time. These are called *global regulons*. While the control of individual operons provides the bacterium with a high degree of specificity in its response to the environment, the control of global regulatory networks allows the cell to coordinate these individual responses. Some well-studied examples of such coordinate regulatory systems are *catabolite repression, stringency,* the *SOS* response, and the *heat shock* response.

Catabolite Repression

Catabolite repression refers to a regulatory system by which the bacterial cell can select its diet of energy-rich compounds from a menu that may be quite extensive. This mechanism involves the positive regulation of a variety of catabolic operons by the *catabolite repressor protein (CRP)* and *cyclic AMP* (an effector). When bound to CRP, cyclic AMP causes a conformational change in the molecule that allows it to bind to the promoter region of the various catabolic operons, allowing for transcription of the catabolite genes in the presence of their inducers. Either CRP or cyclic AMP alone is not sufficient to induce these operons. In the absence of cyclic AMP, the CRP is inactive, and gene transcription of the various catabolic operons is repressed, even in the presence of their inducers.

When *E. coli* grows in the presence of glucose, it utilizes this sugar preferentially as its source of energy, and the enzymes encoded in the various catabolic operons are repressed. The reason for this repression is that as long as *E. coli* utilizes glucose, its intracellular concentration of cyclic AMP is low, thus preventing the activation of the CRP. If, however, glucose is depleted from the environment, cyclic AMP levels increase and the cyclic AMP-CRP complex can ready the various catabolic operons for induction. Thus, catabolite repression provides the cell with the ability to utilize glucose preferentially when it is present in the environment, yet to be able to utilize other available energy sources when glucose is depleted.

Catabolite repression also provides the cell with a mechanism by which it can select which of the available energy sources it will use and in which order. The priority order is set by the differential binding coefficients of the catabolic operons to the CRP–cyclic AMP complex. The catabolic operons with the highest binding affinity for the CRP–cyclic AMP complex will be induced preferentially if its inducer is present. The catabolic operon with the least binding affinity for the CRP–cyclic AMP complex, on the other hand, can be induced only in the absence of the inducers of the other catabolic operons.

Stringency

Stringency describes the response of a bacterial cell when it is faced with amino acid starvation. Its rate of growth is reduced or ceases; it stops manufacturing RNA, protein, chromosomes, and membrane components; and alterations in a variety of other biologic activities occur. This response is clearly economical, since in the absence of protein precursors the cell cannot grow and therefore does not need to synthesize its various components, especially chromosomes, ribosomes, and membranes. Instead, it needs to conserve its energy and wait until the missing amino acid is present again in its environment.

The molecular mechanism of stringency is not completely understood. It is known, however, that the rate of synthesis of the translational machinery (rRNA, tRNA, ribosomal proteins, etc.) is downregulated while the regulation of amino acid biosynthesis and proteases is upregulated. This increases the production of amino acids by degradation of proteins and de novo synthesis and prevents the accumulation of translational machinery, which is unneeded. It is also known that this regulation is mediated by two nucleotides, guanosine tetraphosphate (ppGpp) and guanosine pentaphosphate (pppGpp), previously called magic spots by the discoverers Cashel and Gallent. These regulatory signals are produced by a ribosome-associated stringent factor (a protein) when translation is retarded by the occupancy of an uncharged tRNA in the A site of a ribosome actively engaged in the process of translation. The mechanism by which this intracellular signal effects transcription is unknown.

Heat Shock Response

When *E. coli* is exposed to elevated temperatures, a set of heat shock proteins are induced, which act on a variety of different physiologic pathways. The mechanism by which these genes are turned on involves a sensory protein, *dna*K, which somehow senses the insult, and the product of *htp*R, which replaces the sigma factor, thus allowing the recognition of a different set of promoter sequences by RNA polymerase (the heat shock genes). It is important to note that the *dna*K nucleotide sequence and the heat shock response itself are highly conserved throughout both the animal and plant kingdoms.

SOS Response

This coordinate regulatory system is induced in *E. coli* in response to extensive DNA damage. It involves the derepression of approximately 20 different SOS genes, some of whose products are involved in DNA repair, in blocking cell division. In the undamaged wild-type cell, the SOS regulon genes are repressed by the LexA protein. The products of these genes are synthesized at low constitutive levels. An SOS-inducing signal is somehow generated by DNA damage. This signal, probably portions of single-stranded DNA or DNA degradation products, interacts with the RecA protein, converting it into a protease that, in turn, cleaves the LexA repressor and derepresses the SOS regulon. When the DNA damage is repaired, RecA no longer acts as a protease and LexA represses the SOS genes, which include *lex*A and *rec*A.

Mutation and Variation in Bacteria

Historical Perspectives

Until the mid 1950s, bacteria were regarded as a form of life quite different from that of other organisms. Many believe that bacterial variations resulted from adaptation and that the environment provoked an inheritable alteration in the bacteria exposed to it (e.g., phage resistance resulted from being exposed to the phage). Thus, bacteriology was the last stronghold of Lamarckism (the doctrine of the inheritance of acquired characteristics). Not until such experiments as Luria and Delbruck's fluctuation test (1943), Newcombe's respreading experiment (1949), the Lederbergs' indirect mutant selection by replica plating (1952), and Cavalli-Sforza and Lederbergs' sib-selection studies

(1955) was it widely accepted that spontaneous, preadapted mutations exist in bacteria. Today we recognize that microorganisms, as other organisms, are subject to genotypic variations and that it is through such genetic changes that they have evolved to their present state. There are two basic means by which such genetic variations and the invigoration of the species can come about: *mutation* and *recombination*. In the following section, we shall examine the general ways in which changes in the genotype affect the phenotype and how such changes arise and are dealt with.

Mutation

A mutation refers to any stably inherited *change in genotype* other than the acquisition of genetic information from another individual. Its basis may be change in the DNA constituting a chromosomal gene (i.e., a gene mutation) or other changes such as the deletion or rearrangement of a length of DNA composing more than one gene.

Mutation frequency is the proportion of mutants in a given population of cells. For example, 100 mutants in a population of 100,000,000 would have a mutation frequency of 1/1,000,000, or 1 in 1 million.

Mutation rate is generally defined as the probability of a mutation occurring during some given time interval. It is often calculated as a function of generation or cell doubling time and hence expressed as mutation per cell per cell doubling. The *spontaneous mutation rate* for any gene is relatively low and usually falls between 10^{-5} and 10^{-7} per cell doubling. However, this rate can be greatly increased by the use of various chemical or physical agents called *mutagens*.

Expression of Mutations

Procaryotic cells may contain one or several copies of their chromosomes. However, each copy is derived from the same parent and hence is identical. Thus, *bacteria are haploid* organisms, and therefore any mutation that alters the function of a gene product will eventually be expressed. This expression, however, may or may not occur immediately. After the mutant genome is produced, at least one generation (cell doubling) may be required before the mutant phenotype can be detected. This lag in the time between onset and expression of a mutation may be due to the time required for the segregation of the mutant genome, called *segregational lag,* or for the physiologic expression of the mutant phenotype (e.g., dilution of wild-type enzyme), called *phenotypic lag,* or both.

Classification of Mutations

Mutations can be classified according to their effect on either genotype or phenotype.

Phenotypic Classifications

On the basis of phenotypic changes, *wild type* refers to the normal genetic state of an organism that has all of its genetic functions intact, while mutants that have additional nutritional requirements are called *auxotrophs*. A mutation that occurs in the wild type, causing a change in the phenotype, is called a *forward* mutation. A second mutation that restores the wild-type phenotype is referred to as a *back* mutation. The parents of auxotrophs, as well as *revertants* that are able to regain the nutritional requirements of the wild type, are called *prototrophs*.

Other phenotypic changes include changes in colony morphology (e.g., rough and smooth), antibiotic resistance, phage resistance, colicin resistance, and changes in fermentation capabilities. Another interesting class of phenotypic mutation is the so-called *conditional* mutant, whose phenotypic change is expressed only under a certain set of conditions. The conditions that alter their phenotype include temperature (i.e., temperature-sensitive mutants), osmolarity (osmotic remedial mutants), and pH (pH mutants). The temperature-sensitive mutants produce gene products that are inactive at either high temperature (heat-sensitive mutants) or low temperature (cold-sensitive mutants). The osmotic remedial mutants and pH mutants produce gene products whose expression is influenced by the osmotic strength and pH of the environment, respectively. *Some conditional mutants express a lethal phenotype at the nonpermissive condition.* These mutants are referred to as *conditional lethal mutants* and have played an important role in deciphering complex processes essential to the cell such as DNA replication and cell division.

Genotypic Classifications

Several types of changes can occur at the molecular level of DNA, resulting in changes in the nucleotide sequence of the cell's genome. These mutations fall into several different genetic categories, depending on their effect on DNA structure (neoclotide sequence) and on protein synthesis (transcription and translation of the genetic code).

Classification According to DNA Structural Changes

Any permanent alteration in the sequence of base pairs constitutes a mutation. The possible alterations fall into three categories: (1) *base-pair substitution,* (2) *insertions and deletions,* and (3) *rearrangements,* including transpositions and inversions.

Base-pair substitution (point) mutations result from the change of a single base pair of a nucleotide sequence of a gene. For example, if the base adenine (A) in a strand of DNA, acting as a template during replication, is altered such that it is recognized as cytosine (C), it would pair with guanine (G) instead of thymine (T), resulting eventually in a G–C base-pair substitution for the original A–T base pair. Base-pair substitutions can be divided into two classes: Those in which a purine is replaced by a different purine or a pyrimidine by a different pyrimidine are called *transitions,* and those in which a purine is replaced by a pyrimidine and vice versa are called *transversions.*

Insertions and deletions often result in frameshift mutations that shift the reading frame of a gene so that all codons of the gene downstream (distal) to the mutation site are changed. The result is a grossly altered protein, usually with complete loss of function. An exception would be an insertion or deletion of, for example, three or six bases, which would not shift the reading frame per se and would result in a protein with one, two, etc., amino acids inserted or omitted from the wild-type protein, which may or may not remain functional.

Rearrangements in bacterial chromosomes have been observed, and their mutagenic effect depends on the specific chromosomal alteration encountered. For example, duplications may change gene dosage, while inversions may change the regulation of a particular gene or operon if the inversion occurs between the structural gene and its promoter or regulatory sequence, or the production of a functional gene product if the inversion occurs between genes.

Classification According to Changes in Protein Synthesis

The most important effect of a mutation in a gene is on its translation. Some of the possible effects of a single base-change mutation on translation are as follows:

1. The altered codon may still specify the same amino acid (this is because the genetic code is degenerate and thus more than one codon specifies the same amino acid), resulting in no effect on the phenotype.
2. The altered codon specifies an altered amino acid, called a *missense mutation* (i.e., a mutant codon that is translated into a different, incorrect amino acid is said to contribute to the missense of the message).
3. The codon may be altered to read as a termination signal (amber, ocher, or opal), resulting in a premature polypeptide-chain termination during translation. This type of mutation is referred to as a *non-sense* mutation and usually results in the complete loss of protein function.

Consequences of Mutations

Changes in the nucleotide sequences of DNA may bring about changes in the resulting transcriptional and translational products of the corresponding gene. The effects of such changes on the resulting protein include:

1. An alteration in a catalytic site of an enzyme, resulting in the complete (tight) or partial (leaky) inactivation of the enzyme. Such mutations give rise to auxotrophs or lethal mutants.
2. An alteration in protein structure such that it becomes sensitive to a number of agents such as temperature, osmotic pressure, pH, or various effectors. These mutants include conditional lethal mutants.
3. An alteration in the polypeptide subunit of a polymeric protein that might cause it to undergo abnormal association with its other subunits. Loss of activity or alteration of its allosterism would render the protein sensitive or insensitive to various effectors. Such mutants include *regulatory* mutants.
4. An alteration in a noncritical portion of the polypeptide chain, resulting in no detectable structural or functional change. Such a mutation is called a *silent* mutation.
5. An alteration in a protein involved in the function of several other different proteins (e.g., processing protein or one involved in the secretion of proteins), resulting in two or more phenotypic changes. Such a mutant is said to be *pleiotropic.*

Repair of Mutations

Damage to DNA caused by ultraviolet radiation, ionizing radiation, and radiomimetic chemicals (chemicals whose effects mimic those of radiation) can be repaired. In bacteria, there are three main classifications of repair systems: (1) *direct repair,* (2) *dark repair,* and (3) *post-replication repair.*

Direct Repair

Direct repair involves the reversal of premutational lesions. This process is called *photoreactivation* and is accomplished by specific photoreactivating enzymes capable of recognizing pyrimidine dimers, binding to them, absorbing light energy, and cleaving the bonds that join the adjacent pyrimidines, thereby converting them to monomers.

Dark Repair

Dark repair of pyrimidine dimers in DNA does not require light. In this case, the dimers are excised rather than split. This mechanism requires the participation of at least five proteins: *DNA ligase, DNA polymerase I,* and the gene products of *uvr*A, *uvr*B, and *uvr*C genes. The *uvr*A and *uvr*B gene products bind to the damaged region of DNA, and in the presence of the *uvr*C product, they produce a single-stranded break (nick) in the affected strand at the 5′ end of the damaged region. The dimer is then removed by a specific exonuclease and the resulting gap repaired by DNA polymerase I and DNA ligase.

Microbial Genetics

Postreplication Repair

Postreplication repair occurs if the replication fork passes over the damaged region before it has been corrected by photoreactivation or dark repair. If the replicative fork reaches a damaged region of the chromosome before it is repaired, it skips over the damage and reinitiates DNA synthesis beyond the lesion, leaving the damaged region as single-stranded DNA (i.e., a single-stranded gap). The resulting lesion, therefore, cannot be repaired by excision because it lacks a complementary strand for DNA polymerase I to use as a template. However, this damaged DNA can be repaired by a recombinational event called *postreplication repair*. In this process, the complementary strand to the damaged region (from the recently replicated sister duplex) is inserted across from the damaged DNA, resulting in two repairable lesions: one containing a gap (i.e., where the piece of exchanged DNA once was), which can be repaired by DNA polymerase I and DNA ligase, and one containing the damaged DNA per se with its complementary strand (which it received from its sister through a recombinational event), which can be repaired by the dark-repair system.

Suppression of Mutations

Repair mechanisms reverse genetic damage and restore the original phenotypic expression by restoring the original gene. However, other mechanisms are available that do not correct the original mutation per se, but are capable of restoring the original phenotype. When the effects of a primary mutation are eliminated by altering the translational process, the phenomenon is called *suppression*. There are two types of suppression: *genotypic* suppression and *phenotypic* suppression.

Genotypic Suppression

Genotypic suppression is a genetic term used to describe the effect of a general class of secondary mutations that restore a wild or pseudowild phenotype to a mutant organism in which the primary mutation is still maintained (one of the few cases in which two wrongs make a right). The means by which these compensating mutations suppress the original mutation are manyfold, and these correction mechanisms may operate either during the transcription and translation step of gene expression or at the level of the final gene products. Suppressor mutations can be classified according to their genetic location, as either *intragenic* (within the affected gene) or *extragenic* (outside of the affected gene).

Intragenic Suppressor Mutations

Intragenic suppressor mutations introduce an additional alteration to the affected gene or gene product that completely or partially negates the effect of the primary muta-

tion. For example, an intragenic suppressor mutation may cause an amino acid substitution that compensates for the primary missense mutation and allows the resulting polypeptide to take on a functional conformation. It may also cause an insertion or deletion that compensates for a primary frameshift mutation, or it might even cause a nonsense mutation to code for a sense codon, allowing for a functional protein to be made.

Extragenic Suppressor Mutations

Extragenic suppressor mutations can compensate for the original mutation by providing an alternative metabolic pathway (or enzyme) for the production of the affected metabolic product, or they can act by altering the properties of one of the factors involved in protein synthesis (i.e., transcription and translation). The actual mechanism of suppression can be classified as either direct or indirect depending on whether the consequence of the original mutation is circumvented (indirect) or correct (direct). Extragenic suppressor mutations can also be classified according to the type of mutation they correct and include (1) *non-sense suppressors,* (2) *missense suppressors,* and (3) *frameshift suppressors.*

As already described, a mutation that causes the conversion of an amino acid–specifying codon into one of the three terminator codons, UAG, UAA, and UGA, in an mRNA leads to premature termination of translation and is called a non-sense mutation. The effect of such a mutation can be reversed by secondary extragenic suppressor mutations, called *non-sense suppressors.* These mutations correct non-sense mutations by inserting a substitute amino acid into a polypeptide chain in response to the non-sense codon. If the substituted amino acids allow the resulting protein to function, they restore the wild-type phenotype. These mutations can be further classified according to the non-sense codon on which they act (i.e., amber suppressors read UGA, ocher suppressors read both UAA and UAG, and opal suppressors read UGA). As might be expected, most non-sense suppressor mutations have resulted from an alteration in the anticodon of a tRNA gene. Suppressor tRNA species are often found to be minor members of isoacceptor tRNA families and hence are present in small numbers within the cell.

A missense mutation is a base change in DNA that alters an mRNA codon, resulting in the substitution of a single amino acid in the encoded polypeptide chain. This often alters the function of the gene product. Such a mutation can be corrected by a secondary extragenic suppressor mutation that leads to the insertion of an acceptable amino acid in response to the mutant mRNA codon. These suppressors are called *missense suppressors* and, as is the case with non-sense suppressors, often map in tRNA genes.

Extragenic suppressors called *frameshift suppressor* mutations can correct frameshift mutations by restoring the proper reading frame of translation. Many frameshift suppressor mutations also map in tRNA genes. However, it should be noted that the suppression of missense, non-sense, and frameshift mutations can also be achieved by alterations in the components of ribosomes, since changes in ribosome structure could bring about a range of codon misreadings, which in turn could lead to informational suppression.

Phenotypic Suppression

Mutations can also be corrected by nonmutational alterations of the protein-synthesizing machinery (transcription and translation). For example, sublethal concentrations of streptomycin and other related antibiotics will cause misreading of the genetic code and hence may allow missense or non-sense codons to be read and translated as sense codons. This type of transient, nongenetic suppression is referred to as *phenotypic suppression*. An additional example of phenotypic suppression is the incorporation of base analogues into mRNA, causing its translation to be altered.

Gene Transfer and Recombination in Bacteria

New combinations of genes can arise by mechanisms other than mutation. In eucaryotic cells, for example, a well-developed sexual system for genetic exchange exists. The essential features involve the fusion of two haploid gametes to form a diploid zygote. During the process of gamete formation (meiosis), the diploid number is reduced to a haploid number, and genetic exchanges between homologous chromosomes (derived from both parents) occur. This sexual process contributes not only to the invigoration of the species by allowing reassortment of beneficial traits by genetic recombination but also to speciation by evolutionary progression.

In bacteria, however, zygotes are formed by a more primitive means of genetic exchange, involving three general mechanisms: (1) *transformation,* in which naked DNA is derived from one cell (the recipient); (2) *transduction,* in which a piece of bacterial DNA from the donor is packaged and transferred, through a virus capsid, to the recipient cell, where it may then become incorporated into its genome; and (3) *conjugation,* where the DNA from the donor cell is transferred to the recipient cell through cell-to-cell contact, after which recombination may occur. *All three processes involve a unidirectional transfer of genetic material from donor to recipient.* In the majority of cases, this transfer of chromosomal material is only partial, and it often results in the transient formation of *partial diploids* or what is often called a *meridiploid* or *merozygote.* Such

partial diploids contain the entire genome (*endogenote*) of the recipient cell and the incomplete genome (*exogenote*) of the donor (Fig. 3-6).

Transformation

The discovery of transformation by Griffith in 1928 serves as a landmark in the history of bacterial genetics. His experiments were the first to demonstrate that genetic determinants could be transferred between two bacteria and laid the groundwork for the subsequent recognition that the cell's hereditary material resides in the nucleotide sequence of DNA.

Griffith's original experiments employed *Diplococcus (Streptococcus) pneumoniae,* which causes bacterial pneumonia in humans and produces a fatal disease in mice. The virulence of the pneumococcus is related to its production of a *polysaccharide capsule* that is also responsible for a *smooth-colony* type when the organism is grown on solid media. These capsules can be divided into types based on differences in antigenicity, which are due to slight variations in polysaccharide composition (there are more than 80 different serotypes of pneumococcus capsules). Nonvirulent, *rough mutants* can be isolated from the virulent *smooth strains.* Such mutants are devoid of capsular material. Griffith found that some noncapsulated pneumococcus strains were stable and nonvirulent. However, when he injected mice with a mixture of heat-killed type I capsulated cells and live, noncapsulated cells derived from a type II strain, the mice died. *The causative agent was shown to be a virulent, type I capsulated strain.* In other experiments, the results were reproduced in a test tube. When capsulated (smooth) cells were ground up and added to noncapsulated (rough) cells in a test tube, one could isolate from this mixture viable, capsulated cells. It was the characterization of this in vitro system that led Avery, MacLeod, and McCarthy to identify DNA as the active ingredient of the transforming principle. Since the original discovery of transformation in streptococci, this process has been demonstrated in species of both gram-positive and gram-negative bacteria, including such genera as *Bacillus, Haemophilus, Neisseria, Moraxella, Psychrobacter, Azotobacter, Pseudomonas,* and *Escherichia.*

Transformation, then, is the transfer by naked DNA of a limited amount of genetic information from one bacterium (the donor) to another (the recipient). Recipient bacteria expressing genetic characteristics of the donor bacterium are said to be transformed. This phenomenon has been extensively studied in *Strep. pneumoniae* and *Bacillus subtilis,* and a general model can be described. However, care must be taken in extrapolation to other bacteria. Operationally, transformation can be divided into three steps (Fig. 3-7):

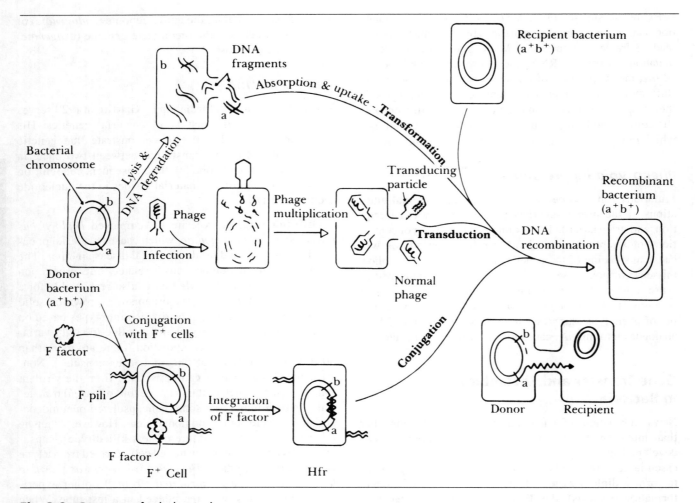

Fig. 3-6   Gene transfer in bacteria.

1. *Absorption* or binding of transforming DNA to the recipient cell surface: In the successful transformation of the recipient cell, double-stranded DNA fragments are bound to its surface. This attachment is mediated by specific receptors located on the external surface of the cytoplasmic membrane. In the case of *Strep. pneumoniae*, there are approximately 80 such binding sites. DNA binding is often accompanied by single-stranded scissions or nicks produced by a membrane-associated endonuclease.

2. *Entry* of the transforming DNA into the recipient cell: This step is often preceded by a second endonuclease cut opposite the first nick, creating double-stranded DNA fragments. A minimum size requirement for the donor DNA exists in most transformation systems and is somewhat species specific. In the *B. subtilis* and pneumococcus transforming systems, one of the strands of the transforming DNA is translocated across the cytoplasmic membrane, while its complementary strand is digested by a membrane-associated exonuclease.

This process of DNA uptake requires metabolic energy and leads to a phenomenon called *eclipse,* where the donor DNA has no transforming activity after uptake until the donor fragment has been incorporated into the recipient's genome. This apparent lack of transforming activity is due to the low transforming activity of single-stranded DNA. In gram-negative transforming systems, the DNA appears to be taken up as a duplex structure with single-stranded regions, and hence the phenomenon of eclipse is not observed.

3. *Incorporation* of the transforming DNA into the recipient cell's genome: The DNA taken up in gram-positive bacteria is single-stranded. If this DNA is homologous with the recipient's DNA, there is a good chance that it will become inserted into the recipient's genome, creating regions in which one strand of the DNA duplex is donor DNA and its complementary strand is recipient DNA. When the two strands of such a heteroduplex structure differ (e.g., as a result of the presence of a mutation in either the donor or recipient DNA), the

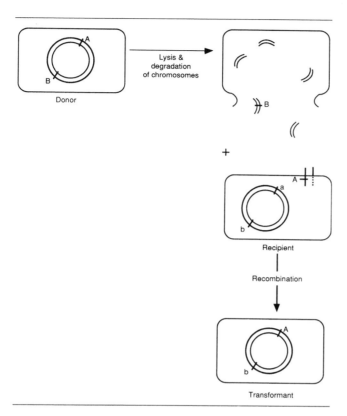

Fig. 3-7 Transformation.

structure is described as *heterozygous.* In both *B. subtilis* and pneumococcus transformation, either complementary strand from the donor may be integrated into the recipient's genome and, at least in the pneumococcus, may be segregated by semiconservative replication (segregational lag). Even in gram-negative bacteria, where the transforming DNA is double-stranded, only one strand is incorporated into the recipient's genome; the other strand and the displaced strand of the recipient DNA are enzymatically degraded.

Cells of a transformable strain are not always transformable. When they are, however, they are said to be *competent.* This physiologic state fluctuates greatly during the growth of a bacterial culture, and for *Strep. pneumoniae,* the maximum competence is usually achieved during the late logarithmic phase of growth. In *Strep. pneumoniae,* competence can be induced by a small protein called a *competence factor,* which causes the cells in the population to synthesize 8 to 10 new proteins. These, in turn, increase the ability of these cells to become transformed. Competence factors are unknown in gram-negative bacteria. However, a culture of *Haemophilus* can become almost 100 percent competent following transfer to nutrient-poor growth media that permit protein synthesis, and *Escherichia coli*

can be artificially induced by suspending the organisms in high concentrations of divalent ions, such as calcium or magnesium. It is thought that such treatments act by altering the outer-membrane structure and unmasking cytoplasmic, membrane-associated, DNA-binding proteins.

Transfection

Transfection is the term used to describe the transformation of naked viral genomes and has played an important role in recombinant DNA technology.

Transduction and Phage Conversion

Before discussing transduction or phage conversion, let us briefly review the life cycle of bacterial viruses. When bacteriophages enter their host, there are two possible outcomes: They can enter the *lytic cycle,* replicate, generate progeny viruses, which leads to the lysis of the bacterial cell and the release of mature phages, or they can enter the *lysogenic cycle,* become integrated into the bacterial chromosome, and be replicated with the bacterial DNA. Bacterial viruses, which exclusively use the lytic cycle, are called *virulent* phages. Bacterial phages in the integrated state are referred to as *prophages,* and the viruses that are capable of this type of life cycle are called *temperate* or *lysogenic* phages. This latter host-virus relationship is called *lysogeny,* and the host is said to be *lysogenized.* In the lysogenic state, the viral genes responsible for phage production are repressed. If this repressed state breaks down and the virus is induced, the virus may enter into the lytic cycle.

Transduction is the transfer of bacterial DNA from one cell to another by means of a virus vehicle. It was discovered by Zinder and Lederberg in 1952. It involves the transfer of a limited amount of genetic information from a lysed donor cell to an intact recipient cell, or, more precisely, that amount of DNA that can be packaged into the bacteriophage protein coat. It is the result of an error that sometimes occurs in the maturation or packaging of the DNA of certain types of bacteriophages. If, during phage development, host (bacterial) DNA or a mixture of host and phage DNA is packaged into the phage capsid (instead of phage DNA alone), then the phage becomes a *transducing particle* and is capable of injecting bacterial DNA of its original host into another bacterium (the recipient). Two different types of errors in phage maturation lead to the formation of transducing particles that are quite different and that are involved in two different types of transduction: *generalized* and *specialized.*

Generalized Transduction

Some transducing particles pick up bacterial host genes in a somewhat random manner so that, theoretically, any gene can be transduced. This process is referred to as generalized transduction (Fig. 3-8). Generalized transducing particles are produced during vegetative growth and multiplication of the phage. A number of bacterial viruses are known to mediate generalized transduction. The aberrant mechanism by which bacterial DNA is packaged into the phage capsid (to produce a generalized transducing particle) is thought to be common to all generalized transducing phages.

Fig. 3-8   Generalized transduction.

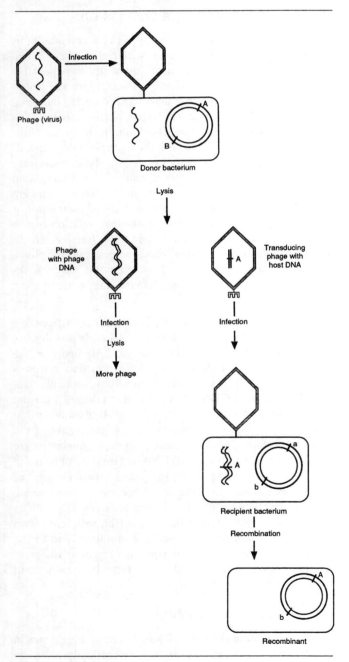

Specialized Transduction

Some bacterial phages preferentially transduce specific regions (genes) of the bacterial chromosome. These phages are referred to as specialized transducing phages and the process as specialized transduction. *Only temperate phages are capable of mediating specialized transduction.* In fact, for specialized transduction to occur, the specialized transducing phage must be integrated into the host chromosome. When this prophage is induced into the lytic cycle, it must excise itself from its host chromosome before it can begin DNA replication and phage production. On a rare occasion, an error is made in the excision process, and some of the adjacent bacterial DNA is excised with the prophage (often with a concomitant loss of some of the phage DNA). The resulting phages are therefore a mixture of phage DNA and specific bacterial DNA (those genes adjacent to the prophage integration site). Because only a specific size of DNA can be packaged into a phage coat, the bacteriophage genome in a specialized transducing particle is usually incomplete, missing that portion replaced by the bacterial genes. Because essential genes for normal bacteriophage functions are usually missing, the bacteriophage is often defective and cannot multiply by itself. Since this excision error is rare, and since most specialized transducing phages are defective and therefore cannot multiply, a lysate obtained by induction normally contains only a few specialized transducing particles and is said to be a *low frequency of transduction (LFT) lysate. A high frequency of transduction (HFT)* lysate can be obtained from a double lysogen containing the defective specialized transducing phage and a helper phage of the same type. The helper phage provides the missing functions of the defective phage by complementation and allows complete maturation of both phages. In such lysates, approximately 50 percent of the progeny phages are specialized transducing phages.

Phage Conversion

The alteration of bacterial phenotype resulting from the presence of a bacterial virus or phage is called *phage conversion.* If it can be demonstrated that this alteration in phenotype is due to the presence of a stable prophage, the term *lysogenic conversion* can be applied. Some medically important examples of phage conversion include (1) diphtheria toxin production by *Corynebacterium diphtheriae* when infected by phage B, (2) botulinum toxin production by *Clostridium botulinum* type C following infection by a phage, (3) the antigenic alterations of somatic O antigen of salmonellae in the presence of a prophage, (4) the erythrogenic toxin production (of scarlet fever) by lysogenic *Streptococcus pyogenes,* and (5) the Shiga-like toxin production by *E. coli* following lysogenization by either of two different bacteriophages (isolated from a pathogen causing hemorrhagic colitis).

Conjugation and Transfer Plasmids

Conjugation in Gram-Negative Bacteria

The discovery of auxotrophic mutations in the 1940s provided a powerful genetic tool for searching for sexual processes in bacteria. Joshua Lederberg made the dramatic discovery of bacterial conjugation in 1946.

Conjugation is the process by which genetic material is passed, unidirectionally, from one bacterium to another. This process is mediated by plasmids termed collectively as *conjugative plasmids* (e.g., fertility factors) in the donor cell. Conjugation occurs in many genera of gram-negative bacteria, including *Escherichia, Proteus, Pseudomonas, Salmonella, Serratia, Shigella, Vibrio,* and *Yersinia.* The plasmids are transferred at high frequency, occasionally mobilizing chromosomal genes as well. The most completely studied of the conjugative plasmids is the *F factor* (fertility factor), which can replicate in *E. coli* and related enteric bacteria, including *Salmonella typhimurium* (Fig. 3-9).

The Nature of the F Factor

The F factor is an autonomously replicating circular heteroduplex of double-stranded DNA with a molecular weight of about 50×10^6 daltons. This plasmid codes for 40 to 60 gene products, some of which are involved in its replication, maintenance, and conjugal transfer. The genetic information necessary for its transfer resides in 13 *transfer (tra) genes,* which make up an operon. The *tra* genes control F-pilus formation and conjugal DNA metabolism. The F *pilus* mediates the adherence of donor and recipient cells during the process of conjugation and may also play a role in DNA transfer. An outer-membrane protein, Omp*A,* of the recipient cell, apparently acts as a receptor site in this process of cell-to-cell adherence.

F$^+$ cells are donor cells that harbor the F plasmid in its autonomous state. When F$^+$ cells are mixed with F$^-$ cells (lacking an F plasmid), all the F$^-$ cells are rapidly converted to F$^+$. However, in such matings the transfer of chromosomal genes is very rare ($<10^{-7}$).

Hfr Cells

Some clones of F$^+$ cells are capable of transferring chromosomal genes with increased efficiency, resulting in a high frequency of recombination (Hfr). *The Hfr cells are the result of the integration of the F plasmid into the bacterial chromosome* (Fig. 3-9). The F factor contains four insertion sequences (IS) that are homologous with IS found on the bacterial chromosome. Recombination between an IS on the bacterial chromosome and one on the F factor leads to the integration of F into the bacterial genome and thus the formation of an Hfr strain. *Hfr cells differ from F*$^+$ *cells in that the entire F factor of the Hfr is*

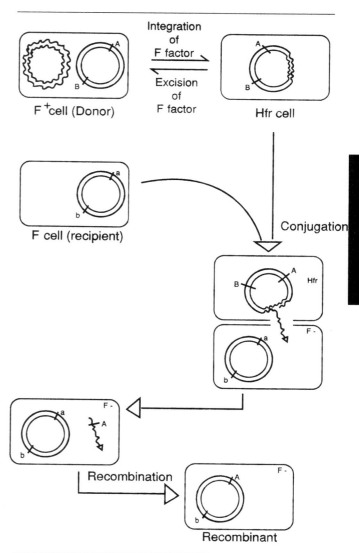

Fig. 3-9 Conjugation.

rarely transferred during conjugation. This is because the IS on F (where F integrates into the chromosome) lie between the origin of transfer (site where the transfer of F-factor DNA is initiated) and the *tra* genes. Therefore, the *tra* genes are transferred only following the transfer of the intervening bacterial chromosome (the bacterial chromosome is circular), which is a very rare event. Consequently, Hfr $\times$ F$^-$ matings differ from those of an F$^+$ $\times$ F$^-$ in that chromosomal markers near the insertion site of F (near the origin of transfer) are transferred with a high frequency, yet the F$^-$ cell (in the Hfr mating) rarely becomes a male (harbors the intact F plasmid).

The location of the integration of the F factor in the bacterial chromosome determines which chromosomal genes are transferred with high frequency. The direction of chromosomal transfer in Hfr cells (clockwise versus counterclockwise) depends on the orientation of F⁻ plasmid integration (i.e., only one strand of the F factor carries the origin of transfer, and, therefore, depending on its orientation in the chromosome, either the Watson or the Crick strand of the heteroduplex molecule will be transferred).

F-Prime Cells

In some Hfr cells, the integrated F plasmid may be excised from the chromosomal DNA, taking with it one or more adjacent bacterial genes (analogous to specialized transduction). *The F factor and its associated bacterial DNA are collectively referred to as an F-prime (F′).* F′ formation generates a chromosomal deletion; the genes carried on the F′ are not duplicated in the chromosome, and hence the cell remains haploid for all genes. Such a cell is termed a *primary F′*. However, the product of an F′ × F⁻ mating, which usually results in the complete transfer of the F′ because of its relatively small size, is a partially diploid cell (a stable merozygote) called a *secondary F′*.

Physiology of Conjugation

When cells that contain an F plasmid are mixed with F⁻ cells, conjugal pairs rapidly form by attachment of the end of the F pilus to the surface of the F⁻ cells. This attachment then triggers a series of events resulting in the transfer of the F factor and any associated chromosomal DNA. This DNA transfer process is initiated from an endonuclease nick in one of the two complementary strands of F (i.e., at the origin of transfer) and serves both as the site at which DNA transfer begins and as the starting point for the replication of the unnicked strand (through a rolling-circle mode of replication). The 5′ end of the nicked strand of F-DNA is the first to enter the recipient cell, with concomitant DNA replication of the complementary strand in the 3′ to 5′ direction in the donor cell. *The DNA transferred during conjugation, therefore, is single-stranded, and its origin contains a 5′ end.* This transfer process continues until the mating pairs break apart or the entire F-associated DNA is transferred to the recipient. The overall process of conjugation has been described as occurring in five distinct stages, according to a model put forward by Roy Curtiss III. These stages are described as follows:

1. *Specific pair formation:* the initial interaction between the donor's F pilus and the recipient cell surface (receptor sites) to form a stable mating pair.
2. *Effective pair formation:* the formation of a bridge between the two mating cells that will allow the transfer of DNA. This stage involves the resorption of the F pili by the donor and the joining of the donor's and recipient's cellular envelopes and is an energy-dependent process.

3. *Chromosomal mobilization:* involves the recognition and nicking of the single-stranded F-DNA sequence corresponding to the origin of transfer.
4. *Chromosomal transfer:* involves the transfer and simultaneous asymmetric replication of the F and associated chromosomal DNA. This replication process is envisioned as providing the driving force for propelling the free 5′ end of the nicked DNA into the recipient cell. As replication is continued in the donor, more of the 5′ end of the F-DNA and associated chromosomal DNA is transferred to the recipient cell.
5. *Recombination:* occurs when the homologous segments of transferred (donor) and recipient DNA pair.

Conjugation in Gram-Positive Bacteria

Conjugation also occurs in gram-positive bacteria, although it is a relatively new discovery. In *Streptococcus faecalis,* for example, a number of conjugative plasmids are capable of self-transfer and of the mobilization of other nonconjugative plasmids and chromosomal genes. Recent studies of this system suggest that it might be quite different from its gram-negative counterpart. For instance, pili play no role in the process, and mating signals between cells are mediated by soluble molecules called *pheromones.* These signal molecules are released from cells that do not carry conjugative plasmids and stimulate those that do to produce an *aggregation substance* on their outer surface. Cells that form this substance form clumps with those that lack it, and plasmids are then transferred between cells within these clumps. Plasmid-linked characteristics transmitted in this manner include hemolysin production and resistance to lincomycin, kanamycin, neomycin, streptomycin, tetracycline, and erythromycin. There are also conjugative transposons involved in transferring antibiotic resistance within the genus *Streptococcus* (see section on transposons).

The Fate of Transferred DNA

Once DNA from a donor bacterium (exogenote) is present in the recipient cell, regardless of the means by which it arrived, it is dealt with in one of the following ways:

1. It may be recognized as foreign and be digested by the host's *restriction enzymes (endonucleases).*
2. It may be incorporated into the recipient cell's genome (endogenote) by means of *recombination.*
3. If the DNA is capable of self-replication (i.e., it is a replicon), it may exist autonomously within the recipient cell, as a plasmid or a defective phage, replicating and segregating with its host's DNA.
4. If the DNA is incapable of replication but is not degraded by the host's restriction system, it will remain in

only one of the resulting progeny cells of the culture. This occurs frequently with specialized transducing phages that do not replicate and in this case is called *abortive transduction*.

Restriction and Modification

The persistence of the exogenote in the recipient cell following DNA transfer depends, to a large extent, on the DNA restriction-modification systems of both the donor and recipient cells. Bacteria have evolved a surveillance or restriction system by which they can recognize and destroy foreign DNA. They do this through the action of *restriction endonucleases*, of which over 200 are presently known. These enzymes *recognize specific nucleotide sequences in DNA and produce double-stranded scissions*, which subsequently lead to their complete degradation. To protect their own DNA, each bacterial strain that possesses a restriction system also possesses a *modification system* to *disguise the restriction sites* recognized by their endonuclease(s). This is accomplished *by methylating the adenine or cytosine residues* contained within these recognition sequences. The DNA sequences recognized by restricting and modifying enzymes vary greatly, and complex patterns of compatibilities exist between bacterial genera, species, and strains. If the transferred DNA comes from a donor cell with a restriction-modification system dissimilar to that of the recipient cell, then it will most likely be degraded. On the other hand, if the exogenote comes from a donor with a similar restriction-modification system, it stands a good chance of persisting. The genetic information for restriction-modification systems may be located on either chromosomes or plasmids.

Recombination

Recombination in bacteria involves the incorporation of the exogenote, or part of it, into the endogenote. Sometimes it involves a reciprocal exchange between these two DNAs. Three basic types of recombination are found to occur in bacteria and their associated phages: (1) *generalized* recombination, (2) *site-specific* recombination, and (3) *illegitimate* recombination. These processes are distinguished by their requirements for nucleotide sequence homology or lack of it.

Generalized Recombination

When the extent of homology between two parental DNA molecules is extensive, the probability of recombination in most bacteria is good, occurring randomly along the region where the two homologies are in register. In *E. coli,* this mechanism *involves a variety of recombination gene products* (*rec*A, *rec*B, and *rec*C genes) as well as various components of the cell's DNA repair system (i.e., an exonuclease, an endonuclease, DNA polymerase I, and DNA ligase). Examples of this type of recombination involve the incorporation of homologous DNA, transferred to donor cells by transduction, transformation, and conjugation.

Site-Specific Recombination

In contrast to general recombination, recombination events can also occur between DNA molecules that share little, if any, homology. When the location of the recombination events is a highly preferred position on one or both of the parental DNA molecules, this is called site-specific recombination. This process in *E. coli is independent of the* rec *gene system*. Examples of this type of recombination are the integration of lambda-phage DNA into the *E. coli* chromosome at minute 17 on its genetic map (lambda-*att* site) and the integration of the F plasmid into the *E. coli* chromosome at IS.

Illegitimate Recombination

Like site-specific recombination, illegitimate recombination *is independent of the* rec *system and requires very little, if any, homology between the parental DNA molecules*. The distinguishing feature of illegitimate recombination is that it *can occur at apparently random sites on the endogenote*. Examples of this type of recombination are the insertions of IS and transposons.

Questions

1. The genetic information of cells:
   A. Was originally thought to reside in tetranucleotides
   B. Was originally thought to reside in proteins
   C. Was originally thought to reside in DNA
   D. Was originally thought to reside in RNA
   E. None of the above
2. The initiation of DNA (chromosome) replication in *E. coli:*
   A. Involves DNA-dependent RNA polymerase
   B. Begins at a genetic locus termed *ter*C
   C. Requires the *tuf* gene product
   D. Requires the *dna*D product
   E. None of the above
3. DNA gyrase:
   A. May be involved in the separation of newly replicated daughter chromosomes
   B. Is a topoisomerase
   C. Alters the topologic state of replicating DNA
   D. Is involved in the replication of the bacterial chromosome
   E. All of the above

4.   The leading strand in DNA replication:
   A. Refers to the continuously replicated strand of DNA at the replicative fork
   B. Proceeds by the addition of nucleotides in the 3′ to 5′ direction
   C. Refers to the discontinuously replicated strand of DNA
   D. Is made up of small Okazaki pieces of DNA joined together by DNA ligase
   E. All of the above

5.   The DNA found in the *E. coli* chromosome:
   A. Is predominantly in the form of "Z-DNA"
   B. Is in the form of a large single-stranded circle
   C. Is highly folded and supercoiled upon itself
   D. Is in the form of a large, linear double-stranded macromolecule
   E. None of the above

6.   Plasmids:
   A. Are bacterial viruses
   B. Are essential for survival
   C. May be involved in the virulence of the host
   D. Are nonreplicating pieces of DNA
   E. None of the above

7.   R factors:
   A. Are found only in gram-negative bacteria
   B. Are found only in gram-positive bacteria
   C. Often consist of two distinct genetic components: the RTF and r determinants
   D. Are linear, double-stranded DNA molecules
   E. None of the above

8.   Transposons:
   A. May contain antibiotic-resistant genes
   B. May contain insertion sequence (IS) elements
   C. Are often found in r determinants
   D. May move from one plasmid to another
   E. All of the above

9.   A mutation:
   A. Is a stably inherited change in the genotype
   B. Is a stably inherited change in the phenotype
   C. Always involves a change in the amino acid sequence of the affected gene product
   D. Is a stably inherited change in both the genotype and phenotype
   E. None of the above

10.   The fate of the exogenote that gains entrance into a bacterial cell may be:
   A. Restriction by exonucleases
   B. Incorporation into the endogenote by recombination
   C. Persistence in a nonreplicative form
   D. Persistence in a replicative form
   E. All of the above

11.   A merizygote:
   A. Is a partial diploid cell

   B. Is represented by a bacterial cell carrying an R factor
   C. Contains the entire genome of both the recipient and donor bacteria
   D. Is a diploid cell
   E. None of the above

12.   A mutation that causes an altered amino acid to be incorporated into mutated gene product is called a:
   A. Non-sense mutation
   B. Frameshift mutation
   C. Amber mutation
   D. Cryptic mutation
   E. None of the above

13. F^+ cells:
   A. Contain the F factor integrated into the bacterial chromosome
   B. Contain F pili on their surfaces
   C. Transfer chromosomal genes at a high frequency
   D. Are also resistant to various antibiotics
   E. None of the above

14.   In generalized transduction:
   A. Only bacterial genes adjacent to the prophage attachment site are transduced by means of special transducing phage
   B. Only bacterial DNA is packaged into the viral capsid
   C. The donor bacteria is called a lysogen
   D. Integration of the phage genome into the bacterial genome is required
   E. None of the above

15.   An intragenetic suppressor mutation:
   A. Can compensate for the original mutation by providing an alternative metabolic pathway (or enzyme) for the production of the affected metabolic product
   B. Can compensate for the original mutation by providing an altered tRNA called a missense suppressor tRNA
   C. May involve codon misreading by ribosomes
   D. Involves a second mutation within the mutated gene
   E. None of the above

16.   Transfection:
   A. Involves the transduction of a virus genome
   B. Involves the conjugation of a virus genome
   C. Involves the transformation of a virus genome
   D. Involves the transposition of a virus genome
   E. None of the above

17.   Restriction endonucleases:
   A. Are involved in the cell's surveillance system for recognizing foreign DNA
   B. Recognize unique nucleotide sequences
   C. May bring about DNA degradation
   D. Are found in many different kinds of bacteria
   E. All of the above

18. If an average gene codes for a polypeptide whose chain length is 350 amino acids long and if 2000 such genes exist in a bacterial chromosome, what would be the probability that a forward mutation would occur in any given gene?
    A. 1/350
    B. 1/3500
    C. 1/700,000
    D. 1/2000
    E. None of the above
19. The probability for a true reversion mutation (back mutation of the original mutation) occurring in the gene in question 18 would be:
    A. About one in 2000
    B. About one in 200,000
    C. About one in 2,000,000
    D. About the same as the original mutation
    E. Greater than the original mutation
20. Which of the following involves the reversal of pre-mutational lesions?
    A. Reversion
    B. Suppression
    C. Photoreactivation
    D. Pseudoreversion
    E. None of the above
21. Non-sense mutations:
    A. Cause the wrong amino acid to be incorporated into the mutant protein
    B. Are the same as "missense" mutations
    C. May be suppressed by an amber suppressor mutation
    D. May be suppressed by an intragenetic suppressor mutation
    E. None of the above
22. DNA transferred between cells by which of the following processes may be degraded by extracellular nucleases?
    A. Conjugation
    B. Transformation
    C. Transduction
    D. Transposition
    E. Translocation

Answers

1. B
2. D
3. E
4. A Once initiated, DNA replication proceeds by poly-nucleotide-chain elongation by the addition of nucleotides in the 5′ to 3′ direction. One strand of the newly made DNA molecule appears to elongate rapidly, copying the template of opposite polarity in a continuous manner. This is called the "leading strand." The other strand of newly made DNA is discontinuously synthesized by the joining of "Okazaki" pieces and is called the "lagging strand."
5. C
6. C While plasmids may confer important characteristics to their bacterial host (attachment pili, toxins, antibiotic resistance, etc.) they are not, under most conditions, essential to cell viability.
7. C R factors are plasmids that are found in both gram-negative and gram-positive bacteria.
8. E
9. A A mutation refers to any stably inherited change in the nucleotide sequence of an organism other than the acquisition of genetic information from another individual. It results in a change in genotype but may or may not result in a change in phenotype.
10. E
11. A Merizygote or partial diploids are the result of the unidirectional transfer of genetic material from a donor bacterial cell to a recipient bacterial cell via transformation, transduction, or conjugation. They contain the entire genome (endogenote) of the recipient cell and the incomplete genome (exogenote) of the donor cell.
12. E The question defines a missense mutation, which is not included as a choice.
13. B F^+ cells are donor cells that harbor the F plasmid in its autonomous state and may transfer this conjugative plasmid efficiently to F^- recipients. F^+ cells, however, transfer chromosomal genes only rarely. Since the F plasmid carries the F-pili gene, F^+ cells have F pili.
14. B Generalized transducing phages are produced when the host bacterial DNA is mistakenly packaged into the phage capsid.
15. D Intragenic suppressor mutations introduce an additional alteration (second mutation) to the affected gene or gene product that completely or partially negates the effect of the primary mutation.
16. C
17. E
18. D Since mutations are random events, and since we are dealing with a hypothetical "average gene size," then each gene has the same probability of being mutated. Hence, since there are 2000 genes, the probability of a particular gene being mutated is 1/2000.
19. B The reversion of the original mutation to wild type would target a specific (single) base pair of the genome coding for 2000 genes. The average gene would have 3 × 350 or 1050 base pairs. Since there are 2000 genes in the genome, the target would be

$1/2000 \times 1050$ or $1/2,100,000$ base pairs. Hence, the frequency of a true reversion for a particular gene would be far less than the frequency for a forward mutation in the same gene.

20. C

21. C Non-sense mutations are the result of an altered codon (mutation) that is read as a termination signal during translation (amber, ocher, or opal), resulting in a truncated protein. Such mutations can be suppressed by extragenic suppressor mutations called non-sense suppressors, which are also often classified according to the non-sense codon they suppress (amber, ocher, or opal).

22. B Transformation refers to the transfer by naked DNA from one bacterium (the donor) to another (the recipient). Such "naked DNA" is vulnerable to extracellular nucleases until it is taken up by competent recipient cells.

Suggested Reading

Friefelder, D. *Microbial Genetics*. Boston: Jones and Bartlett Publishers, 1987.

Ingraham, J. L., Low, K. B., Magasanik, B., Schaechter, M., and Umbarger, H. E. (eds.). *Escherichia coli and Salmonella typhimurium Cellular and Molecular Biology*. Washington, D.C.: American Society for Microbiology, 1987.

Joklik, W. K., Willett, H. P., Amos, D. B., and Wilfert, C. M. *Zinsser Microbiology* (20th ed.). Norwalk, CT: Appleton and Lange, 1992.

Kornberg, A., and Baker, T. A. *DNA Replication*. New York: Freeman, 1991.

Puhler, A., and Timmis, K. N. *Advanced Molecular Genetics*. New York: Springer-Verlag, 1984.

Pathogenic Bacteriology

Mechanisms of Bacterial Pathogenicity

David C. Straus

Pathogenicity indicates the ability of an organism to produce pathologic changes or disease in the host. Virulence is the degree of pathogenicity of the organism. The number of microorganisms necessary to cause a disease is directly related to virulence. If 10 bacteria of organism A, introduced into the peritoneal cavity, are sufficient to cause a bacteremia in an experimental animal, that is a highly virulent organism. If 10^7 bacteria of organism B are injected into the peritoneal cavity of a similar experimental animal, and no disease results, organism B is relatively avirulent. Virulence can be measured by several factors, such as the fatality rate associated with a certain bacterial infection or the ability of the bacterium to invade host tissue.

Variation in Virulence

The virulence of a pathogenic bacterium can be increased or decreased in a variety of ways. Virulence can be increased by passage of the organism through a host system that allows for the rapid proliferation of the organism, such as passing *Streptococcus pneumoniae* in mice. Virulence can also be increased by the acquisition by the organism of special factors; for example, acquisition of the beta phage by *Corynebacterium diphtheriae* induces production of the diphtheria toxin by this organism.

Virulence can be decreased by passage of the organism through a host system that does not normally favor the rapid proliferation of the organism. For example, growth of the organism at a temperature that is less than optimal (e.g., growth at 42°C when the organism favors 37°C is the way in which Louis Pasteur attenuated the anthrax bacillus). Finally, loss of certain virulence factors, such as cessation of toxin production by virtue of the loss of the beta phage of *C. diphtheriae,* results in a decrease in the virulence of this bacterium.

Major Components of Virulence

The most important components of virulence include invasiveness, adherence, and toxigenicity. The ability of different bacteria to invade host tissue runs a gamut of varying degrees. These include (1) an inability to colonize host tissue (nonpathogens), (2) local colonization with no overt pathology associated with host tissue (normal flora), (3) local colonization with local pathology (organism cannot survive in host tissue, no systemic invasion, little diffusion of toxin; e.g., cholera), (4) local colonization with local pathology (no invasion of tissue, diffusion of toxin causes systemic involvement; e.g., diphtheria), (5) local colonization followed by systemic involvement (development of foci of disease in tissue distant from the point of original introduction; e.g., meningococcal meningitis), (6) penetration of normal defense barriers without local colonization (establishment of pathogens in host organ systems, rare in bacterial infections; e.g., leptospiral infections), and (7) local or systemic infection following predisposing factors (e.g., a cold of the upper respiratory tract predisposes the host to pneumonia produced by *Strep. pneumoniae*).

Genetics of Pathogenesis

The ability of bacteria to cause a certain disease in a specified host involves the production of one or several virulence factors. The loss of one virulence factor usually does not result in an avirulent state but it is possible (e.g., loss of ability to produce toxin results in an avirulent *C. diphtheriae* strain). During the course of an infection by a pathogen, each of the various virulence factors play an important role in the disease process. These factors are, of course, coded for by genes. The genes that code for virulence factors reside on plasmids, bacterial chromosomes, or bacteriophages; however, most virulence genes are located on bacterial chromosomes. Another interesting genetic phenomenon is related to the human host. It appears that acquired immunity, natural immunity, and susceptibility to certain diseases are directly influenced by the

Table 4-1   Characteristics of Endotoxins and Exotoxins

Endotoxins	Exotoxins
Produced only by gram-negative bacteria	Produced by both gram-negative and gram-positive bacteria
Actively excreted by living bacteria and upon their lysis	Actively excreted by living bacteria and upon their (rarely) lysis
Lipopolysaccharide in composition	Protein in composition
Toxicity resides in lipid A component	Toxicity due to the biologic action of the protein
Immunogenic in mammalian systems	Immunogenic in mammalian systems
Heat stable (can withstand autoclaving and still be toxic)	Most are heat labile (denatured by exposure to 100°C)
Toxic in mg quantities in humans (not highly toxic)	Toxic in μg quantities in humans (highly toxic)
Cannot be made to form a toxoid	Can be made to form a toxoid
Antibodies neutralize their toxicity	Antibodies neutralize their toxicity
Produce fever in experimental animals	Rarely produce fever in experimental animals
Always contain ketodeoxyoctonate (KDO)	Never contain KDO

genetic makeup of an individual. Susceptibility to certain diseases correlates with the presence of the major histocompatibility complex. Two excellent examples of this are the association of late onset, juvenile arthritis and ankylosing spondylitis with the HLA-B27 complex. The reason for this association is not clear.

Aggressins

Aggressins are factors that contribute to the invasiveness of pathogenic bacteria. They can usually be divided into one of three categories: adherence factors, antiphagocytic mechanisms, and spreading factors. Examples of adherence factors are the pili of *Pseudomonas aeruginosa* and *Escherichia coli* and the lipoteichoic acids of *Streptococcus pyogenes*. There are several important antiphagocytic mechanisms. Capsules represent one of these and are usually carbohydrate in nature, such as the polysaccharide capsules of *Strep. pneumoniae* and *Klebsiella pneumoniae*. An important exception to this is the D-glutamic acid capsule of *Bacillus anthracis*. Some bacteria (e.g., *Staphylococcus aureus*) possess antiphagocytic structures composed of protein and carbohydrate. Other important antiphagocytic structures that pathogenic bacteria possess are cell-wall proteins that render the organism difficult to ingest. The M protein of *Strep. pyogenes* and protein A of *Staph. aureus* represent two such structures. Another major antiphagocytic mechanism is leukocidin, which is a substance that is toxic for white blood cells. Two excellent examples of leukocidins are the Panton-Valentine leukocidin of *Staph. aureus* and the streptolysin O produced by *Strep. pyogenes*.

Spreading factors represent another class of bacterial aggressins, and these compounds are usually referred to as exoenzymes, that is, enzymes that are excreted by the organism. These enzymes, which allow the bacteria to spread throughout the host tissue, are represented by examples such as hyaluronidase of *Strep. pyogenes*, lecithinase (alpha toxin) of *Clostridium perfringens*, and fibrinolysin of *Strep. pyogenes*. Finally, we must consider as a virulence factor the truly remarkable ability of some pathogenic bacteria to survive inside of phagocytic cells. Organisms that have acquired this ability include *Mycobacterium tuberculosis*, *Salmonella typhi*, and *Brucella abortus*.

Toxigenicity

Most pathogenic bacteria produce toxins that are capable of damaging host tissues by a variety of different mechanisms. Bacterial toxins can usually be divided into two distinct groups: exotoxins and endotoxins (Table 4-1) Exotoxins are produced by both gram-positive and gram-negative organisms. Exotoxins differ from endotoxins in that they are usually heat labile, are usually released into the surrounding medium without cell lysis, and are highly potent in comparison to the markedly lower potency of endotoxin. The following is a list of some of the most important bacterial exotoxins, the organisms that produce them, and some of their properties.

Exotoxins

1. Botulism toxin *(Clostridium botulinum)*
   a. Attaches to presynaptic terminals of cholinergic nerves, where it blocks release of acetylcholine
   b. This results in a flaccid paralysis of the victims
   c. Victim dies of respiratory failure
2. Tetanus toxin *(Clostridium tetani)*

a. Attaches to the anterior horn cells of the spinal cord and brain stem, where it blocks release of inhibitory transmitter from inhibitory terminals

b. This results in hyperflexia and spasm of skeletal muscle

c. Victim dies of respiratory failure

3. Alpha toxin *(C. perfringens)*

a. Breaks down lecithin in host cell membranes, which results in cell death and spread of the organism throughout host tissue

b. This toxin is lethal, necrotizing, and hemolytic

4. Diphtheria toxin *(C. diphtheriae)*

a. Causes cessation of mammalian protein synthesis by inactivating elongation factor 2 (EF-2) of eucaryotic cells

b. Production coded for by a bacteriophage (lysogen)

c. Nicotinamide adenine dinucleotide (NAD$^+$) is required for its activity

5. Anthrax toxin *(B. anthracis)*

a. Composed of edema factor (an adenylate cyclase that increases cyclic adenosine monophosphate [cyclic AMP] concentrations in eucaryotic cells), protective antigen, and lethal factor

b. Active against the central nervous system (CNS) and leukocytes

6. Erythrogenic toxin *(Strep. pyogenes)*

a. Responsible for the rash of scarlet fever

b. Production coded for by a bacteriophage (lysogen)

7. Alpha toxin *(Staph. aureus)*

a. Acts on cell membranes, causing cell lysis

b. May act in a manner similar to complement

8. Exfoliatin *(Staph. aureus)*

a. Causes exfoliation in infants and neonates

b. Disease is called staphylococcal scalded skin syndrome (SSSS) in infants or Ritter's disease in neonates

9. Enterotoxins *(Staph. aureus)*

a. Protein toxins

b. Affect the emesis control centers of the CNS

10. Heat-labile toxin *(E. coli)*

a. Activates adenylate cyclase, resulting in an accumulation of cyclic AMP in the epithelial cells of the mucosal lining

b. This causes a marked ion and water transport into the intestinal lumen and resultant diarrhea

11. Heat-stable toxin *(E. coli)*

a. Activates guanylate cyclase, resulting in an increase in cyclic guanosine monophosphate in the epithelial cells of the mucosal lining

b. The resultant ion and water transport into the small intestine produces diarrhea in the patient

12. Neurotoxin *(Shigella dysenteriae)*

a. Attacks the CNS by an unknown mechanism

b. Also acts as an entertoxin (causes secretion of fluids into the intestinal lumen)

c. Inactivates 60S ribosomal subunits in vitro and in vivo, resulting in cessation of mammalian protein synthesis

13. Cholera toxin *(Vibrio cholerae)*: same mode of action as *E. coli* heat-labile toxin

14. Exotoxin A *(P. aeruginosa)*: same mode of action as *C. diphtheriae* toxin

15. Cytotoxin *(Legionella pneumophila)*

a. Kills several types of tissue culture cells by an unknown mechanism

b. Selectively inhibits the activation of polymorphonuclear leukocyte oxidative metabolism, allowing the organism to survive intracellularly

Superantigen Toxins

Certain bacterial toxins have been shown to serve as immunomodulators of the host defense system. Examples of these toxins are the staphylococcal enterotoxins, the streptococcal pyrogenic toxins (erythrogenic toxins), the staphylococcal pyrogenic toxins, and the staphylococcal toxic shock syndrome toxin. These toxins are referred to as superantigens because of their ability to stimulate T-cell proliferation in minute concentrations.

Endotoxins

Endotoxin is also commonly referred to as lipopolysaccharide (LPS). Lipopolysaccharide is an integral part of the cell wall of gram-negative bacteria. Its chemical structure is as follows:

Lipid A—ketodeoxyoctonate (KDO)—
R core (polysaccharide)—O polysaccharide

from the innermost section of the bacterial cell wall on the left to the outer portion. It is very heat stable (can withstand autoclaving) as compared to the more heat-labile exotoxins. The toxicity of LPS is relatively low as compared to most exotoxins. It is toxic in milligram quantities, while most exotoxins are toxic in microgram quantities. The toxicity of the LPS molecule has been shown to reside in the lipid A portion.

Koch's Postulates

With the large number of pathogenic bacteria and their myriad virulence factors, how can we be sure that a given bacterial strain produces disease? This question was resolved by Robert Koch, a German physician, in the late 1800s. Koch devised four conditions (postulates) that must be met before a particular microorganism is said to cause a disease. They are: (1) The organism must be isolated from most patients who have the disease; (2) the organism must be grown in pure culture, preferably in vitro; (3) when a pure culture of the organism is introduced into a normal susceptible animal, disease must result; and (4) the organism must be isolated from the diseased experimental animal. These postulates served well for nearly 100 years, but we recently have had to modify them, particularly in the cases of viruses that grow in humans but not in other animal species.

Indigenous Flora

David J. Hentges

Almost all surfaces of the human body are colonized by a diverse group of bacteria that are called normal or indigenous flora. These bacteria do no harm by their presence; on the contrary, there is evidence that they are beneficial to the host by stimulating development of the immune system and interfering with the establishment of populations of pathogenic bacteria. In cases in which host defenses are impaired or breaches occur in the skin or mucous membranes, however, flora components are capable of producing infections and may even cause death.

In the uterus, the fetus is bacteriologically sterile, but during the process of birth, microorganisms impinge on it, and the process of colonization begins. Most of the microorganisms with which the infant comes into contact are unsuccessful colonizers, and only those that are able to propagate and persist under the environmental conditions present on the surfaces become established. Many flora components are capable of adhering to specific epithelial cell receptor sites. Adherence is often tissue specific. Its selective nature plays an important role in determining the composition of the flora of a particular region of the body.

In considering the flora of body surfaces, we are concerned only with those regions in which microorganisms appear in appreciable numbers and are actively multiplying. They include the skin and mucous surfaces contiguous with it, and the nose, throat, mouth, intestine, vagina, and outer portion of the urethra. The rule in the other regions, such as the trachea, bronchi, esophagus, stomach, and upper urinary tract, is either sterility or the presence of a limited number of transient organisms.

Skin

The skin presents a region of varied habitats for the support of microorganisms. The most superficial layer consists of flat, scalelike plaques, the stratum corneum, which are continuously shed, carrying away the bacteria associated with them. The uneven surface of the skin is interrupted at

intervals by two orifices, the ducts of the sweat glands and the hair follicles. Sebaceous glands empty into the hair follicles. Their waxy secretion mixes with sweat and spreads over the skin surface to provide nutrients for resident microorganisms.

The dominant members of the cutaneous community are gram-positive cocci and rods, of which *Staphylococcus epidermidis* and diphtheroids are most common. *Staphylococcus aureus* inhabits the skin of some individuals. Diphtheroids consist of aerobic rods of the genus *Corynebacterium*, which are present on the skin surface, and anaerobes of the genus *Propionibacterium*, which are found primarily in the hair follicles. Gram-negative bacteria are present on the skin in smaller numbers, inhabiting primarily moist areas such as the axilla and toe webs.

Microorganisms other than bacteria that constitute a portion of the skin flora include yeasts of the genera *Pityrosporum* and *Candida* and the most unusual inhabitant, a tiny mite, *Demodex folliculorum*, which lives in the hair follicles and sebaceous glands of the face of most adults.

Nose

Like the skin, the predominant aerobic flora of the nose consists of gram-positive diphtheroids and cocci, particularly *Staph. epidermidis*. *Propionibacterium* species are the predominant anaerobes. It is well known, however, that nasal "carriers" of pathogenic bacteria are common, harboring organisms such as *Staph. aureus*, beta-hemolytic streptococci, and *Corynebacterium diphtheriae*.

Mouth

The flora of the mouth is complex. This is not surprising considering the variety of structures it contains that are capable of supporting microbial populations. These include the gingival crevices around the teeth, where the oxygen concentration is low; the rough surfaces of the tongue; and the relatively smooth surfaces of the teeth, cheeks, palate, and gums. In addition, saliva contains microorganisms. The flora differs somewhat in these regions. Normally present in the mouth are several species of streptococci, *Actinomyces*, lactobacilli, *Haemophilus*, a great variety of both gram-positive and gram-negative anaerobic bacteria, and spirochetes. The anaerobes are found in the gingival crevices and the crypts of the tongue.

Dental plaque develops as a consequence of the colonization of tooth surfaces with bacteria. The plaque contains streptococci that are capable of synthesizing water-insoluble carbohydrate polymers (glucan) to which both aerobic and anaerobic bacteria attach. Plaque bacteria produce organic acids as metabolic end products of carbohydrate metabolism. The acids dissolve tooth enamel and cause caries.

Pharynx

The flora of the pharynx is similar to that of the mouth except that staphylococci, *Neisseria,* and diphtheroids are also present. Anaerobes reside in tonsillar crypts. Some individuals harbor, in their throats, pathogens such as pneumococci, *Haemophilus influenzae, Neisseria meningitidis,* and *Corynebacterium diphtheriae* without apparent symptoms of disease.

Gastrointestinal Tract

The esophagus and empty stomach are essentially free of microorganisms. After a meal, however, microorganisms reach the stomach in the food, saliva, and nasopharyngeal secretions, and counts of 10^5 per milliliter of gastric juice are obtained. As a result of the high acidity, digestive enzymes, and rapid emptying, the organisms soon disappear, and within 60 minutes the stomach is once again sterile.

The upper small intestine contains no apparent resident flora, although after a meal, bacteria can be detected in its contents. In the terminal ileum, bacterial populations of 10^6 to 10^8 organisms per milliliter are observed, representing the flora of the region. It consists of enterobacteria, streptococci, lactobacilli, and anaerobic bacteria, such as *Bacteroides* and bifidobacteria.

The colon contains the largest concentration of bacteria of any region of the body. In healthy individuals, total bacterial populations exceed 10^{11} organisms per gram colonic content, consisting of more than 400 species. Because of the highly reducing conditions of the region, 90 to 99 percent of the bacteria are anaerobic. The flora is made up of both gram-positive and gram-negative cocci and rods, some of which inhabit the mucosal layer. The predominant organisms are *Escherichia coli,* enterococci and other streptococci, *Bacillus* species, *Bacteroides fragilis,* eubacteria, bifidobacteria, clostridia, and anaerobic cocci.

Urinary Tract

The flora of the urinary tract is much less complex than the colonic flora. The outermost portions of both the male and female urethra are colonized with bacteria commonly found in the skin (*Staph. epidermidis* and diphtheroids) and, in addition, lactobacilli, nonpathogenic streptococci, and occasionally aerobic and anaerobic intestinal bacteria. The upper part of the urethra near the bladder is free of microorganisms. Its sterility is maintained primarily by the flow of urine during the evacuation of the bladder.

Vagina

The type of flora present in the vagina varies with the individual's age. At birth, the vagina is sterile, but within 24 hours it is colonized with bacteria. Estrin, passively transferred from mother to infant, induces the deposition of glycogen in the vaginal lining, resulting in a temporary flora that resembles that of an adult. It consists of *Lactobacillus acidophilus,* diphtheroids, staphylococci, streptococci, and the anaerobes *Bacteroides,* bifidobacteria, *Veillonella,* fusobacteria, *Peptococcus,* and *Peptostreptococcus.* The pH of the area is about 4.5. Glycogen secretion ceases at about 1 month of age and *Staph. epidermidis,* diphtheroids, *E. coli,* and streptococci predominate at the higher pH of approximately 7.0. At puberty, glycogen secretion resumes, the pH drops, and the adult flora becomes established and remains until menopause. After menopause, less glycogen is secreted, the pH rises again, and the flora resembles that of prepubescent girls.

Protective Activity of the Indigenous Flora

Perhaps the single most important function of the indigenous flora is to provide protection against infectious diseases originating on mucous membranes. This is accomplished by stimulating, nonspecifically, immune responsiveness and by interfering with the establishment of populations of pathogenic microorganisms. Exogenous colonization by pathogens is blocked by a variety of mechanisms that are called, collectively, bacterial interference. Interference has been attributed to production of bacteriocins, maintenance of an inhospitable environment, and generation of toxic metabolic products by the flora. Competitions between pathogens and flora components for limiting nutrients or attachment sites have also been proposed as interference mechanisms.

Antimicrobial Agents

Rial D. Rolfe

The feasibility of using chemical compounds as chemotherapeutic agents is dependent on the principle of *selective toxicity:* A substance must be harmful to parasites but relatively innocuous to host cells. Selective toxicity is based on specific differences between the metabolism or structure of the host cell and that of the parasite. Antimicrobial agents can interfere at a number of vulnerable sites in the bacterial cell (Table 4-2). They can interfere with (1) cell-wall synthesis, (2) membrane function, (3) protein synthesis, (4) nucleic acid function, and (5) intermediary metabolism.

Pathogenic Bacteriology

Table 4-2   Major Antimicrobial
Agents and Their Mechanisms of Action

Inhibition of cell-wall synthesis
Penicillins
Cephalosporins
Monobactams
Penems and carbapenems
Vancomycin
Bacitracin
Novobiocin
Cycloserine
Inhibition of protein synthesis
Aminoglycosides
Tetracyclines
Chloramphenicol
Erythromycin
Clindamycin
Nitrofurans
Inhibition of nucleic acid function
Metronidazole
Rifampin
Quinolones
Inhibition of folic acid synthesis
Sulfonamides
Sulfones
p-Aminosalicylic acid
Trimethoprim
Damage to cell membrane
Polymyxins
Unknown mechanism of action
Isoniazid
Ethambutol

Antimicrobial Agents that Inhibit Cell-Wall Synthesis

In contrast to eucaryotic cells, bacteria possess a rigid cell wall that consists principally of a complex peptidoglycan. Agents that damage the cell wall or inhibit its synthesis can lead to lysis and death of the microorganism. Inhibitors of cell-wall synthesis include beta-lactam antibiotics (penicillins, cephalosporins, monobactams, penems, carbapenems), vancomycin, bacitracin, novobiocin, and cycloserine.

Penicillins

Pharmacology

All penicillins have in common a 6-aminopenicillanic acid nucleus and a condensed side chain. The nucleus consists of a five-membered *thiazolidine ring* and a *beta-lactam ring* that carries a free amino group at the carbon 6 position (Fig. 4-1). *Penicillin G* and *penicillin V* are naturally occurring penicillins derived from strains of the mold

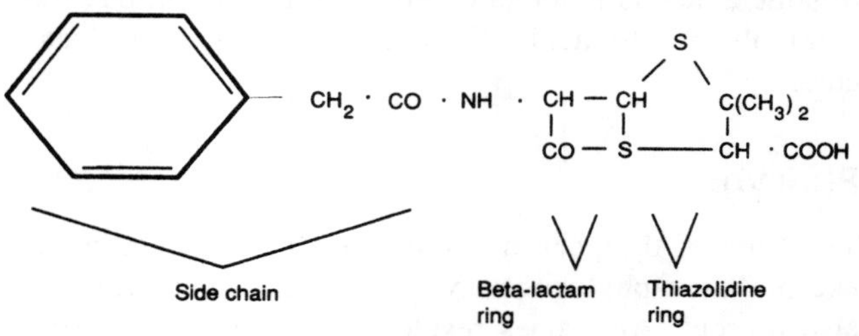

Fig. 4-1   Structure of benzylpenicillin (penicillin G).

Penicillium. Different side chains can be added chemically to the free amino group to produce a variety of *semisynthetic penicillins* (e.g., ampicillin, carbenicillin, methicillin). The side chain determines the antibacterial spectrum and pharmacological properties of a particular penicillin. Most penicillins are much more active against gram-positive than gram-negative bacteria. However, ampicillin and carbenicillin have similar activity against both groups of bacteria.

Mechanism of Action

All penicillins interfere with the biosynthesis of bacterial cell walls. Penicillin-binding proteins located on the cell membrane tightly bind to penicillins. These proteins are *transpeptidases* and *carboxypeptidases* that are involved in the terminal cross-linking of linear glycopeptides into the peptidoglycan complex. When penicillins bind to these proteins they inhibit their enzymatic activity. In addition, *autolytic enzymes* are activated in penicillin-treated cells. These enzymes then hydrolyze portions of the peptidoglycan layer resulting in lysis of the bacterial cell. Lysis only occurs when the bacterial cells are actively multiplying.

Mechanisms of Resistance

The most important mechanism of bacterial resistance to penicillins is enzymatic hydrolysis of the amide bond present in the beta-lactam ring by *beta lactamases* (penicillinases). This hydrolysis results in the formation of penicilloic acid and loss of antimicrobial activity (Fig. 4-2). Synthesis of beta lactamases can be either chromosomal or plasmid mediated and either constitutive or inducible. *Beta-lactamase inhibitors* (e.g., clavulanic acid and sulbactam) irreversibly bind to and inactivate beta lactamases. These inhibitors, which have little intrinsic antibacterial activity, can be administered simultaneously with penicillins (or cephalosporins) to inhibit hydrolysis of the beta-lactam ring.

Beta lactamases are only one mechanism of resistance to beta-lactam compounds. Some bacterial mutations can

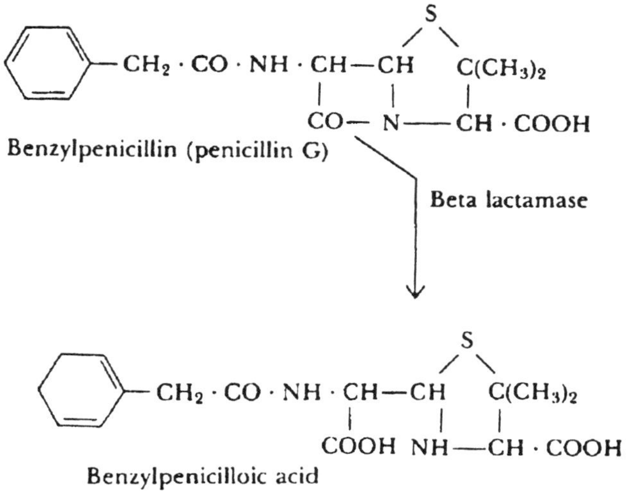

Fig. 4-2   Site of beta-lactamase activity.

result in alterations of the mucopeptide structure, resulting in the inability of penicillins to reach the binding proteins on the cell membrane. Mutational alterations in penicillin-binding proteins may lead to the inability of penicillin to bind to these target sites. *Tolerance* is another mechanism of penicillin resistance. Tolerant strains of bacteria are resistant to the bactericidal activity of beta-lactam antibiotics but are not resistant to the bacteriostatic activity of these agents. Penicillin fails to activate the autolytic enzymes in tolerant bacteria. Tolerance appears to be plasmid mediated.

Toxicity

Beta-lactam antimicrobial agents possess less direct toxicity to humans than does any other group of antimicrobial agents. The major adverse effects of the penicillins are *hypersensitivity reactions*, which occur in 1 to 10 percent of patients and range in severity from a mild rash to immediate anaphylactic shock. Degradation products of penicillin (e.g., penicilloic acid) can act as haptens to combine with proteins contaminating the antimicrobial solution or with human proteins to result in an immediate hypersensitivity reaction mediated by immunoglobulin E (IgE) antibody. All the penicillins are cross-sensitizing and cross-reacting. Skin testing can be performed to detect hypersensitive individuals, and it is possible to desensitize individuals. However, it is usually preferable to select an antimicrobial agent in another class for therapy.

Gastrointestinal disturbances, primarily in the form of diarrhea, can occur during use of any of the penicillins, but are most pronounced with ampicillin. Very high doses of penicillin can also produce CNS toxicity in the form of myoclonic seizures.

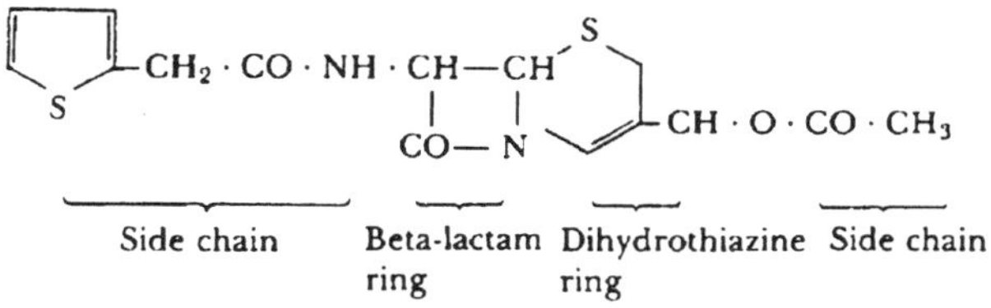

Fig. 4-3   Structure of cephalothin.

Cephalosporins

Pharmacology

Cephalosporins resemble the penicillins in that they possess a *beta-lactam ring*. The five-membered thiazolidine ring characteristic of the penicillins is replaced by a six-membered *dihydrothiazine ring* in the cephalosporins (Fig. 4-3). The nucleus of cephalosporins, 7-aminocephalosporanic acid, can be modified with different side-chain radicals to create a whole family of *semisynthetic cephalosporin* antibiotics with high therapeutic activity and low toxicity (e.g., cephalothin, cephalexin, cefazolin, cefamandole, cefoxitin).

Mechanism of Action

The cephalosporins are active against both gram-positive and gram-negative bacteria and have a *bactericidal* mode of action like that of the penicillins.

Mechanisms of Resistance

Resistance to the cephalosporins is mediated by the same mechanisms as described for the penicillins. *Cephalosporinases* are a subgroup of beta lactamases that can disrupt the cephalosporin beta-lactam ring and render the antimicrobial agent inactive.

Toxicity

The cephalosporins are relatively safe antimicrobial agents. They can induce *hypersensitivity reactions* identical to those produced by the penicillins, and there is some *cross antigenicity* between the penicillins and the cephalosporins. Approximately 10 percent of individuals allergic to penicillins will also be allergic to cephalosporins. Additional side effects include thrombophlebitis following intravenous administration and rare instances of bone marrow depression and nephrotoxicity.

Monobactams

The monobactams (e.g., aztreonam) constitute a unique family of antimicrobial agents that are characterized by a *beta-lactam ring* without an adjacent fused ring structure. These agents have very good activity against gram-nega-

Pathogenic Bacteriology

tive bacteria but are generally inactive against gram-positive and anaerobic bacteria.

Penems and Carbapenems

Penems and carbapenems are beta-lactam drugs that are stereochemically different from penicillins and cephalosporins. *Imipenem* (N-formimidoylthienamycin), a currently used carbapenem, has a broad spectrum of antimicrobial activity and is resistant to most beta lactamases.

Vancomycin

Vancomycin is a complex glycopeptide that is unrelated to any other antimicrobial agent. Vancomycin is a *bactericidal* antibiotic primarily active against gram-positive bacteria. This agent inhibits the early stages of peptidoglycan synthesis. Vancomycin is useful in treating serious infections caused by strains of gram-positive bacteria resistant to beta-lactam antimicrobial agents (e.g., methicillin-resistant *Staphylococcus aureus*). It is also used in the treatment of antibiotic-associated colitis caused by *Clostridium difficile*. Organisms resistant to vancomycin are either deficient in autolysins or impermeable to the agent.

The most frequent adverse reaction to vancomycin is *neurotoxicity* manifested by auditory nerve damage and hearing loss. Additional undesirable side effects include thrombophlebitis, skin rashes, fever, chills, and kidney damage.

Bacitracin

Bacitracin is a polypeptide that interferes with peptidoglycan synthesis. This antibiotic is *bactericidal* against many strains of gram-positive bacteria. Bacitracin is not used in systemic therapy because of its nephrotoxicity. However, in combination with polymyxin B or neomycin, bacitracin is useful for *topical application* to skin and mucous membranes. Bacitracin is also administered orally for the treatment of *Clostridium difficile*–associated intestinal disease.

Novobiocin

Novobiocin is a *bacteriostatic* antibiotic that inhibits the synthesis of *teichoic acid* at the cell membrane. Because of frequent undesirable side effects (e.g., fever, skin rashes, granulocytopenia, jaundice, and impaired renal function), there is no clear-cut indication for the use of this agent.

Cycloserine

Cycloserine interferes with peptidoglycan synthesis by inhibiting reactions involving incorporation of D-alanine in the pentapeptide. Cycloserine has found clinical use only in the treatment of *tuberculosis*. However, because of its *CNS toxicity,* its use is limited to re-treatment in drug-resistant cases, where it is administered as one of a three-or-more drug combination.

Antimicrobial Agents that Inhibit Protein Synthesis

A variety of antimicrobial agents inhibit bacterial protein synthesis. The most useful of these agents include the aminoglycosides, the tetracyclines, chloramphenicol, erythromycin, clindamycin, and nitrofurans. These antimicrobial agents do not have a major effect on mammalian protein synthesis because of differences in the structure and function of bacterial and mammalian protein ribosomes. The *bacterial 70S ribosome* consists of a 30S subunit and a 50S subunit. The *30S ribosomal subunit* is the site of binding of the charged aminoacyl–transfer ribonucleic acid (tRNA) to messenger RNA (mRNA). The *50S ribosomal subunit* is the site of linking together incoming amino acids with the growing peptide chain. Most antimicrobial agents that inhibit protein synthesis are directed against either the 30S or 50S ribosomal subunit.

Aminoglycosides (Aminocyclitols)
Pharmacology

The aminoglycosides (aminocyclitols) are a large group of clinically important antimicrobial agents that share many chemical, antimicrobial, pharmacologic, and toxic characteristics. Seven aminoglycosides are currently available for clinical use: *streptomycin, neomycin, kanamycin, gentamicin, tobramycin, amikacin,* and *spectinomycin.* All aminoglycosides except spectinomycin are rapidly *bactericidal* and have a relatively broad antibacterial spectrum, with activity directed against many gram-positive as well as most gram-negative microorganisms. Spectinomycin exerts only bacteriostatic antimicrobial activity.

Mechanism of Action

Aminoglycosides bind irreversibly to the *30S subunit* of bacterial ribosomes. This results in faulty translation of the mRNA. Improper amino acids are inserted in the peptide chain, and the resulting non-sense sequence of amino acids creates a nonfunctional, structurally abnormal protein. Evidence suggests that amikacin, neomycin, and gentamicin also attach to the 50S ribosomal subunit.

Mechanisms of Resistance

Bacterial resistance to aminoglycosides is achieved by several mechanisms. The most common type of resistance is the production of periplasmic enzymes, which modify the aminoglycosides by *phosphorylation, acetylation,* or *adenylation.* The enzymatically modified aminoglycosides are not transported into the cell. The production of these enzymes is plasmid mediated and bacteria that develop this type of resistance to one aminoglycoside usually continue to be susceptible to inhibition by the other aminoglycosides. Aminoglycoside-resistant bacterial strains can also occur by mutation. A *mutation* can result in the loss or alteration of a specific protein on the 30S ribosomal subunit, which in turn prevents aminoglycoside attachment to the ribosome. Specific mutations can also prevent the *active transport* of aminoglycosides into bacteria. Aminoglycoside-resistant bacterial mutants are usually refractory to all of the aminoglycosides.

Oxygen is required for the active transport of aminoglycosides into bacterial cells. Therefore, these agents are inactive against anaerobic bacteria and are frequently less effective against facultative microorganisms multiplying under anaerobic conditions.

Toxicity

The most serious adverse reactions associated with aminoglycoside use are *neuromuscular paralysis, nephrotoxicity,* and *ototoxicity.* Nephrotoxicity can result from prolonged therapy or from excessively high serum levels and is usually reversible within 4 to 5 months after the discontinuation of drugs. The toxic effects of aminoglycosides on the *eighth cranial nerve* can result in loss of hearing and loss of balance. Early damage is usually reversible over a period of time. However, once significant damage occurs, permanent residua frequently remain. Hypersensitivity to streptomycin can result in fever, skin rashes, and other allergic manifestations.

Tetracyclines

Pharmacology

Naturally occurring tetracycline is produced by a species of *Streptomyces.* Side chains can be added synthetically to this tetracycline to produce many different *semisynthetic tetracyclines* (oxytetracycline, chlortetracycline, demethylchlortetracycline, doxycycline, minocycline). All the tetracyclines are primarily *bacteriostatic* and have a broad spectrum of inhibitory activity, which includes both grampositive and gram-negative bacteria. They penetrate mammalian cell membranes and are effective in the treatment of infections caused by some obligate intracellular parasites.

Mechanism of Action

Tetracyclines enter bacterial cells by an energy-dependent process and bind reversibly to the *30S ribosomal subunit.* This in turn inhibits protein synthesis by blocking the binding of the charged aminoacyl-tRNA to the acceptor site on the mRNA-ribosome complex.

Mechanisms of Resistance

Bacterial resistance to tetracyclines can be either plasmid mediated or under chromosomal control. Bacteria develop resistance to the tetracyclines predominantly by becoming *less permeable* to the antibiotic. Bacterial resistance to one tetracycline usually implies resistance to all the tetracyclines.

Toxicity

Tetracyclines rarely give rise to serious toxicity. However, they avidly bind to developing *bone structures* and may be associated with hypoplasia of the enamel and depression of skeletal growth in premature infants. Tetracyclines also cause a gray-brown to yellow discoloration of teeth in children who take these agents. Therefore, tetracyclines should not be administered to *children* under the age of 8 years. In addition, the tetracyclines cross the placenta and should not be administered during *pregnancy. Hypersensitivity* reactions occur with the tetracyclines but are uncommon. An individual who is allergic to one tetracycline should be considered allergic to all the tetracyclines. *Photosensitivity* reactions consisting of a red skin rash on areas exposed to sunlight may occur in individuals who receive these agents. The tetracyclines produce varying degrees of gastrointestinal upset following oral administration. Colonization of the host by tetracycline-resistant organisms (especially *Candida*) is a frequent occurrence during tetracycline therapy.

Chloramphenicol

Pharmacology and Mechanism of Action

Chloramphenicol is a *bacteriostatic* antimicrobial agent with essentially the same broad antibacterial spectrum as the tetracyclines. This antimicrobial agent binds to the *50S ribosomal subunit* at a locus that prevents the attachment of the amino acid–containing end of the aminoacyl-tRNA to the ribosome. This interferes with the binding of the amino acids to the nascent peptide chain, and protein synthesis is prevented.

Mechanisms of Resistance

Bacterial resistance to chloramphenicol is often associated with the production of an enzyme, *chloramphenicol acetyltransferase,* which acetylates the antibiotic to an inactive diacetyl derivative. The production of this enzyme is under the control of a plasmid. Bacteria also develop resistance to chloramphenicol by becoming impermeable to the agent, although this only rarely occurs in clinical medicine.

Toxicity

The most important toxic effects of chloramphenicol are related to the bone marrow and can be divided into two

Pathogenic Bacteriology

types. The first is a reversible depression of *bone marrow*. This type of toxicity is common in patients receiving prolonged therapy and results in abnormalities in early forms of red cells, elevated serum iron, and anemia. These changes are dose related and are reversible upon discontinuation of the agent. The second type of toxicity is a rare but generally fatal depression of bone marrow function. This type of toxicity is most frequently manifested as *aplastic anemia* and is not necessarily dose related. Chloramphenicol-induced aplastic anemia can occur weeks to months following completion of therapy. It is estimated to occur in about 1:30,000 to 1:60,000 patients.

Neonates receiving chloramphenicol may experience abdominal distention, vomiting, cyanosis, circulatory collapse, and death. This side effect, referred to as the *gray syndrome*, results from high serum levels of chloramphenicol due to diminished ability of neonates to conjugate and excrete chloramphenicol. Prolonged chloramphenicol therapy may cause optic neuritis resulting in decreased visual acuity, but these symptoms are generally reversible following discontinuation of therapy. Primarily because of the toxicity of chloramphenicol to bone marrow, this antimicrobial agent should not be administered when an alternative form of therapy is available.

Erythromycin

Pharmacology

Erythromycin consists of a macrocyclic lactone ring attached to two sugar moieties. This antimicrobial agent is primarily active against gram-positive bacteria, although some activity is exhibited against gram-negative bacteria. Erythromycin is a useful alternate agent in cases of penicillin allergy. Depending on the drug concentration, bacterial species, phase of growth, and density of the inoculum, erythromycin may be *bacteriostatic* or *bactericidal*.

Mechanism of Action

Erythromycin inhibits bacterial protein synthesis by reversibly binding to the *50S ribosomal subunit* resulting in blockage of the transpeptidation or translocation reactions.

Mechanisms of Resistance

Resistance to erythromycin may be the result of decreased *permeability* of the cell wall to the drug (chromosomal mutation) or of an *alteration* in a single 50S ribosomal protein at the erythromycin receptor site, leading to reduced erythromycin binding (chromosomal mutation or plasmid mediated). Cross resistance occurs between erythromycin and clindamycin.

Toxicity

Erythromycin is one of the safest antibiotics in clinical use and untoward reactions are not life threatening. Undesirable side effects include fever, mild gastrointestinal upsets, cholestatic hepatitis, allergic reactions (skin rashes and eosinophilia), and transient hearing loss.

Clindamycin

Pharmacology

Clindamycin resembles erythromycin in mode of action and antibacterial spectrum but is chemically unrelated. Probably the most important indication for clindamycin is in the treatment of severe *anaerobic infections*.

Mechanisms of Action and Resistance

Clindamycin binds to the *50S subunit* of bacterial ribosomes at the same site as erythromycin. Clindamycin-resistant microorganisms have an altered protein on the 50S ribosomal subunit that prevents attachment of the antibiotic.

Toxicity

The major side effect of clindamycin is *diarrhea*. Additional side effects include reversible hepatoxicity, allergic reactions, and reversible bone marrow depression.

Nitrofurans

The nitrofurans (e.g., nitrofurazone, nitrofurantoin, furazolidone) are synthetic compounds that are bactericidal for many gram-positive and gram-negative bacteria as well as certain fungi and protozoa. They inhibit protein synthesis by blocking initiation of *translocation*. Nitrofurans have no effect on systemic infections but are effective agents in the treatment of uncomplicated *urinary tract infections*. Nitrofurans are also used topically.

Gastrointestinal intolerance is the most common side effect of orally administered nitrofurans. Occasionally, hemolytic anemia, skin rashes, and pneumonitis have been observed.

Antimicrobial Agents that Inhibit Nucleic Acid Function

Metronidazole

Pharmacology

Metronidazole has selective antimicrobial activity against obligate *anaerobic bacteria*, some microaerophilic bacteria, and certain protozoan pathogens (e.g., *Trichomonas vaginalis, Giardia lamblia, Entamoeba histolytica*). All of these microorganisms are anaerobic and share certain metabolic pathways crucial to the activity of metronidazole.

Mechanism of Action

Metronidazole enters cells by passive diffusion. The nitro group of metronidazole is then reduced, leading to the production of short-lived *cytotoxic intermediates* that soon decompose into biologically inactive end products. The reduction of metronidazole is achieved by redox systems that are of great significance in the metabolism of anaerobes but play only a minor role, if any, in other microorganisms. The toxic intermediates attack multiple sites in the bacterial cell. However, the interaction of these reactive intermediates with *deoxyribonucleic acid* (DNA) is thought to be responsible for the bactericidal activity of metronidazole.

Mechanisms of Resistance

Resistance to metronidazole occurs infrequently and is due to a diminished ability of bacteria to reduce this agent.

Toxicity

Peripheral *neuropathy* is the most serious side effect of metronidazole therapy. Resolution of the neuropathy usually occurs upon discontinuation of the agent. Relatively minor side effects include nausea, headache, and dry mouth.

Rifampin

Pharmacology

Rifampin (rifampicin) is a semisynthetic derivative of rifamycin, an antibiotic produced by *Streptomyces*. The principal use of rifampin is in the treatment of *tuberculosis*. Rifampin is administered concurrently with another antituberculosis agent to delay the emergence of rifampin-resistant mycobacteria. Rifampin is also used for *prophylaxis* in close contacts of patients with meningitis caused by either *N. meningitidis* or *H. influenzae*.

Mechanism of Action

Rifampin specifically inhibits bacterial *DNA-dependent RNA polymerase*.

Toxicity

Occasional adverse effects include rashes and thrombocytopenia.

Quinolones

Quinolones are bactericidal agents that block DNA synthesis by inhibiting *DNA gyrase*. *Nalidixic acid* was the first agent of this group to be introduced and was used primarily in the treatment of uncomplicated urinary tract infections

caused by gram-negative bacteria. However, the newer quinolones (e.g., *norfloxacin* and *ciprofloxacin*) have largely replaced nalidixic acid because of their broader spectrum of activity.

Antimicrobial Agents that Inhibit Folic Acid Synthesis

Sulfonamides

Pharmacology

The sulfonamides are a large group of antimicrobial agents derived from the parent compound sulfanilamide. The substitution of various side-chain radicals on sulfanilamide results in a series of compounds of varying physical, pharmacologic, and antibacterial properties. Sulfonamides can be classified as (1) short- or medium-acting sulfonamides (sulfisoxazole, sulfamethoxazole, sulfacytine, sulfadiazine), (2) long-acting sulfonamides (sulfamethoxypyridazine, sulfameter), (3) sulfonamides limited to the gastrointestinal tract (sulfaguanidine, phthalylsulfathiazole, salicylazosulfapyridine), and (4) topical sulfonamides (mafenide acetate, sulfacetamide). Sulfonamides exhibit *bacteriostatic* activity against a broad spectrum of gram-positive and gram-negative bacteria, chlamydiae, *Nocardia*, and some protozoa. However, because other antibiotics are generally more effective and less toxic, sulfonamides are recommended for the treatment of only a limited number of infections.

Mechanism of Action

All sulfonamides share the same mechanism of action; interference with microbial *folic acid* synthesis. Folic acid serves as an important intermediate in the synthesis of nucleotides. Sulfonamides inhibit competitively the incorporation of *para-aminobenzoic acid (PABA)* into *tetrahydropteroic acid* (Fig. 4-4). Sulfonamides are structural analogues of PABA and have a higher affinity for *tetrahydropteroic acid synthetase* than does PABA (Fig. 4-5). These antimicrobial agents result in the formation of nonfunctional analogues of folic acid and inhibit bacterial growth. Sulfonamides do not inhibit cells that cannot synthesize folic acid, including mammalian cells, and those bacteria that can use performed folic acid for growth.

Mechanisms of Resistance

Mutational resistance to sulfonamides results in either increased microbial production of PABA or the production of tetrahydropteroic acid synthetase, which has a higher affinity for PABA than do the sulfonamides. Plasmid-mediated resistance results in decreased permeability to sulfonamides.

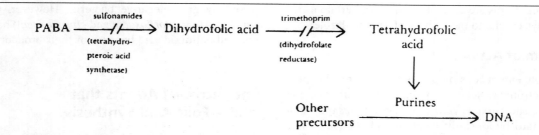

Fig. 4-4   Action of sulfonamides and trimethoprim on the pathway of folic acid synthesis.

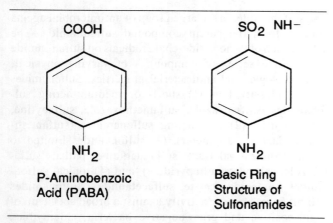

Fig. 4-5   Structural similarities between PABA and sulfonamides.

Toxicity

The most serious adverse reaction to sulfonamides is *bone marrow* depression, leading to hemolytic anemia, aplastic anemia, agranulocytosis, thrombocytopenia, and leukopenia. Sulfonamides may also cause gastrointestinal disturbances, fever, headache, depression, jaundice, and hepatic necrosis. Significant hypersensitivity reactions (skin rashes, erythema nodosum, and erythema multiforme) may occur when sulfonamides are administered by any route.

Sulfones

The sulfones are synthetic compounds that are structurally similar to the sulfonamides; their mode of action is also similar. The major antimicrobial agent in this group is *diaminodiphenylsulfone (DDS)*. This agent is used only in the treatment of *leprosy*, where it arrests the course of the disease if employed in the early stages.

p-*Aminosalicylic Acid (PAS)*

This agent is also structurally similar to the sulfonamides and has the same mode of action. PAS is used primarily as a second-line drug for treatment of *tuberculosis*.

Trimethoprim

Pharmacology and Mechanism of Action

Trimethoprim is a structural analogue of *dihydrofolic acid*. This antimicrobial agent inhibits bacterial *dihydrofolic acid reductase*, resulting in an inhibition of folic acid and ultimately purine and DNA synthesis (see Fig. 4-4).

Trimethoprim is frequently used in combination with sulfamethoxazole. This combination is called *co-trimoxazole*. The simultaneous use of a sulfonamide with trimethoprim results in the inhibition of sequential metabolic steps in folic acid synthesis thereby decreasing the incidence of bacterial resistance to either agent and increasing the spectrum of activity over each agent used individually. Co-trimoxazole is used in the treatment of urinary tract infections, enteric fever, and other bacterial and parasitic infections.

Mechanisms of Resistance

Bacteria resistant to co-trimoxazole bypass the blocked metabolic steps of folic acid production by using nucleotides or related substances that are available in the environment.

Toxicity

The toxic and undesired side effects of co-trimoxazole include all those described for the sulfonamides. In addition, impaired folic acid utilization may be seen during prolonged co-trimoxazole administration.

Antimicrobial Agents that Damage the Cell Membrane

Polymyxins

Pharmacology

Polymyxins A, B, C, D, and E are related cyclic polypeptides characterized by a limited antimicrobial spectrum. The polymyxins are active almost exclusively against gram-negative bacilli. All but polymyxins B and E are too toxic for therapeutic use in humans. *Colistin* is the same as polymyxin E.

Mechanisms of Action

The polymyxins are *bactericidal* against both resting and multiplying bacteria. These agents function as *cationic detergents*. They increase cell permeability by interacting with phospholipids of the cell membrane. This damage permits intracellular constituents to escape from the cell, and death ensues. Selective chemotherapeutic activity is possible because the cytoplasmic membrane of bacteria is more readily disrupted by polymyxins than is the cell membrane of eucaryotic cells.

Mechanisms of Resistance

Microorganisms resistant to polymyxins have cell walls that prevent access of the agent to the cell membrane. However, resistance rarely develops during therapy.

Toxicity

The two most important side effects of polymyxins are *neurotoxicity* and *nephrotoxicity*. These side effects have limited the use of polymyxins to serious infections caused by susceptible bacteria and to topical applications.

Antimicrobial Agents with Unknown Mechanisms of Inhibition

Isoniazid

Isoniazid is a bactericidal antimicrobial agent that has limited inhibitory activity against most bacteria but is very active against *mycobacteria,* especially *Mycobacterium tuberculosis.* Isoniazid is used in combination with other antimycobacterial agents (e.g., rifampin and ethambutol) to reduce the emergence of resistant tubercle bacilli. The mode of action of isoniazid is unknown, but it possibly exerts competitive antagonism against *pyridoxine*-catalyzed reactions in bacteria. The most important side effects of isoniazid are related to its *hepatotoxicity* and toxicity for the peripheral and *central nervous systems.*

Ethambutol

Ethambutol is a narrow-spectrum antimicrobial agent with activity primarily directed against *Mycobacterium tuberculosis.* Ethambutol is given in combination with other antituberculosis drugs to delay the emergence of ethambutol-resistant mycobacteria. The mechanisms of action of ethambutol are unknown.

The most common side effects of ethambutol therapy are visual disturbances, including reduction in visual acuity

and optic neuritis. These are usually reversible when ethambutol therapy is discontinued.

Special Aspects of Antimicrobial Therapy

Superinfections

One of the most serious and frequent complications of antimicrobial therapy is superinfection with an organism resistant to the agent being used. Antimicrobial agents affect not only pathogenic bacteria but also susceptible members of the *normal microbial flora.*Quantitative relationships between species of the normal flora can be disturbed, and naturally excluded species can become established as a result of the loss of the normal biologic competition.

Three of the more common types of superinfections include (1) *candidiasis* due to proliferation of *Candida albicans,* (2) *Clostridium difficile*–associated gastrointestinal disease, and (3) systemic infections resulting from *translocation* of bacteria from the intestinal tract to healthy tissue.

Chemoprophylaxis

Antimicrobial chemoprophylaxis is the administration of an antimicrobial agent to prevent the establishment of pathogenic microorganisms in the host. Chemoprophylaxis is usually limited to the action of a specific agent against a specific microorganism and is likely to be successful only when the microorganism rarely gives rise to mutants resistant to the agent employed.

Antibacterial chemoprophylaxis is an accepted clinical procedure for the prevention of group A streptococcus, meningococcus, and plague infection. It has also found wide application in the reduction of the lower-bowel flora before bowel surgery. Penicillin is frequently administered prophylactically to individuals with valvular heart damage who are undergoing procedures that are likely to result in bacteremia to prevent the development of bacterial endocarditis.

Combined Therapy

Preference should always be given to the treatment of infections with a single agent, but there are certain indications for the use of combinations (usually two) of antimicrobials. Combinations of antimicrobial agents may be rationally used for the following reasons:

1. Prevention of the emergence of resistant microorganisms: Combination therapy has been clearly documented as effective in preventing the development of resistance during treatment of tuberculosis.

2. *Synergism*: The use of synergistic combinations of antimicrobial agents to treat infections is another indication of combined therapy. Examples of these synergistic combinations include the use of penicillin and streptomycin in the treatment of certain types of bacterial endocarditis and the use of gentamicin and carbenicillin in treating systemic *Pseudomonas* infections.

3. Polymicrobial infections: Certain polymicrobial infections require the use of more than one antimicrobial agent to eliminate all the infecting organisms.

4. Infections in impaired hosts: Combined broad-spectrum therapy is frequently required to treat infections occurring in patients with abnormalities of host defense systems.

5. Life-threatening infections: Combined therapy may be helpful in emergency treatment of serious infections before a precise diagnosis can be established.

The inappropriate use of antimicrobial combinations may have important adverse effects. The activity of two agents against a microorganism that is susceptible to both is not necessarily additive. For example, bacteriostatic drugs, such as tetracycline and chloramphenicol, interfere with the bactericidal action of drugs that block synthesis of the bacterial cell wall, such as penicillin and vancomycin. Combination therapy may also increase the frequency of resistant pathogens in the environment. The chances of toxic reactions developing during therapy is increased when more than one agent is used.

Susceptibility Testing

Since microorganisms vary in their susceptibility to antimicrobial agents, it is imperative that the means are available for determining the susceptibility of an infecting microorganism as a guide to effective chemotherapy. The principal methods used by the clinical laboratory to determine the antimicrobial susceptibility of a microorganism include *dilution tests*, such as the broth tube and agar plate procedures, and the *disk agar diffusion technique.*

Dilution tests are performed by inoculating a standardized suspension of a microorganism into serial dilutions of an antimicrobial agent prepared in broth or agar. After a suitable period of incubation, the minimal concentration of antimicrobial that *inhibits* growth of the microorganism is determined *(minimal inhibitory concentration [MIC])*. With minor additions, the tube dilution technique can be adapted to determine the minimal concentration of an antimicrobial required to *kill* the microorganism *(minimal bactericidal concentration [MBC])*.

The most widely used technique for antimicrobial susceptibility testing is the disk agar diffusion procedure, also

referred to as the disk method or the *Bauer-Kirby technique*. In this procedure, filter-paper disks impregnated with appropriate concentrations of antimicrobial agents are placed on an agar culture plate that has been inoculated with a culture of the microorganism to be tested. After incubation, the diameter of the clear zone surrounding the disk is taken as a measure of the inhibitory power of the antimicrobial against the particular test organism.

Disinfection and Sterilization

David J. Hentges

Sterilization is an absolute term implying the inactivation of all forms of life. When applied to microbiology, it means inactivation of microorganisms so that they can no longer reproduce, often referred to as the death of microorganisms. The microorganisms may be structurally intact and may even be able to perform biosynthetic activities, but they are unable to multiply. Some substances, which are termed bactericidal, cause the death of bacteria (permanently prevent multiplication), whereas other substances, termed bacteriostatic, interrupt multiplication as long as they are in contact with bacteria, but multiplication resumes when they are removed.

Disinfection, as distinct from sterilization, is the process of eliminating disease-producing, rather than all microorganisms, from an area. Disinfectants are used on inanimate objects but are frequently too toxic to be applied to living tissue. Antiseptics which serve the same purpose as disinfectants, can be applied to living tissue because they are less toxic. Over the years, the distinction between the terms disinfectant and antiseptic has become blurred, however, and the two are frequently used interchangeably (i.e., skin disinfectant).

The term *septic* means the presence of microorganisms in an environment and the term *aseptic* means the absence of microorganisms.

Various physical and chemical processes are available for the sterilization or disinfection of materials. Physical agents, including heat, radiation, and filtration, function exclusively to sterilize substances. Chemical agents, on the other hand, function to either sterilize or disinfect.

Physical Agents
Heat

Heat is the most effective method of sterilization and whenever possible should be the method of choice. The time required for sterilization with heat is inversely related to the temperature of exposure. Objects can be sterilized either by dry heat applied in an oven or by moist heat provided as steam. Of the two methods, moist heat is preferred because of its more rapid killing due to the penetration of steam and its condensation to release heat. Steam, under 15 lb. per square inch pressure at 121°C, will kill vegetative cells and spores within 20 minutes. Autoclaves used for sterilization in microbiology laboratories or hospital clinical laboratories provide these conditions. It must be kept in mind, however, that in order to be effective the steam must come into contact with all materials to be sterilized. Hermetically sealed or very dense or water-resistant substances are not effectively sterilized by autoclaving. When this is the case, sterilization by dry heat is used. Effective sterilization with dry heat requires a temperature of 180°C for 2 hours for killing all organisms, including sporeformers. Moist heat is used for sterilizing surgical bandages, moisture-resistant instruments, and bacteriologic culture media and dry heat for sterilizing glassware, powders, and oily substances such as ointments, which are insoluble in water and impervious to steam.

Radiation

Heat-labile substances can be sterilized by radiation. The two types of radiation used for sterilization are ionizing radiation (x-rays and gamma rays) and ultraviolet light. X-rays and gamma rays are at a much higher energy level than ultraviolet light and consequently have much greater penetrating power and capacity to produce lethal effects on microorganisms. The optimal bactericidal wavelength for ultraviolet light is approximately 260 nm, which corresponds with the absorption maximum of DNA. The major lethal action of ultraviolet light on microorganisms is attributed to damage to DNA. However, because of its low energy, the penetrating power of ultraviolet light is poor and it is effective in sterilizing surfaces only.

Filtration

Heat-labile solutions can be sterilized by filtration. A number of different types of filters have been devised to sterilize solutions, but the type that is most commonly used is the membrane filter. Membrane filters are cellulose ester disks of various pore sizes. A pore size of 0.22 μ is effective in removing most bacteria, but it should be remembered that viruses and even mycoplasmas will pass through a filter of this pore size. Membrane filters are used to sterilize drugs, solutions containing serum, or plasma and sugar solutions.

Chemical Agents

Chemical agents kill microorganisms either by damaging cell membranes or by irreversibly modifying functional groups of enzymes, cell walls and membrane proteins, and nucleic acids.

Agents that Damage Cell Membranes

Surface-active agents are examples of chemical compounds that damage cell membranes. They possess both water-attracting (hydrophilic) and water-repelling (hydrophobic) groups on the same molecule. The hydrophobic portion of the molecule is a fat-soluble, long-chain hydrocarbon whereas the hydrophobic portion is an ionizable cationic or anionic group. The most important antibacterial surface-active agents are cationic compounds in which a long-chain hydrophobic residue is balanced by a positively charged hydrophilic group. Quaternary ammonium compounds, such as benzalkonium chloride (Zephiran), are the best-known surface-active agents of this type. When microorganisms are exposed to these agents, the positively charged portion of the molecule associates with the phosphate groups of the membrane phospholipids while the uncharged hydrophobic portion penetrates the lipid-rich interior of the membrane, causing distortion and leakage of essential metabolites from the cell. Soap is considered an anionic detergent because, when dissociated, it yields a negatively charged ion. Anionic detergents, such as soap, do not effectively kill microorganisms but are useful in removing them from surfaces.

Phenolic compounds also cause microbial membrane damage. As a practical disinfectant phenol (carbolic acid) has been replaced by less toxic phenol derivatives containing alkyl or chloro groups and by the diphenyls. The simplest of the alkyl phenols are the cresols. Ortho-, meta-, and paracresol are appreciably more active than phenol and are usually employed as a tricresol mixture emulsified in soap. Lysol is an example of such a mixture. In addition to the cresols, chlorinated diphenyl compounds, such as hexachlorophene and chlorhexidine, are useful disinfectants.

Alcohols represent the third class of compounds that interfere with microbial cell membrane activity. They penetrate into the hydrocarbon region of the lipid membrane and, in addition, denature cellular proteins. Short-chain aliphatic alcohols, primarily ethanol and isopropyl, are commonly used as skin antiseptics.

Agents that Modify Functional Groups of Proteins and Nucleic Acids

Soluble salts of mercury, arsenic, silver, and other heavy metals poison enzyme activity by forming mercaptides with the sulfhydryl groups of cysteine residues. Various forms of mercury and silver have been employed in medicine for many years. The organic mercurials nitromersol (Metaphen), thimerosal (Merthiolate), and merbromin (Mercurochrome) are useful antiseptic agents. Silver nitrate is highly bactericidal for gonococci and is routinely used as a 1% solution for the prophylaxis of ophthalmia neonatorum in newborn infants.

In addition to the heavy metals, halogens and hydrogen peroxide are effective as disinfectants and antiseptics. Hydrogen peroxide, an oxidizing agent, is used as a mild antiseptic. The mode of action of the halogens is due to their oxidative activities and their ability to halogenate proteins. Elemental chlorine serves as an effective water disinfectant and chlorine-releasing compounds are used as sanitizing agents. When elemental chlorine reacts with water, hypochlorous acid, a powerful oxidizing agent, is formed. Iodine, a common skin antiseptic, is applied in a tincture that is an aqueous alcoholic solution of 2% I_2 and 2.4% sodium iodide. It causes some tissue damage, but this problem has been circumvented by binding iodine to surface-active carrier molecules, which increases solubility and provides for a sustained, gradual release of the halogen. These complexes are called iodophores. The best-known iodophore is povidone-iodine (Betadine).

Alkylating agents that serve as disinfectants include formaldehyde, glutaraldehyde, and ethylene oxide. Formaldehyde and glutaraldehyde are applied as liquids and ethylene oxide as a gas. The lethal effects of these compounds on microorganisms result from their alkylating action on proteins. Alkylation is the replacement of a hydrogen atom on a carboxyl, hydroxy, or sulfhydryl group of a protein with a hydrocarbon radical. Formaldehyde as a 37% aqueous solution is called formalin. Formalin is used in embalming fluid, in the preparation of vaccines, and for preserving fresh tissue. Glutaraldehyde, which is 10 times more effective than formaldehyde and is considerably less toxic, is used as a cold sterilant for surgical instruments. Because it is applied as a gas, ethylene oxide has excellent penetrating power. It is not difficult to recognize the value of this agent for sterilizing delicate pieces of hospital equipment or plastic items that would be damaged by heat or liquid sterilization procedures.

Gram-Positive Bacilli

David C. Straus

Corynebacterium diphtheriae

Morphology

Corynebacterium diphtheriae tends to be club-shaped when grown on artificial media. It is gram positive, nonsporeforming, and approximately 2 to 6 μm in length and 0.5 to 1.0 μm in diameter. When the organisms divide, they tend to stick together in patterns resembling Chinese letters in stained smears.

Diphtheria Toxin

The toxin is responsible for the clinical symptoms observed with diphtheria. An infecting beta phage (lysogen) is required for toxin production; however, the toxin's production is controlled by the metabolism and physiologic state of the bacterium. Toxin is secreted in high concentrations by bacteria of abnormally low iron content. The toxin is a heat-labile protein (molecular weight 62,000) whose mechanism of action is inactivation of translocase factors (EF-2) of eucaryotic cells. The toxin is composed of A (active; mol wt 23,000) and B (binding; mol wt 39,000) fragments. Nicotinamide adenine dinucleotide is a required cofactor for fragment A activity. Fragment A catalyzes the following reaction intracellularly:

$$NAD + EF\text{-}2 \xrightarrow{\text{\textit{fragment A}}} \text{adenosine diphosphoribosyl–} \\ EF\text{-}2 \text{ (inactive)} + \text{nicotinamide} + H^+$$

When EF-2 is inactivated by this reaction, protein synthesis stops and cells begin to die.

Pathogenicity

Natural infection is demonstrable only in humans. *Corynebacterium diphtheriae* is commonly spread through airborne droplets. Diphtheria in humans usually begins when the organism colonizes the upper respiratory tract. There it elaborates toxin, which results in epithelial cell necrosis. The ensuing inflammatory response causes the production of the pseudomembrane, composed of dead epithelial cells, dead polymorphonuclear leukocytes, fibrin, and bacteria. This pseudomembrane can sometimes cause suffocation of the patient. Cutaneous diphtheria (mucosal surfaces) can occur and causes ulcerating skin lesions but no systemic effects.

Immunity and Epidemiology

Acquired immunity to clinical diphtheria is due to the presence of circulating antitoxin antibody. Because of the high degree of susceptibility in childhood, artificial immunization at an early age is highly recommended. The DTP vaccine (diphtheria toxoid, tetanus toxoid, and heat-killed *Bordetella pertussis*) is commonly used in the United States. Immunity lasts for several years, but booster shots are highly advisable. Some neurologic damage has been reported associated with the whole-cell portion *(B. pertussis)* of the DTP vaccine. However, it is clear that the theoretical risks of immunization are far less than the documented risks inherent with the actual disease (whooping cough).

Treatment and Prevention

Once circulating diphtheria toxin has penetrated a susceptible cell, antitoxin is no longer effective. Therefore, in suspected cases of diphtheria, antitoxin therapy must be administered as soon as possible. Since antitoxin is normally of horse origin, a test for hypersensitivity to horse serum proteins should be performed first. Antibiotic therapy (penicillin) should never be relied on alone in the treatment of diphtheria. The disease is rare in the United States because of the DTP vaccine, because humans are the only important reservoir, and because all strains produce the same antigenic type of toxin.

Bacillus anthracis

Morphology

Bacillus anthracis, the causative agent of anthrax, is a very large (3–7 μm in length), gram-positive, nonmotile, spore-forming rod. The organism is found singly or in short chains in smears from infected tissue. Spores are usually formed under adverse conditions that tend to be unfavorable for the continued multiplication of the vegative form. Spores are relatively resistant to heat and disinfectants, and can remain viable for years in dry earth and for months in animal hides. Colonies have a "Medusa's head" appearance under a hand lens.

Important Antigens and Pathogenicity

Bacillus anthracis produces an antiphagocytic capsule composed of D-glutamic acid and an exotoxin that is made up of three antigenically distinct thermolabile proteins. The three proteins are an edema factor (an adenylate cyclase in an inactive form), a protective antigen, and a lethal factor. Anthrax is primarily a disease of animals with which humans are accidentally infected. The most common form of the disease in humans is the cutaneous variety (malignant pustule); however, systemic involvement can occur and is frequently fatal. Inhalation anthrax (woolsorter's disease) can lead to hemorrhagic mediastinitis and death.

Immunity, Treatment, and Prevention

Second attacks of anthrax are rare; however, vaccines composed of killed bacilli are not effective. Acquired immunity is due to antibodies against the capsule and toxin. The drug of choice for cutaneous anthrax is penicillin, but chemotherapy is usually ineffective against respiratory anthrax. Animal anthrax can be partially controlled by immunization of animals with attenuated vaccines and disposal of dead animals by cremation or burial. "High-risk" humans should be vaccinated with the protective antigen portion of the toxin.

Bacillus cereus

Morphology

Bacillus cereus is quite similar in cell morphology to *B. anthracis.* In contrast to *B. anthracis,* it is motile and insensitive to penicillin.

Pathogenicity and Treatment

This organism is an infrequently diagnosed cause of food poisoning in the United States. It can cause two distinct clinical syndromes. One has an incubation period of 4 hours and is characterized by severe nausea and vomiting. The other syndrome has a longer incubation period (20 hours) and is characterized clinically by diarrhea and abdominal cramping. Food poisoning due to these bacteria is due to spore survival during cooking and resultant spore germination and enterotoxin production. In addition to food poisoning, *B. cereus* is found in serious infections associated with impairment of host defense mechanisms, primarily by foreign bodies, prosthetic devices, or restricted blood supply. In patients with serious underlying disease such as leukemia, overwhelming bacteremia, endocarditis, or meningitis can develop. Clindamycin is the drug of choice but *B. cereus* is also sensitive to erthromycin, vancomycin, and tetracycline.

Listeria monocytogenes

Morphology

Listeria monocytogenes receives its name from the striking monocytic blood reaction (an increase in the number of circulating monocytes) it produces in the infected host. It is a small gram-positive coccobacillus that has a tendency to grow in short chains. The organism is actively motile by peritrichous flagella.

Pathogenesis and Treatment

The virulence of *L. monocytogenes* appears to be dependent on successful parasitism of phagocytic cells. In humans, listeriosis is characterized by widely disseminated abscesses or granulomas of the liver, spleen, and central nervous system. Meningitis in the adult is the most commonly recognized form of listeriosis. Genital tract infection in the gravid woman, with infection of the offspring, is the most characteristic of the infections caused by *L. monocytogenes.* The organism can also cause intrauterine infections and premature delivery. The fatality rate is very high in untreated cases of septicemia and meningitis. Penicillin is the drug of choice.

Gram-Positive Pyogenic Cocci: Staphylococci and Streptococci

David C. Straus

Staphylococci

Morphology

Staphylococci are gram-positive, nonmotile cocci with a diameter of 1.0 μm. They grow in clusters on solid media and in short chains (rarely containing more than four members) and clusters in liquid media.

Metabolism

Staphylococci are one of the hardiest of all nonsporeforming bacteria. Most strains are relatively heat stable, withstanding temperatures as high as 60°C for 30 minutes. Staphylococci are facultative anaerobes and produce the enzyme catalase that catalyzes the following reaction:

$$2H_2O_2 \rightarrow 2H_2O + O_2 \uparrow$$

The two most important species of staphylococci are *Staphylococcus aureus* and *Staphylococcus epidermidis*. All strains of *Staph. aureus* produce coagulase, an enzyme that clots citrated plasma. *Staphylococcus epidermidis* does not produce coagulase and is of relatively low pathogenicity compared to *Staph. aureus*. *Staphylococcus aureus* also ferments mannitol and produces lipolytic enzymes, which render these organisms resistant to the antibacterial lipids of the skin. A third species of staphylococci has recently been gaining in prominence. This coagulase-negative organism, *Staph. saprophyticus,* is a common cause of urinary tract infections. It is second only to *Escherichia coli* in its frequency in causing urinary tract infections in young, sexually active females. There are about 10 species of coagulase-negative staphylococci. They include *Staph. hominus, capitus, haemolyticus,* and *saprophyticus.*

Staphylococcal Toxins

Pathogenic staphylococci release a number of different toxins, such as hemolysins, a leukocidin, six enterotoxins, and exfoliatin. The hemolysins are referred to as alpha, beta, gamma, and delta. The alpha toxin, which is dermonecrotic when administered subcutaneously in rabbits and is lethal in mice and rabbits when given intravenously, is the only hemolysin of clinical importance. The nonhemolytic Panton-Valentine leukocidin is thought to kill white blood cells by causing them to degranulate. The staphylococcal enterotoxins (type A, B, C_1, C_2, D, E, F) are proteins of 35,000 mol wt that cause emesis and diarrhea. Exfoliatin is a protein of approximately 24,000

mol wt that is heat stable and is responsible for SSSS in neonates, also known as Ritter's disease. The staphylococci also produce a toxin that has been shown to be associated with toxic shock syndrome (TSS). This protein is now referred to as TSS-toxin 1 (TSST-1).

Toxic Shock Syndrome

Clinical findings in TSS are hypotension, fever, scarlet-fever rash, desquamation of the skin on recovery, and multisystem involvement in the absence of disseminated infection. This suggests the involvement of one or more toxins. TSST-1 has been identified as a major factor in the pathogenesis of TSS, but its role is unclear. Antibodies to TSST-1 are produced in patients, and appear to be protective, but they are produced poorly by women recovering from menstrual TSS. Also, the fact that only approximately 90 percent of the *Staph. aureus* strains isolated from women with menstrual TSS and 85 percent of the strains isolated from individuals with nonmenstrual TSS produce TSST-1 indicates that other toxins may be involved.

Enzymes and Antigens

Staphylococcus aureus appears to be the most important organism that produces extracellular coagulase. There is also a cell-bound coagulase that is serologically distinct from the free coagulase. Coagulase-positive strains elaborate several other enzymes that may be involved in pathogenicity (staphylokinase, lipase, hyaluronidase, and DNAase). *Staphylococcus aureus* strains also produce protein A, a small, basic antiphagocytic protein that reacts with the Fc fragment of mammalian IgG. Some *Staph. aureus* strains appear to produce carbohydrate antiphagocytic capsules.

Typing

Serologic typing of *Staph. aureus* has proved to be quite difficult because of the prevalence of anti–*Staph. aureus* antibodies. Most typing laboratories use the less difficult procedure of phage-typing of *Staph. aureus* strains. Suspensions of the phage are divided into five host ranges, and single drops of these suspensions are placed on plates heavily seeded with *Staph. aureus*. Clear zones of lysis indicate phage susceptibility.

Pathogenicity

The most noteworthy aspect of staphylococcal disease is suppuration. Much of the localized tissue damage is irreversible, and scarring can result. Staphylococcal septicemia is a life-threatening disease, and we are quite fortunate that only rarely does this organism break through the localizing barriers and invade the lymphatics and bloodstream. Invasive infections, however, do occur, most often as a result of complications of accidental trauma and chronic debilitating diseases.

Virulence of Staph. aureus

Staphylococcus aureus is thought to be decidedly more virulent than *Staph. epidermidis* for a variety of reasons: (1) *Staph. aureus* is more resistant to phagocytosis than is *Staph. epidermidis* (only *Staph. aureus* produces protein A and capsule); (2) as much as 5 percent of a population of *Staph. aureus* can survive in phagocytic cells, whereas *Staph. epidermidis* cannot; (3) only *Staph. aureus* produces alpha toxin; (4) only *Staph. aureus* can produce staphylococcal enteritis when the organism invades the bowel wall of patients whose normal flora has been depressed by antibiotics; and (5) only *Staph. aureus* produces enterotoxins and staphylococcal food poisoning, as well as the toxic shock syndrome. *Staphylococcus epidermidis*, however, can also be pathogenic and has been shown to infect prosthetic heart valves and venous catheters and to cause subacute bacterial endocarditis.

Laboratory Diagnosis

Staphylococci cannot be differentiated from other gram-positive cocci on purely morphologic grounds. Exudates should always be cultured on blood agar because this supports better growth of other pathogens, promotes pigment formation by staphylococci, and permits direct detection of hemolysins. *Staphylococcus aureus* strains usually produce a golden-yellow pigment, but pigment production alone is not an adequate indicator of virulence. The properties that correlate best with pathogenicity are elaboration of DNAase and coagulase.

Immunity and Treatment

Humans have a high degree of natural resistance to staphylococci. Following serious staphylococcal infection, the antibody titer of the serum to *Staph. aureus* usually rises, but the presence of antistaphylococcal antibodies in the serum is not always fully protective. In treatment, one should always keep in mind that *Staph. aureus* strains that produce penicillinase occur frequently. Therefore, the drug sensitivity of the infecting organism should be determined quickly and the patient treated vigorously. Penicillinase-producing strains are resistant to ordinary penicillins but may be susceptible to semisynthetic penicillins.

Streptococci

General Features

The streptococci are catalase-negative gram-positive cocci that characteristically grow in chains or as diplococci.

They are approximately 1 μm in diameter. They are capable of causing a wide variety of diseases, including "strep" sore throat, rheumatic fever, scarlet fever, acute glomerulonephritis, pneumonia, tooth decay, endocarditis, and other diseases.

Classification

The streptococci are classified serologically or on the basis of their hemolytic reactions on blood agar plates. The alpha-hemolytic streptococci produce a green discoloration on blood agar as a result of incomplete hemolysis. The beta-hemolytic streptococci cause complete destruction of red blood cells, and the zones around the colonies are clear. The gamma-hemolytic streptococci produce no hemolysis, either within the agar or on the surface. Serologically, the streptococci can be classified on the basis of group-specific carbohydrate antigens on their cell walls (Lancefield classification). The various groups are designated A through O. Table 4-3 lists medically important streptococci and some of the distinguishing features of each.

Group A Beta-Hemolytic Streptococci

The genus-species name for the group A beta-hemolytic streptococcus (GAS) is *Streptococcus pyogenes*. These are medically the most important streptococci.

Cellular Antigens

The GAS organisms are surrounded by a capsule composed of hyaluronic acid. This polysaccharide surface antigen has antiphagocytic properties but is not immunogenic in humans due to its similarity to human hyaluronic acid. The GAS possess a group-specific antigen (the group A carbohydrate) in their cell wall. This antigen is found in all strains of *Strep. pyogenes*. Antibodies to this antigen are not protective in humans. The GAS also possess a cell-wall–associated protein referred to as the M protein, or type-specific antigen. In the GAS, there are more than 60 different serologic types based on the cell-wall M protein. An M-protein–covered GAS has the capability of eluding phagocytic cells, but anti–M protein antibody is protective. It has recently been shown that adherence to buccal epithelial cells of the upper respiratory tract of humans is mediated by the lipoteichoic acids produced by these organisms.

Extracellular Products

The GAS produce a wide variety of extracellular products. One of these, the erythrogenic toxin, is responsible for the rash observed in scarlet fever. The production of this toxin is coded for by a bacteriophage genome (lysogen), as is the production of diphtheria toxin by *Corynebacterium diphtheriae*. The GAS produce two hemolysins, called strep-

Table 4-3   Medically Important Streptococci

Species	Lancefield group	Hemolysis	Important facts about streptococci
Streptococcus pyogenes	A	Beta	M-protein antiphagocytic structure; hyaluronic acid antiphagocytic structure; highly sensitive to penicillin; 60 serotypes
Streptococcus agalactiae	B	Beta	Carbohydrate antiphagocytic capsule; leading cause of neonatal gram-positive bacterial meningitis; 6 serotypes
Streptococcus zooepidemicus, equi, equisimilis, dysgalactiae	C	Beta	Hyaluronic acid antiphagocytic structure; group C streptococci are important causes of animal disease and are not infrequently associated with human diseases
Enterococcus (Streptococcus) faecalis	D	Alpha, beta, or gamma	Normal flora; infection results from invasion by normal flora; frequently associated with endocarditis, urinary and bilary tract infections
Streptococcus pneumoniae	None	Alpha	Carbohydrate antiphagocytic capsule; important cause of bacterial lobar pneumonia; 80 different serotypes
Viridans streptococci (includes *Strep. mitis, mutans, salivarius, MG intermedius*)	None	Alpha	Normal flora of the upper respiratory tract; normally nonpathogenic; can infect the endocardium following rheumatic fever and cause subacute bacteria endocarditis (SBE); important cause of SBE

tolysins S and O. Streptolysin S is responsible for beta hemolysis observed on blood agar plates. It is stable in air and is not immunogenic in humans. Streptolysin O is inactivated by the presence of molecular oxygen. It is immunogenic in humans and anti-streptolysin O (ASO) antibodies are normally found in the sera of those individuals recovering from a GAS infection. The GAS also produce a streptokinase that promotes lysis of human blood clots and a hyaluronidase that is referred to as the "spreading factor."

Streptococcal Disease

The diseases produced by the GAS can be divided into two distinct groups: suppurative, or pus forming, and nonsuppurative sequelae. The suppurative diseases include streptococcal pharyngitis and all suppurative complications, such as otitis media, cervical adenitis, mastoiditis, peritonsillar abscesses, meningitis, pneumonia, and peritonitis. Also included in this category are puerperal sepsis, cellulitis, impetigo, and erysipelas. Scarlet fever occurs as a complication of GAS disease. Hyaluronic-acid capsule and M protein play a combined antiphagocytic role in pathogenesis. The nonsuppurative sequelae are disease states that exist after the primary GAS infection has been resolved. The two most important nonsuppurative sequelae are acute glomerulonephritis (AGN) and rheumatic fever (RF). Acute glomerulonephritis results from infections caused by a limited number of GAS types. The

majority of nephritogenic strains are type 12; others include types 1, 4, 6, 49, and 52. Acute glomerulonephritis is characterized by hematuria, edema, and hypertension. These symptoms usually appear about a week after the onset of the GAS infection. Acute glomerulonephritis is thought to be an autoimmune disease, and the resulting inflammatory response is probably due to the fixation of complement. Rheumatic fever, on the other hand, may follow pharyngeal infection by any type of GAS. Rheumatic fever is a syndrome characterized by carditis, arthritis, chorea, and electrocardiographic abnormalities. Beginning in 1984, there was a resurgence of RF in the U.S. It appears possible that there may indeed be specific rheumatic strains responsible for these outbreaks, but the significance of this is unclear. The latent period between the onset of the acute GAS pharyngitis and the symptoms of RF is usually 2 to 3 weeks. It is not clear how immunologic reactivity to streptococcal products causes the recurrent cardiac, joint, and skin lesions, but immunologic cross reactions have been described between streptococcal antigens and human heart tissue.

Immunity to GAS Disease

Only anti–M protein antibody is protective against the GAS. No individual is likely to become immune to all group A streptococcal types because there are 60 kinds. Only a few types of GAS are nephritogenic; therefore, an initial attack of AGN greatly reduces the probability of a second attack. However, a wide variety of streptococcal types may cause RF. Therefore, an initial attack of RF does not reduce the probability of a second attack. Immunity to scarlet fever is associated with the presence of antierythrogenic toxin antibodies. Since there are three immunologically distinct erythrogenic toxins, second attacks of scarlet fever are possible.

Laboratory Diagnosis, Treatment, and Prevention

Suspected GAS isolates are plated on blood containing agar, and the plates are examined for beta-hemolysis. Diagnosis is facilitated by the fact that GAS are more sensitive to the antibiotic bacitracin than are other groups of streptococci. We are fortunate that GAS are among the most susceptible of all pathogenic bacteria to the action of antimicrobial drugs, with penicillin being the drug of choice. For prevention of GAS infections, penicillin is often given continually in small doses to patients with RF. Additionally, penicillin is used to eradicate nephritogenic GAS from the families of patients with AGN.

Beta-Hemolytic Streptococci of Other Groups

The group B streptococci (Streptococcus agalactiae) are now known to be an important cause of neonatal disease. They are divided into six serotypes (Ia, Ib/c, Ia/c, II, III, and IV) by virtue of carbohydrate type-specific antigens. Sixty percent of all group B streptococcal neonatal infections are caused by serotype III. Antibodies to these carbohydrate antigens are protective. Group B streptococci can cause "early-onset" disease, which occurs within several days postpartum where there is an association with sepsis, lung involvement, and meningitis. "Late-onset" disease occurs after a week and up to a month postpartum. This syndrome is primarily associated with meningitis. Streptococcal strains of groups C, E, G, H, K, and O are also beta-hemolytic and can often be isolated from the respiratory tract, but these strains are rarely pathogenic for humans. Probably the most important of these strains, medically, are the group C streptococci. The species most often involved with human infections is Streptococcus equisimilis. It has been shown to be an infrequent cause of pneumonia, pharyngitis, and bacteremia in humans.

Viridans Streptococci

Often referred to as the alpha-hemolytic streptococci, viridans streptococci include such organisms as Streptococcus mitis, mutans, sanguis, and salivarius. They have a relatively low degree of virulence and often colonize the upper respiratory tract within the first few hours after birth. Unlike the pneumococci (Streptococcus pneumo-

niae), they are neither bile soluble nor sensitive to ethylhydrocupreine (optochin). They are the leading cause of subacute bacterial endocarditis, an infection of a serious nature greatly enhanced by the difficulty encountered in treatment. Subacute bacterial endocarditis results from the colonization and infection of an endocardial surface already damaged by RF or congenital heart disease.

Pneumococcus (Strep. pneumoniae)

Pneumococcal organisms are encapsulated, lancet-shaped, gram-positive, alpha-hemolytic diplococci. They have been in the past and continue to be extremely important pathogens.

Morphology

In sputum, pus, serous fluid, and body tissue, Strep. pneumoniae may be found in short chains and occasionally as individual cocci. It is normally gram positive up to and including the exponential phase of growth, but eventually becomes gram negative, as a result of the production of autolytic enzymes. Autolysis is stimulated by surface-active agents such as bile salts, and this test for bile solubility is useful in identifying the pneumococci.

Antigenic Structure and Pathogenic Role of the Capsule

More than 80 serologically different types of Strep. pneumoniae have been identified by their distinct polysaccharide capsule. Pneumococcal capsules are composed of large polysaccharide polymers that form hydrophilic gels on the surface of the bacteria. Only smooth or encapsulated strains are pathogenic for humans. Active or passive immunization against a specific polysaccharide capsular antigen produces a high level of protection. Virulence has been shown to be related to capsular size, and the type 3 organism, which produces the largest capsule, is the most virulent. These capsules are thought to act as virulence factors because they impede phagocytosis.

Pathogenesis of Pneumococcal Pneumonia

Approximately 40 percent of normal adults carry Strep. pneumoniae in their throats. However, we are fortunate that epidemics of pneumococcal pneumonia rarely occur. This is no doubt due to the defense barriers of the lower respiratory tract. These include the epiglottal reflex, the sticky mucus lining the airway, the cilia of the respiratory epithelium, the cough reflex, the lymphatics that drain the terminal bronchi and bronchioles, and the alveolar macrophage. However, when pneumococcal pneumonia develops, it usually follows some predisposing factor, such as a viral infection (e.g., a cold or trauma to the throat).

Immunity

Type-specific anticapsular antibody is not demonstrable until the fifth or sixth day following infection. Fortunately, 70 percent of all untreated patients go on to complete recovery. Recurrent attacks are usually due to infection by a new serotype.

Laboratory Diagnosis

Pneumococcal pneumonia is rapidly demonstrable by a Gram's stain of the sputum. The sputum should also be cultured on blood agar for conclusive identification. Pneumococci are often confused with the viridans streptococci, but can be differentiated from these organisms by their bile solubility and Optochin sensitivity. The pneumococci can also be identified by the quellung reaction, in which the cells are suspended in homologous type-specific antiserum, which combines with the capsular polysaccharide and renders it visible under the light microscope.

Treatment and Prevention

Penicillin is the drug of choice in the treatment of pneumococcal pneumonia, while secondary choices include erythromycin and lincomycin. Prophylactic measures are rarely indicated; however, immunization with type-specific polysaccharide is useful in closed communities where the likelihood of an epidemic might exist.

Neisseriaceae

Rial D. Rolfe

Neisseria is one of five genera included in the Neisseriaceae. The other genera included in this family are *Branhamella*, *Kingella*, *Moraxella*, and *Acinetobacter*. *Neisseria* are aerobic, small, gram-negative cocci that are nonmotile and nonsporeforming. They characteristically grow in pairs with adjacent sides flattened. The two principal pathogens of the genus are *Neisseria gonorrhoeae* (gonococcus) and *Neisseria meningitidis* (meningococcus). This genus also includes relatively nonpathogenic species (*Neisseria flavescens, mucosa, subflava,* and *sicca*) that are frequently part of the *normal flora* and may be confused with meningococci and gonococci. Despite their lack of general pathogenicity, these species occasionally cause disease (e.g., endocarditis and meningitis).

Neisseria species can be differentiated by a variety of tests. The inability of *N. gonorrhoeae* and *N. meningitidis* to grow at *22°C* and their fastidious nutrient requirements distinguish these two species from most of the "nonpathogenic" species of *Neisseria*. The distinction between *N. gonorrhoeae* and *N. meningitidis* usually is based on the metabolism of *carbohydrates*. *Neisseria meningitidis* produces acid from both glucose and maltose, whereas *N. gonorrhoeae* produces acid from glucose only. All species of *Neisseria* contain high levels of *cytochrome oxidase* and *catalase*.

Neisseria gonorrhoeae

Epidemiology

Gonorrhea, the most common reportable infectious disease in the United States, is almost always *venereally* transmitted and ordinarily produces a mild infection at the site of inoculation. *Neisseria gonorrhoeae* may also be transmitted by *oral-genital* contact (pharyngeal gonorrhea) and *rectal intercourse* (rectal gonorrhea), both of which are prevalent among homosexual men. The majority of individuals with pharyngeal or rectal gonorrhea are asymptomatic.

Pathogenic Mechanisms

Neisseria gonorrhoeae produces several virulence factors. All pathogenic strains of *N. gonorrhoeae* are piliated, whereas the nonpathogenic strains lack these surface structures. *Pili* aid in the attachment of gonococci to human mucosal surfaces and also inhibit phagocytosis. Another gonococcal surface constituent that promotes adherence is the outer membrane protein *PII*. All gonococcal strains (as well as meningococcal strains) produce extracellular proteases that inactivate the *IgA1* subclass of IgA by specifically cleaving the immunoglobulin heavy chain. Since IgA is the major immunoglobulin on mucosal surfaces, this enzyme enables the gonococci to evade the effects of secretory antibody. The gonococcus also produces a *cytotoxic factor* that damages ciliated epithelial cells. The *endotoxin* of *N. gonorrhoeae* is probably responsible for much of the toxicity associated with this microorganism.

Clinical Manifestations

The site of primary infection in women is usually the *cervix*, and the majority of infected women are *asymptomatic*. Some women may develop salpingitis, pelvic peritonitis, and other local complications from ascending genital infections originating at the endocervix. *Infertility* is the major complication of ascending genital infection in women. The principal site of primary infection in men is the *urethra*, and greater than 90 percent of infected men are *symptomatic* with purulent urethral discharge or dysuria. Gonococcal infection may spread by direct extension from the male urethra to produce prostatitis, urethral stricture, and epididymitis.

Gonococci infecting the genitalia, pharynx, or rectum may invade the bloodstream and be carried to various parts of the body to give rise to a variety of syndromes collectively called *disseminated gonococcal infection (DGI)*. The gonococci invading the bloodstream usually share certain characteristics *(DGI biotype)*, which include resistance to killing by serum, sensitivity to penicillin, and fastidious growth requirements. The two most common clinical manifestations of DGI are acute septic *arthritis* and *dermatitis*. The skin lesions associated with gonococcal dermatitis are typically few in number and located on the distal dorsal surfaces of the wrists, elbows, and ankles. Additional complications of DGI include *perihepatitis* (Fitz-Hugh-Curtis syndrome), endocarditis, myocarditis, glomerulonephritis, and meningitis.

In addition to venereal transmission, *N. gonorrhoeae* may be transmitted by nonsexual contact. *Gonorrheal ophthalmia* of the newborn occurs when the eyes of neonate are infected during passage through the birth canal. This disease was once a common cause of blindness in the United States, but is largely prevented today by the instillation of 1% *silver nitrate* (Credé's procedure) or an *erythromycin*-containing ointment in the conjuctival sac of the infant shortly after birth. *Neisseria gonorrhoeae* can also cause purulent *conjunctivitis* in adults following direct inoculation of the conjunctiva. Gonococcal *vulvovaginitis* in prepubescent girls is transmitted by the use of common bed linens, bathtubs, toilets, and other inanimate objects. The disease usually is self-limited but occasionally progresses to invasion of the fallopian tubes or to peritonitis. *Neisseria gonorrhoeae* vaginal infection is not seen after the onset of puberty because the vaginal epithelium becomes resistant to infection with gonococci.

Diagnosis

The laboratory diagnosis of gonococcal infection is based primarily on the identification of *N. gonorrhoeae* in infected sites by microscopic examination and by culture. The finding of gram-negative diplococci within or closely associated with *polymorphonuclear leukocytes* in purulent urethral exudate strongly suggests the diagnosis of gonorrhea in men. However, a similar finding in exudates from women is of limited diagnostic value because the Gram's stain is often falsely negative in women. To confirm the gram's stain or to establish the diagnosis, *N. gonorrhoeae* must be isolated and identified. Material for culture should be obtained from the pharynx, anorectal area, and urogenital tract. Blood should also be obtained for culture when gonococcemia is suspected. Material from sites that are normally sterile (e.g., blood, joint fluid, and spinal fluid) is cultured on nonselective media such as *chocolate agar* containing added glucose and other defined supplements.

Chocolate agar is prepared by heating blood agar to release hemoglobin. Specimens from sites that harbor a normal flora (e.g., rectum and pharynx) are cultured on *Thayer-Martin medium*, which contains antibiotics (vancomycin, colistin, nystatin, and trimethroprim) to inhibit the growth of microorganisms other than *N. gonorrhoeae*. All media are incubated at 37°C under an atmosphere of increased carbon dioxide tension. Identification of *N. gonorrhoeae* is performed by carbohydrate fermentation and fluorescent-antibody staining.

Treatment

Standards for treatment of gonococcal infection are revised regularly. For uncomplicated infections of mucosal surfaces, *ceftriazone* is now the treatment of choice. Alternate therapeutic agents include cefoxitin, spectinomycin, trimethoprim-sulfamethoxazole, ciprofloxacin, and cefuroxime. Simultaneous treatment of *Chlamydia trachomatis* with tetracycline is recommended since mixed infections are common.

Neisseria meningitidis

Epidemiology

Meningococcal disease occurs both sporadically and as large-scale epidemics throughout the world. The peak incidence of *N. meningitidis* infections is in *children* between the ages of 6 months and 24 months of age. The only known reservoir of meningococcal infection is the nasopharynx of humans. Meningococci are transmitted from person to person by *airborne droplets* of nasopharyngeal secretions.

Pathogenic Mechanisms

Nine *serogroups* of *N. meningitidis*, designated A, B, C, D, X, Y, Z, W-135, and 29-E, have been identified on the basis of immunologic specificity of capsular polysaccharides. Organisms in groups A, B, and C are most often responsible for clinically recognized disease. The capsular polysaccharides contribute to the invasiveness of *N. miningitidis* by inhibiting *phagocytosis*. Protective antibodies are directed against the capsular polysaccharide. *Neisseria meningitidis* endotoxin causes fever and shock, and has been implicated in the vascular damage commonly seen in meningococcemia. All strains of every *N. meningitidis* serogroup produce an *IgA1* protease that is excreted into the extracellular environment. The ability of *N. meningitidis* to utilize *transferrin-bound iron* as a sole iron source has also been implicated as a virulence factor since nonpathogenic *Neisseria* species lack the ability to use iron from transferrin.

Clinical Manifestations

Upon reaching a susceptible host, the meningococci localize in the nasopharynx and multiply. Disease develops in few individuals colonized with *N. meningitidis* because of the high degree of natural immunity in the general population. The incidence of *natural immunity* increases with age and this accounts for the greater prevalence of disease in children than in adults. Asymptomatically colonized individuals may serve as reservoirs in transmitting the disease to susceptible hosts. When *N. meningitidis* invades the bloodstream, it results in a spectrum of diseases, ranging from benign transient bacteremia to a fulminating acute systemic infection accompanied by high fever, shock, widespread purpura, disseminated intravascular coagulation, adrenal insufficiency, and rapid death (*Waterhouse-Friderichsen* syndrome). Dissemination of meningococci via the bloodstream can result in metastatic lesions in various areas of the body, such as the skin, meninges, joints, eyes, and lungs. The clinical manifestations vary depending on the site of colonization. The most common clinical manifestation of meningococcemia is a petechial *skin lesion* that develops on the trunk and lower portions of the body. The two most frequent complications of meningococcemia are *arthritis* and *meningitis*.

Diagnosis

Specimens of blood, cerebrospinal fluid, and nasopharyngeal secretions should be examined for the presence of *N. meningitidis* in cases of suspected meningococcal disease. Additional sites from which the meningococcus may be isolated include joint fluid, transtracheal aspirates, pericardial fluid, and skin petechiae. A tentative diagnosis of meningitis due to *N. meningitidis* can be made by demonstrating the presence of intracellular gram-negative diplococci in smears of *cerebrospinal fluid*. The same media and incubating conditions used in the isolation of *N. gonorrhoeae* are used in the isolation of *N. meningitidis*. Countercurrent immunoelectrophoresis, latex agglutination, or coagglutination employing staphylococcus with protein A can be used to detect meningococcal polysaccharide in specimens such as cerebrospinal fluid, synovial fluid, and urine.

Treatment

Penicillin is the antimicrobial agent of choice in the treatment of patients with meningococcal disease. Patients allergic to penicillin are treated effectively with spectinomycin or tetracycline. *Chemoprophylaxis* is effective in disrupting the spread of meningococcal infection in closed environments by eliminating the organism from the upper respiratory tract of asymptomatic carriers. Penicillin, however, is unsatisfactory for the prophylactic treatment of carriers. *Rifampin*, minocycline, and the sulfonamides effectively eliminate meningococcus from the nasopharynx.

Vaccination with purified group-specific meningococcal *capsular polysaccharide* is an effective means of preventing epidemics of *N. meningitidis* infection and reducing the carrier state. Group A, C, Y, and W-135 meningococcal vaccines are licensed and available. The vaccine does not contain the group B polysaccharide because it is poorly immunogenic in humans.

Other Genera in the Family Neisseriaceae

Branhamella

Branhamella is a significant cause of otitis media in children and respiratory infection in adults.

Acinetobacter

Acinetobacter species are gram-negative coccobacillary rods that cause disease chiefly in compromised, hospitalized patients. Sepsis, pneumonia, and urinary tract infections are the most frequent manifestations.

Small Gram-Negative Bacilli

Rial D. Rolfe

Haemophilus

Bacteria belonging to the genus *Haemophilus* are a heterogeneous group of small, gram-negative bacilli that are nonmotile and nonsporeforming. These microorganisms are part of the human *normal flora* of the upper respiratory tract and oral cavity. Blood contains two factors necessary for the growth of many *Haemophilus* species: a heat-stable substance *(X factor)* and a heat-labile substance *(V factor)*. The X factor has been identified as *hematin*, and the V factor can be replaced by *NAD* or *NADP*. The internal subdivision of *Haemophilus* into species depends in part on demonstrating the requirement for one or both of these growth factors. Several microorganisms (e.g., staphylococci) excrete the V factor into the surrounding environment. The ability of certain *Haemophilus* species to grow in the immediate vicinity of V factor–producing microorganisms on solid media deficient in this factor is called the *satellite phenomenon*.

Haemophilus influenzae

Epidemiology

Naturally acquired *H. influenzae* infection occurs only in humans and is more common and more serious in children than adults. In infants and young children, it causes acute

Table 4-4 Nonzoonotic Gram-Negative Bacteria

Species	Primary mode of transmission	Primary clinical manifestations
Haemophilus influenzae	Respiratory secretions	Respiratory tract infection Meningitis
Haemophilus influenzae biogroup aegyptius	Inanimate objects	Conjunctivitis
Haemophilus ducreyi	Sexual intercourse	Chancroid
Bordetella pertussis	Respiratory secretions	Whooping cough
Actinobacillus	Opportunistic from normal flora	Endocarditis Granulomatous lesions
Bartonella bacilliformis	Sand fly	Hemolytic anemia Cutaneous lesions
Calymmatobacterium granulomatis	Sexual intercourse	Granuloma inguinale
Cardiobacterium hominis	Opportunistic from normal flora	Endocarditis
Chromobacterium	Contaminated soil and water	Necrotizing metastatic lesions Diarrhea
Flavobacterium meningosepticum	Environmental contaminant	Meningitis
Gardnerella vaginalis	Genitourinary tract	Vaginitis
Plesiomonas shigelloides	Surface water	Gastroenteritis
Eikenella corrodens	Opportunistic from normal flora	Head and neck infections
Capnocytophaga	Opportunistic from normal flora	Periodontal disease

bacterial meningitis and several other pediatric diseases. In adults, it is primarily associated with chronic pulmonary disease. The principal mechanism of transmission is *person to person* by the respiratory route (Table 4-4).

Pathogenicity

The virulence of *H. influenzae* for humans is directly related to capsule formation. The *polysaccharide capsule* enables the organism to resist the action of complement. Six antigenically distinct capsular types, designated a through f, have been described. Virtually all strains of *H. influenzae* isolated from invasive infections belong to *serotype b,* whereas other strains can also cause disease but are usually noninvasive. The type b capsule is made up of a polymer of ribose, ribitol, and phosphate *(polyribophosphate [PRP])*. The capsular carbohydrates of *H. influenzae* evoke antibodies that protect against infection. Most adults possess these antibodies in their blood, whereas they are usually absent in young children. *Haemophilus influenzae* does not produce an exotoxin and there is no evidence that endotoxin plays a significant role in pathogenicity. Some strains of *H. influenzae* produce an enzyme that specifically cleaves *IgA1.*

Clinical Manifestations

Haemophilus influenzae enters the host by way of the respiratory tract and usually produces asymptomatic nasopharyngeal colonization or a mild nasopharyngitis. Oc-

casionally, *H. influenzae* may spread contiguously to produce suppurative infections involving the sinuses, middle ear, or bronchi. A preceding or concomitant viral infection of the upper respiratory tract predisposes a patient to infection with *H. influenzae*. This microorganism is the leading cause of *obstructive epiglottitis* in children, a potentially lethal disease. *Haemophilus influenzae* invasion of the bloodstream may result in *meningitis,* endocarditis, suppurative arthritis, or osteomyelitis. *Haemophilus influenzae* (serotype b) is the leading cause of meningitis in young children. Approximately one third of infants who recover from *H. influenzae* meningitis have permanent, residual neurologic defects.

Diagnosis

Cultures are the most accurate means for diagnosing *H. influenzae* infections. Depending on the clinical manifestations, specimens can consist of nasopharyngeal swabs, pus, blood, and spinal fluid. *Haemophilus influenzae* is a fastidious organism and requires both *X* and *V* factors for growth as well as an increased atmospheric concentration of *carbon dioxide. Haemophilus influenzae* is identified by performing selected biochemical tests. Immunofluorescence can be used to identify the organism directly in clinical specimens. Counterimmunoelectrophoresis and latex-particle agglutination and enzyme-linked immunosorbent assay can be used to identify the presence of *H. influenzae* type b antigens in body fluids.

Treatment

Serious complications, including death, can occur when *H. influenzae* type b infections are not treated or are improperly treated. The initial therapy for suspected systemic disease caused by *H. influenzae* is *ceftriaxone*. *Haemophilus influenzae* respiratory tract infections, such as otitis media and sinusitis, are treated with either ampicillin or a cephalosporin. However, ampicillin resistance due to plasmid-mediated beta-lactamase production has become increasingly prevalent during the last few years.

Prevention

Vaccines consisting of the *capsular polysaccharide* of *H. influenzae* type b conjugated to diphtheria toxoid or other carrier proteins are very effective in preventing disease due to *H. influenzae* type b. The vaccines can be given to children as young as 2 months of age.

Haemophilus influenzae Biogroup *Aegyptius*

Haemophilus influenzae biogroup *aegyptius* (Koch-Weeks bacillus) is the cause of *pinkeye,* an acute, purulent, and highly communicable form of conjunctivitis recognized throughout the world (Table 4-4). This disease can occur in epidemics, especially in tropical and subtropical climates. The disease is transmitted from person to person by hands, towels, handkerchiefs, and other objects that contact the face and eyes. *Haemophilus influenzae* biogroup *aegyptius* requires both *X and V factors* for growth. Definitive diagnosis is dependent on isolation of the organism from conjunctival scrapings. The conjunctivitis usually responds to topically applied *sulfonamides.*

Certain strains of *H. influenzae* biogroup *aegyptius* cause *Brazilian purpuric fever,* a life-threatening childhood infection characterized by purpura and shock.

Haemophilus ducreyi

Haemophilus ducreyi is the etiologic agent of an ulcerative venereal disease known as *chancroid.* Chancroid is a highly contagious disease usually transmitted by sexual intercourse, but it can be transmitted by inanimate objects (Table 4-4). An ulcer (chancroid or soft chancre) forms at the site of inoculation. The infection remains localized and spreads no further than the neighboring lymphatics, which may become swollen and painful.

Diagnosis of chancroid is made by cultivating the organism from the ulcer or from lymph node aspirates.

Oral *erythromycin* is regarded as the antimicrobial agent of choice in the treatment of chancroid.

Haemophilus parainfluenzae

Haemophilus parainfluenzae is occasionally implicated in upper respiratory tract infections and subacute bacterial endocarditis. It requires only the V factor for growth.

Haemophilus aphrophilus

Infections due to *H. aphrophilus* are infrequent but include endocarditis, septicemia, brain abscess, meningitis, and pneumonia. This microorganism does not require the V factor for growth and is variable in X-factor requirement.

Haemophilus paraphrophilus

Haemophilus paraphrophilus has been reported as a cause of endocarditis.

Haemophilus Haemolyticus

Haemophilus haemolyticus can cause upper respiratory tract infection in children and requires both X and V factors for growth.

Yersinia

The genus *Yersinia* contains three species of pathogenic importance to humans: *Yersinia pestis, Yersinia enterocolitica,* and *Yersinia pseudotuberculosis.* These microorganisms are small, aerobic, gram-negative bacilli that do not form spores. They show a marked tendency toward bipolar staining (i.e., they resemble a safety pin, with a central clear area).

Yersinia pestis

Epidemiology

Yersinia pestis is the etiologic agent of *plague.* Although plague is no longer as prevalent as it was in the past, sporadic cases still occur in many parts of the world, including the United States. Plague is primarily an infectious disease of rodents, especially rats, and humans are accidental hosts (Table 4-5). The disease is endemic among the wild rodents (e.g., ground squirrels, prairie dogs) of the southwestern United States. *Yersinia pestis* infection in these rodents is referred to as *sylvatic plague.* The disease is transmitted from rodent to rodent through the bite of *fleas* that have become infected by sucking the blood of an infected animal. Transmission of plague from rodents to humans can take any one of the following routes: (1) Humans may acquire the disease from the bite of a flea that has previously fed on an infected rodent, (2) the disease may be transmitted from an individual with *pneumonic plague* to a susceptible individual by infectious droplet secretions, (3) humans may contract the disease by han-

Table 4-5 Zoonoses Caused by Gram-Negative Bacteria

Species	Disease	Source of human infection	Modes of transmission to humans
Brucella species	Brucellosis	Goats, pigs, cattle, dogs	Ingestion of infected milk, milk products, or meat Inhalation of infected droplets Contact with infected animal tissue
Yersinia pestis	Plague	Rodents, humans	Rodent to human by flea Respiratory secretions from pneumonic plague Handling infectious tissue Person to person by flea
Yersinia pseudotuberculosis and *Yersinia enterocolitica*	Yersinioses	Wild and domestic animals	Contaminated food and water
Francisella tularensis	Tularemia	Wild animals	Rodent to human by arthropod vector Ingestion of contaminated water or tissue Contact with infective aerosols
Pasturella multocida	Pasteurellosis	Cats, dogs	Bites and scratches
Streptobacillus	Rat-bite fever	Rodents	Rodent bite
Rochalimaea henselae	Cat-scratch fever	Cats	Bites and scratches

dling tissue of an infected animal, and (4) the flea can transmit plague from person to person.

Mechanisms of Pathogenicity

The virulence of *Y. pestis* is due to several factors. *Fraction 1*, a protein envelope antigen, renders the organism resistant to phagocytosis. Antibodies to fraction 1 are protective in humans. Another antiphagocytic component of *Y. pestis* is the *VW antigen*. *Yersinia pestis* produces two toxins of pathogenic importance. The first of these is an *endotoxin* that is responsible for many of the clinical manifestations of plague. The other toxin, referred to as the *murine toxin*, is protein in nature and acts primarily on the vascular system to cause hemoconcentration and shock. *Yersinia pestis* also possesses *coagulase* and *fibrinolytic* activities, which enhance the invasiveness of this microorganism.

Clinical Manifestations

Infection due to *Y. pestis* can occur in any one of three clinical forms: bubonic, septicemic, and pneumonic. In *bubonic plague*, which is the most common form of *Y. pestis* infection, the microorganisms enter the host through the skin and are carried by the lymphatics to the lymph nodes, where they form abscesses. There is usually no discernible cutaneous lesion at the portal of entry. After an incubation period of 2 to 5 days, there is a sudden onset of high fever and the regional lymph nodes become painful and swollen. The infected lymph nodes, or *buboes,* are usually located in the groin or axilla area. Without adequate treatment, death usually occurs in 3 to 4 days.

Yersinia pestis infection may progress to the bloodstream, resulting in *septicemic plague.* Occasionally, a high level of bacteremia may occur early in the course of the disease before local buboes evolve. The bacteria rapidly disseminate to all organs, especially the spleen, liver, and lungs, resulting in purulent and necrotic lesions. The patient usually dies of endotoxic shock unless effective therapy is administered early in the course of the disease.

Pneumonic plague results either from involvement of the lungs during the course of bubonic and septicemic plague *(secondary pneumonic plague)* or from inhalation of infected droplet secretions *(primary pneumonic plague).* Pneumonic plague is a rapidly progressive infection and untreated patients rarely survive longer than 3 days.

The majority of individuals who recover from plague have a relatively solid and permanent immunity to subsequent infection.

Diagnosis

The laboratory diagnosis of plague is made by demonstrating the bacilli in tissue and by serologic tests. Rapid diagnosis of plague is extremely important because of the rapid progression of untreated disease. *Yersinia pestis* grows well on many different types of culture media. Direct fluorescent antibody permits rapid identification of *Y. pestis* in isolated cultures and clinical specimens. Antibodies to the fraction 1 antigen may be detected by use of an agglutination test or a complement fixation test.

Treatment and Prevention

The case fatality rate of untreated bubonic plague is 50 to 60 percent, whereas that of pneumonic plague approaches 100 percent. If adequate therapy is begun early in the course of the disease, however, the mortality can be dramatically reduced. The treatment of choice is *streptomycin* either alone or in combination with tetracycline.

Immunization of humans with a plague vaccine reduces the incidence and severity of disease. However, immunization is only recommended for laboratory personnel who work directly with the microorganism and for other individuals who are likely to be exposed to endemic plague. The plague vaccine licensed for use in the United States contains *formalin-killed Y. pestis.*

Yersinia pseudotuberculosis and *Yersinia enterocolitica*

Epidemiology

Yersinia pseudotuberculosis and *Y. enterocolitica* are closely related microorganisms that cause a variety of *zoonotic* enteric illnesses collectively referred to as *yersinioses*. Both microorganisms are worldwide in distribution and have been recovered from many wild and domestic animals. The majority of human cases can be attributed to contact with water or food contaminated with the excreta of infected animals (Table 4-5). The gastrointestinal tract is the portal of entry in most cases of yersinioses. Infection due to these two *Yersinia* species most often occurs in children under 15 years of age.

Mechanisms of Pathogenicity and Clinical Manifestations

Yersinia pseudotuberculosis and *Y. enterocolitica* invade epithelial cells of the gastrointestinal tract to produce intestinal disease in animals and people. *Yersinia enterocolitica* also produces a heat-stable enterotoxin that contributes to the symptoms of gastroenteritis.

The most common clinical presentation of *Y. enterocolitica* infection is an acute *enteritis* with watery *diarrhea*. Acute *mesenteric adenitis* is the most common clinical presentation of *Y. pseudotuberculosis* infection. Intestinal infections caused by either organism are generally self-limiting and resolve within 5 to 10 days. If septicemia develops, however, suppurative lesions may occur in many different organs, and the condition is no longer benign and self-limiting. Septicemia most commonly occurs in patients who are immunocompromised and the mortality is high.

Diagnosis

Yersinioses can be differentiated from other intestinal diseases by isolating the etiologic agent from blood, liver, spleen, lymph nodes, or feces and by demonstrating the presence of specific serum antibodies. Both microorganisms multiply at *4°C*, and this ability is used to facilitate recovery of *Yersinia* from specimens heavily contaminated with other microorganisms (e.g., feces).

Treatment

Yersinia pseudotuberculosis and *Y. enterocolitica* are usually quite sensitive to *aminoglycosides* and *trimethoprim-sulfamethoxazole*. However, the value of antimicrobial therapy in any of the enteric yersinioses is unclear, since these infections appear to run their course independent of antimicrobial therapy.

Brucella

Epidemiology

Brucellosis, principally a disease of the genitourinary tract of domestic animals, is caused by bacteria of the genus *Brucella*. Brucellae are fastidious, aerobic, nonmotile, nonsporeforming, gram-negative bacilli that display bipolar staining. Four species of *Brucella* cause human disease: *B. abortus, B. suis, B. melitensis,* and *B. canis*. These four species are pathogenic in a wide range of mammals, and each has a preferred host (Table 4-6). Brucellae tend to localize in the pregnant uterus (frequently causing abortion) and mammary glands of their animal reservoir. The predilection of brucellae for placental tissue (*viscerotropism* or *organotropism*) is due to the presence of a growth stimulant, *erythritol*. Human placentas, which lack erythritol, are not especially susceptible to brucellosis.

Brucellosis in humans is a *zoonosis* that is usually acquired either directly or indirectly from infected domestic animals (see Table 4-5). Infection is widespread among goats, cattle, and pigs. Animals usually recover spontaneously but excrete the bacteria for varying intervals of time in vaginal secretions, urine, and milk. Cows can become carriers and excrete brucellae in their milk for many years. Within the U.S., infection in humans is primarily from *occupational exposure* and is seen most often in abattoir employees, farmers, and veterinarians. The most common routes of infection in humans are the *gastrointestinal tract* (ingestion of infected milk, milk products, or meat), *mucous membranes* (inhalation of infected droplets), and *skin* (contact with infected tissues of animals).

Pathogenic Mechanisms

Brucella species do not produce exotoxin, but they do elaborate *endotoxin*, which contributes to the pathogenesis of the disease. Virulent strains of brucellae are capable of intracellular multiplication in cells of the reticuloendothelial system.

Table 4-6 Characteristics of *Brucella* species

| *Brucella* species | Preferential host | Growth in presence of: | | Carbon Dioxide requirement | Hydrogen Sulfide production | Hydrolysis of urea |
		Thionine	Basic fuchsin			
B. abortus	Cattle	+ / −	+	+ / −	+ / −	Slow
B. melitensis	Goats	+	+	−	−	Slow
B. suis	Swine	+	+ / −	−	+ / −	Rapid
B. canis	Dogs	+	−	−	−	Slow

Key: + = all strains positive; − = all strains negative; + / − = variable response amongst strains

Clinical Manifestations

The pathogenic species of brucellae are highly invasive, and once gaining entrance into the host they multiply *intracellularly* in polymorphonuclear leukocytes and are carried through the lymphatics to the thoracic duct and bloodstream. The incubation period before onset of symptoms is highly variable and relatively long (weeks or months). The clinical manifestations of human brucellosis can be classified into several types:

1. *Asymptomatic brucellosis*: The majority of infections with brucellae are asymptomatic.
2. *Acute brucellosis*: Symptoms of an acute febrile illness develop in these patients.
3. *Relapsing brucellosis (undulant fever)*: This form of brucellosis is characterized by febrile periods alternating with afebrile periods.
4. *Brucellosis localized in various organs*: Brucellae can attack essentially every organ and tissue of the human body, although they tend to localize within the *reticulo-endothelial system* (bone marrow, liver, spleen, and lymph nodes). Other sites of localization include the lungs, genitourinary tract, central nervous system, cardiovascular system, and joint tissue. The tissue reaction in brucellosis leads to the development of small granulomatous nodules that may develop into abscesses.
5. *Strain 19 vaccine disease*: *Brucella abortus* strain 19 is a live, attenuated vaccine used in the immunization of cattle. A mild form of brucellosis can occur when veterinarians are accidentally inoculated with strain 19 through the skin, conjunctiva, or gastrointestinal tract.

Symptomatic brucellosis can continue for several months, and relapses of disease during convalescence commonly occur. Reinfection in patients who recover from brucellosis usually results in a very mild, febrile illness.

Diagnosis

A definitive diagnosis of brucellosis is dependent on isolation of the organism and serologic tests. Attempts should be made to isolate the organism from blood, feces, urine, bone marrow, and lymph nodes. Primary isolation of brucellae from clinical specimens usually requires prolonged incubation on enriched media. Bacteria that resemble brucellae are identified and speciated on the basis of a number of tests (see Table 4-6). Each *Brucella* species possesses two heat-stable surface antigens, designated *A* and *M*, but in different proportions. It is possible to differentiate *B. melitensis* from the other two species by agglutination reactions based on these surface antigens. However, *B. abortus* and *B. suis* cannot be differentiated in this way. The presence of brucellae in clinical material or culture may also be detected by fluorescent antibody staining.

An agglutination test using standardized *B. abortus* antigen can also be used to aid in the diagnosis of brucellosis. Patients recovering from an attack of brucellosis may continue to show a positive agglutination reaction for months or years. Therefore, a positive agglutination reaction test is only suggestive of active disease.

Treatment and Prevention

Doxycycline plus *rifampin* is the combination of choice for the treatment of brucellosis. Prevention of brucellosis in humans involves pasteurization of milk, controlling the disease in animals through immunization, and preventing humans from coming in contact with sick animals.

Francisella tularensis

Epidemiology

Francisella tularensis is a small, nonsporeforming, gram-negative bacillus. This bacterium is nonmotile and may display bipolar staining. *Francisella tularensis* is the etiologic agent of *tularemia* (rabbit fever), an acute infectious disease of wild animals, especially rodents, transmitted from animal to animal by biting fleas and ticks (see Table 4-5). Tularemia is transmitted to humans from lower animals by the bite of an infected *arthropod* (chiefly ticks and deer flies in the United States), by direct contact with tissues or body fluids of an infected animal, by ingestion of contaminated water or inadequately cooked contaminated meat, or by contact with or inhalation of infective aerosols. The main sources of human disease in the United States are *rabbits* and *hares*.

Clinical Manifestations

Four clinical types of tularemia are recognized in humans: ulceroglandular, oculoglandular, typhoidal, and pneumonic. The incubation period for tularemia ranges from 3 to 10 days. In *ulceroglandular tularemia,* the most common form of the disease, an ulcerating papule develops at the portal of entry in the skin or mucous membrane. From the site of inoculation, the organisms are carried by the lymphatics to the regional lymph nodes, which become enlarged and tender. The organisms may enter the bloodstream and spread to parenchymatous organs, particularly the lungs, liver, and spleen, where they form granulomatous lesions that later undergo necrosis. Those who recover from ulceroglandular tularemia are incapacitated for weeks or months.

Oculoglandular tularemia usually results from inoculation of the conjunctiva with a hand contaminated with infective tissue fluid or from infectious aerosols. This type of tularemia can lead to permanent blindness and is characterized by a unilateral, painful, purulent conjunctivitis.

Pneumonic tularemia is produced by either inhalation of infective aerosols or by hematogenous dissemination from localized infections.

The *typhoidal* form of tularemia usually results from ingestion of the organism but may occur following intradermal or respiratory inoculation. The disease resembles typhoid fever with gastrointestinal manifestations, fever, and toxemia. Penetration of *F. tularensis* into the oropharynx can result in an acute exudative or membranous pharyngotonsillitis.

Immunity following recovery from tularemia is usually lifelong.

Diagnosis

Diagnosis of tularemia is seldom made by culture of *F. tularensis* because of the requirement of special media with added *sulfhydryl* compounds and frequent overgrowth by other microorganisms. Furthermore, many laboratories do not attempt to isolate *F. tularensis* because of the high rate of laboratory-acquired disease. Fluorescent antibody techniques can be used to identify the microorganism directly in exudates and tissue.

Most cases of tularemia are diagnosed serologically. Agglutinins appear during the second or third week of illness.

Treatment and Prevention

Streptomycin is the antimicrobial agent of choice in the treatment of all forms of tularemia.

A *live, attenuated strain* of *F. tularensis* is available to immunize both animals and humans. This vaccination does not provide complete protection but the severity of the disease is reduced in vaccinated individuals. At present, vaccination is indicated only for individuals at high risk of contracting the disease, such as laboratory personnel.

Pasteurella

Epidemiology

Members of the genus *Pasteurella* are small, nonmotile, gram-negative bacilli that often display bipolar staining. There are four species of *Pasteurella* of medical importance: *P. multocida, P. pneumotropica, P. ureae,* and *P. haemolytica. Pasteurella multocida* is the species most frequently isolated from human infections, although infections due to the other *Pasteurella* species are clinically indistinguishable from diseases caused by *P. multocida.*

Pasteurella species are normal inhabitants of the upper respiratory and gastrointestinal tracts of lower animals. Humans become infected through cat or dog *bites* and *scratches* or through contact with a diseased carcass (see Table 4-5). Approximately 25 percent of animal bites become infected with this microorganism.

Clinical Manifestations

Pasteurella infection in humans usually manifests in one of three ways: focal *soft tissue infection, chronic respiratory infection,* or *bacteremia* with or without metastatic lesions. Local soft tissue infections have an acute onset of erythema, pain, and swelling. Abscess formation may occur in some patients. Local complications of soft tissue infections include osteomyelitis, cellulitis, and inflammation of the tendon sheath.

Pasteurella may invade the bloodstream, resulting in a variety of infections, including meningitis, brain abscess, septic arthritis, and liver abscess. Respiratory tract infections include sinusitis, empyema, and bronchiectasis. Fatal infections due to *Pasteurella* rarely occur in the absence of underlying illness.

Diagnosis

Specimens for isolation of *Pasteurella* depend on the clinical manifestations but may include sputum, abscess aspirates, blood, and spinal fluid. *Pasteurella* species grow readily on medium enriched with blood.

Agglutinins in the sera of patients with generalized *Pasteurella* infection can be detected by a hemagglutination assay.

Treatment

Penicillin is considered the treatment of choice for *Pasteurella* infections.

Bordetella

The genus *Bordetella* encompasses three species that are pathogenic for humans: *B. pertussis*, *B. parapertussis*, and *B. bronchiseptica*. All three species are small, nonspore-forming, gram-negative bacilli. *Bordetella bronchiseptica* is the only motile species and *B. pertussis* is the only species that is encapsulated. *Bordetella pertussis* is a fastidious microorganism that requires a complex medium for growth, whereas the other two species grow on simple nutrient agar.

Bordetella pertussis

Epidemiology

Bordetella pertussis is the etiologic agent of pertussis *(whooping cough)*, a highly communicable upper respiratory tract infection. Naturally acquired *B. pertussis* infection occurs only in humans. Pertussis is most common in *children*, although clinical disease does occur among adults. The disease is especially dangerous within the first 6 months of life since *maternal antibody* offers little or no protection against disease. Pertussis is transmitted from person to person by aerosolized upper respiratory tract secretions, by fomites contaminated with nasal or oral secretions, and by direct contact (see Table 4-4).

Mechanisms of Pathogenicity

The *capsule* of *B. pertussis* is an important virulence factor. When first isolated from a patient, *B. pertussis* is encapsulated and fully virulent. In vitro laboratory passage leads to the selection of organisms that are not encapsulated and not virulent. *Bordetella pertussis* also produces other factors that are responsible for the clinical manifestations. These factors include a heat-stable *endotoxin*, a heat-labile *exotoxin*, and a *lymphocyte-stimulating factor* (also known as histamine-sensitizing factor and islet-activating protein). The lymphocyte-stimulating factor produces leu-

kocytosis and lymphocytosis. *Bordetella pertussis* has two *hemagglutinins* that mediate adherence of these bacteria to mammalian respiratory cilia. *Bordetella pertussis* possesses a cell-wall antigen *("protective antigen")* that induces immunity to infections.

Clinical Manifestations

Upon entering the respiratory tract of a susceptible host, *B. pertussis* localizes on the ciliated epithelium of the bronchi and trachea. After an incubation period of 7 to 10 days, the disease occurs in three stages: (1) the catarrhal, prodromal, or preparoxysmal stage; (2) the paroxysmal stage; and (3) the convalescent stage.

The *catarrhal stage* is characterized by a mild cough and symptoms of a minor upper respiratory tract infection. *Communicability* is greatest during this stage of the illness, which usually lasts about 2 weeks.

Pertussis progresses in severity to a *paroxysmal stage* characterized by rapid consecutive coughs and a deep *inspiratory whoop*. The inspiratory whoop is caused by air drawn forcibly through a narrowed glottis. The paroxysmal stage lasts 4 to 6 weeks.

The *convalescent stage* is characterized by a reduction in the frequency and severity of the cough and usually lasts 3 to 4 weeks. Reversion from the convalescent to the paroxysmal stage is common in infants.

Bordetella pertussis rarely penetrates the mucous membranes of the respiratory tract and complications of pertussis are usually due to *secondary bacterial infections*. The most common of these complications include otitis media and lobar pneumonia. Rarely, serious and occasionally fatal involvement of the central nervous system may occur.

Naturally acquired immunity to pertussis is not permanent but second attacks are usually mild and pass unrecognized.

Diagnosis

The bacteriologic diagnosis of pertussis is made by recovering the organism from respiratory secretions. This is best accomplished by passing a *nasopharyngeal swab* through the nose to the posterior pharyngeal wall, where it is allowed to remain in place until the patient coughs. The swab is then removed and inoculated onto *Bordet-Gengou medium* (potato-glycerol-blood agar). *Bordetella pertussis* can be identified directly in nasopharyngeal specimens by fluorescent antibody staining.

Treatment and Prevention

Antimicrobial therapy administered during the paroxysmal stage of the disease has very little effect on the clinical course of pertussis since elimination of the bacterium does not always result in clinical improvement. However, *erythromycin* may eliminate *B. pertussis* from these patients and, in doing so, render them noninfectious. Susceptible contacts with a positive nasopharyngeal smear for *B. pertussis* should receive chemoprophylaxis with erythromycin to abort or attenuate the illness.

Active *immunization* with whole-cell pertussis vaccine is the only effective method of control. These vaccines do not confer complete protection. However, the disease in immunized individuals is appreciably milder. The vaccine is usually administered in combination with diphtheria and tetanus toxoids.

Bordetella parapertussis

Bordetella parapertussis is occasionally isolated from patients with acute respiratory tract infections resembling mild whooping cough. Pertussis vaccine offers no protection against *B. parapertussis*. However, a parapertussis vaccine is available in areas where the disease is prevalent.

Bordetella bronchiseptica

Bordetella bronchiseptica occasionally causes a pertussis-like disease in humans but is mainly a pathogen of animals.

Miscellaneous Gram-Negative Bacilli

Actinobacillus

Actinobacillus species are small, nonmotile, nonspore-forming, gram-negative bacilli. *Actinobacillus actinomycetemcomitans*, the principal pathogen in this genus, is part of the normal oral and gastrointestinal flora of humans and is an *opportunistic* pathogen (see Table 4-4). It has been isolated from patients with endocarditis, localized purulent granulomatous lesions, abscesses in soft tissues, septicemia, urinary tract infections, and osteomyelitis.

Bartonella bacilliformis

Bartonella bacilliformis is a small, motile, gram-negative bacillus that is the etiologic agent of *Oroya fever*, a severe febrile hemolytic anemia, and *verruga peruana*, a disease characterized by benign cutaneous erythematous nodular eruptions. These two clinical manifestations are stages of the same bacterial infection called *Carrión's disease*. *Bartonella bacilliformis* infection is confined geographically to inhabitants of the river valleys of the Andes Mountains of Peru, Colombia, and Ecuador. The organism is transmitted from individual to individual by the bite of an infected *sand fly* (see Table 4-4). Humans are the only known reservoir of this disease.

Laboratory diagnosis of Carrión's disease is based on microscopic demonstration of *B. bacilliformis* within the erythrocytes and isolation of the organism from blood or cutaneous nodules.

Chloramphenicol is the antibotic of choice in the treatment of Oroya fever. The effectiveness of antibiotics on the verruga peruana stage of the disease is doubtful.

Calymmatobacterium granulomatis

Calymmatobacterium granulomatis is a short, nonmotile, gram-negative bacillus that causes a venereal disease known as *granuloma inguinale* (also called granuloma venereum and donovanosis) (see Table 4-4). The disease is not highly communicable and repeated exposure is necessary for the development of most clinical cases. This disease occurs most often in tropical and subtropical environments.

Granuloma inguinale is characterized by an indurated nodule in the skin and subcutaneous tissues of the groin and genitalia. The nodule may erode to form a granulomatous ulcer that can slowly spread by direct extension to destroy large areas of skin about the anus and genitalia. Metastatic hematogenous spread to bones, joints, and liver occasionally occurs.

Diagnosis of granuloma inguinale depends on the demonstration of encapsulated, oval bodies *(Donovan bodies)* in the cytoplasm of large histiocytic endothelial cells.

Although therapy of granuloma inguinale may be difficult, *tetracycline* is the most effective agent in the treatment of this disease.

Cardiobacterium hominis

Cardiobacterium hominis is a pleomorphic, gram-negative bacillus that is part of the indigenous flora of the human upper respiratory and gastrointestinal tracts (see Table 4-4). Endocarditis is the most frequent manifestation of *C. hominis* infection.

Penicillin and ampicillin are considered the antimicrobial agents of choice to treat patients with endocarditis caused by this bacterium.

Chromobacterium

Chromobacterium violaceum is the only species in this genus that produces infection in humans. It is found primarily in the soil and water of tropical and subtropical climates (see Table 4-4). The microorganism usually gains entrance to the host through skin abrasions and causes septicemia and necrotizing metastatic lesions primarily on the liver. *Chromobacterium violaceum* may also gain entrance through the gastrointestinal tract and has been associated with diarrhea.

Chromobacterium violaceum is sensitive to chloramphenicol, gentamicin, and tetracycline.

Flavobacterium meningosepticum

Flavobacterium meningosepticum is the species of primary clinical importance in this genus. This microorganism is a long, thin, nonmotile, gram-negative bacillus. *Flavobacterium meningosepticum* is widely distributed in nature, and the hospital environment is frequently contaminated with this organism (see Table 4-4). It is most frequently associated with nosocomially acquired meningitis in neonates.

Flavobacterium meningosepticum is usually resistant to a wide range of antimicrobial agents and therapy must be based on susceptibility testing results.

Gardnerella vaginalis

Gardnerella vaginalis is frequently recovered from the female genitourinary tract and probably plays an etiologic role in *vaginitis* (see Table 4-4). A characteristic of vaginal infection with this microorganism is the presence of *"clue cells,"* which are vaginal epithelial cells covered with bacteria. This microorganism has also been reported to cause neonatal sepsis, postpartum bacteremia, and nonspecific urethritis.

Plesiomonas shigelloides

Plesiomonas shigelloides is a gram-negative, motile bacterium whose natural habitat is warm surface water and mud (see Table 4-4). It most frequently causes a self-limited gastroenteritis, although it has been reported as a cause of cellulitis and septicemia. This microorganism is sensitive to cephalosporins, aminoglycosides, imipenem, and ciprofloxacin.

Eikenella corrodens

Eikenella corrodens is a gram-negative rod that is a part of the normal flora of the mouth and upper respiratory tract as well as other mucosal surfaces of the human body (see Table 4-4). It is usually associated with infections involving the head and neck or abdominal area. However, hematogenous spread from these primary infection sites can lead to establishment of foci in other body sites. In addition, *E. corrodens* can cause infection following human bites.

Capnocytophaga

There are three species in this genus that infect humans: *C. ochracea, C. sputigena,* and *C. gingivalis.* These are gram-negative fusiform-shaped rods. They have been associated primarily with periodontal disease, but have also been identified as a cause of bacteremia in immunocompromised granulocytopenic patients (see Table 4-4).

Streptobacillus

Streptobacillus moniliformis is one cause of *rat-bite fever;* the other is *Spirillum minus* (see section on spirochetes). *Streptobacillus moniliformis* is a nonencapsulated, nonmotile, gram-negative, filamentous bacillus that is present as part of the normal flora of the nasopharynx of rats and other rodents (see Table 4-5). Rat-bite fever due to *Strep. moniliformis* is worldwide in occurrence, although it is associated primarily with poor or primitive living conditions with a large rat population. The disease is usually acquired by the bite of a rat or other rodent. However, it can be transmitted by milk, water, and food contaminated by rats.

An inflamed lesion commonly develops at the site of the bite, followed by an abrupt onset of chills, fever, vomiting, headache, and severe pain in the joints. A maculopapular rash frequently develops that involves the palms, soles, and extremities. Severe forms of the disease can lead to endocarditis, pneumonia, and multiple abscesses in many organ systems.

Diagnosis is made by isolation of *Strep. moniliformis* from the blood or joint fluids.

Penicillin is very effective in treating rat-bite fever caused by *Strep. moniliformis.*

Rochalimaea henselae

Cat-scratch fever is characterized by localized lymphadenopathy in a person who reports being in contact with or being scratched by a cat (see Table 4-5). Symptoms can also include skin or eye rashes and temporary blindness. *Rochalimaea henselae* is the most likely etiologic agent of this disease, although this is controversial. The disease is usually self-limited and no antibiotic therapy is recommended.

Enteric Bacteria

David J. Hentges

The enteric bacteria are gram-negative, nonsporulating, facultatively anaerobic rods that are present in the intestinal tracts of humans and many animals. Most of these bacteria belong to the family Enterobacteriaceae, although similar bacteria classified in other families are also considered to be enteric bacteria because of their intestinal habitat. Enteric bacteria are differentiated on the basis of DNA homology and cultural, biochemical, and antigenic characteristics. There are three major classes of antigens associated with these bacteria: the O or cell-wall antigens, the K or capsular antigens, and the H or flagellar antigens. The O-antigen complexes are located in the outer membrane of the cell walls of enteric bacteria (Fig. 4-6). They are lipopolysaccharide in composition. The O-specific side

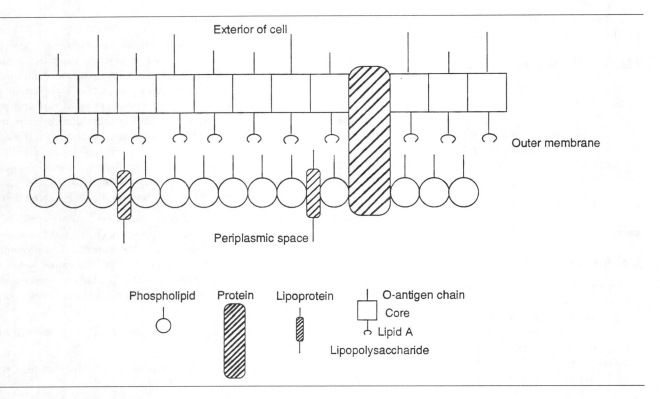

Fig. 4-6 Structure of the outer membrane of the cell wall of Enterobacteriaceae.

chains, which extend out from the surface of the cell walls, consist of polymers of repeating oligosaccharide units of three or four monosaccharides. O-antigenic variation among enteric bacteria is attributed to differences in sugar composition, sequence, linkage groups, and additional substituents of the repeating oligosaccharide units. The H antigens are proteins, and the K antigens are polysaccharides.

Endotoxin

The substance responsible for endoxicity of enteric bacteria is the lipid A component of the lipopolysaccharide, which can be cleaved from the core of the complex by mild acid hydrolysis (Fig. 4-6). Rough mutants of these bacteria lack O-specific side chains and may also lack a portion of the core. However, they do possess lipid A and therefore have endotoxic activity.

Infections

The majority of enteric bacteria are components of the indigenous intestinal flora and, under normal circumstances, do not produce disease in the intestinal tract. However, some enteric bacteria, which do not reside in the intestinal tract of healthy individuals, are capable of severe disease production if they gain entrance to and multiply in the intestine. They represent the intestinal pathogens, a second category of enteric bacteria, which are discussed in the next section. This section focuses on the indigenous flora components that produce a variety of infections in humans if displaced from their natural habitat. Extraintestinal infections produced by enteric bacteria include:

1. Urinary tract infections
2. Pneumonia
3. Wound infections
4. Bacteremia
5. Meningitis
6. Abscesses
7. Endocarditis

These infections are frequently hospital acquired. Between 40 and 50 percent of nosocomial infections are caused by enteric bacteria. The organisms are responsible for a majority of nosocomial urinary tract infections and a large percentage of bacteremias, respiratory tract infections, and surgical wound infections.

Escherichia coli

E. coli, the prime nosocomial pathogen, is a major cause of urinary tract infections and bacteremias. Since the intestinal tract is its only natural habitat, its presence in environmental samples is considered proof of fecal contamination. The identification of *E. coli* is based on colony morphology on differential and selective media, biochemical reactions, and serologic reactions to determine antigenicity. *Escherichia coli* strains characteristically ferment carbohydrates, including lactose, with the production of acid and gas. *E. coli* strains with K antigens 1, 2, 3, 5, 12, and 13 are found with high frequency in extraintestinal infections.

Other Coliform Organisms

The genera *Klebsiella, Enterobacter, Serratia,* and *Citrobacter* share biochemical properties in common with *E. coli* and, along with *E. coli,* are referred to as coliform organisms. Unlike *E. coli,* these organisms are widely distributed in nature and are isolated from soil, water, and food, as well as from the intestinal tract. Most of them ferment lactose. They have been incriminated in hospital-acquired infections, sometimes causing bacteremia and frequently infections complicating burns. They are also involved in infections following intravenous or urinary tract catheterization or respiratory tract manipulations such as tracheotomy or use of inhalation therapy equipment. One organism of this group, *Klebsiella pneumoniae,* which is heavily encapsulated, is responsible for severe respiratory tract infections in debilitated individuals.

Proteus

The genus *Proteus* and related organisms *Morganella morganii* and *Providencia rettgeri* (formerly classified as *Proteus morganii* and *Proteus rettgeri*) do not ferment lactose and are not considered to be coliform organisms. They possess the enzyme urease, which characterizes them and aids in their identification. Urea is hydrolyzed by this enzyme to produce carbon dioxide and ammonia. Ammonia production causes an increase in pH. Hydrolysis of urea in urine by one of these organisms during a urinary tract infection causes alkalinization and decreased solubility of calcium and magnesium phosphates. This leads to formation of stones, which trap bacteria and protect them from antimicrobials. The ammonia produced may also directly damage urinary tract epithelium. In addition to urinary tract infections, surgical wound infections, lower respiratory tract infections, and occasionally bacteremia are caused by these organisms.

Pseudomonas aeruginosa

P. aeruginosa is sometimes present in the intestinal tract of humans. It is grouped with the enteric bacteria, although it belongs to the family Pseudomonadaceae rather than Enterobacteriaceae. The genus *Pseudomonas* encompasses more than 140 species. Of medical importance, in addition to *P. aeruginosa,* are *Pseudomonas pseudomallei,* which causes melioidosis, and *Pseudomonas mallei,* which causes glanders. These diseases are uncommon, however. *Pseudomonas aeruginosa* seldom produces infection in healthy individuals, but poses a major threat to hospitalized patients with underlying diseases such as cystic fibrosis or cancer. Cancer patients, who are frequently immunocompromised and receive antimicrobial therapy prophylactically, are particularly prone to infections with antibiotic-resistant *P. aeruginosa.* Susceptible patients may develop pneumonia, urinary tract infections, bacteremia, and various localized infections following surgery or burns. *Pseudomonas aeruginosa* is also responsible for outbreaks of folliculitis (infection of hair follicles) in individuals who use hot tubs or whirlpool baths.

Pseudomonas aeruginosa is ubiquitous. Almost any site in the hospital environment may harbor the organism, especially if moisture is present, including sinks and taps, respirators, drinking vessels, and hospital food. The organism is a nonfermentative aerobe that derives its energy in the oxidation of organic compounds and therefore grows on the surface of liquid media as a pellicle. Most strains of *P. aeruginosa* produce characteristic blue-green pigments, pyocyanin, and fluorescein, which facilitate identification.

A variety of substances associated with *P. aeruginosa* contribute to its virulence. These include endotoxin, the polysaccharide slime layer, leukocidin, enzymes such as proteases and phospholipase C, and a specific toxin called exotoxin A. Exotoxin A blocks protein synthesis in eucaryotic cells by ribosylating and therefore inactivating elongation factor 2, which is required for translocation of polypeptidyl transfer RNA from acceptor to donor sites on the ribosome. *Pseudomonas aeruginosa* strains isolated from the respiratory tract of patients with cystic fibrosis produce colonies that are frequently very mucoid.

Intestinal Pathogens

David J. Hentges

The organisms that produce enteric diseases in humans gain entrance to the body by the oral route and multiply in the intestinal tract. Some of the pathogens produce enteric disease by excreting exotoxins (called enterotoxins because of the site of activity), while others are invasive, penetrating intestinal epithelial cells and passing into intestinal tissue and in some cases into other areas of the body (Table 4-7). A few enteric pathogens are both toxigenic and invasive.

Pathogenic Bacteriology

Table 4-7   Three Types of Intestinal
Infections Produced by Enteric Bacteria

Mechanism	Enterotoxin production	Superficial ulceration (mucosal)	Penetration (systemic)
Site of infection	Proximal small bowel	Distal small bowel or colon	Distal small bowel or colon
Illness	Watery diarrhea	Dysentery	Extraintestinal spread
Organisms responsible	*Vibrio cholerae*	*Shigella* species	*Salmonella* species
	Enterotoxigenic *Escherichia coli*	Enteroinvasive *E. coli* *Vibrio parahaemolyticus*	*Campylobacter jejuni* *Yersinia enterocolitica*

Toxigenic Enteric Pathogens

Vibrio cholerae

Vibrio cholerae is the classic toxigenic enteric pathogen. There are five species within the genus *Vibrio,* of which *V. cholerae* and *Vibrio parahaemolyticus* are the major pathogens. However, other vibrios, known variously as nonagglutinable vibrios or noncholera vibrios, are capable of producing diarrhea in humans and have been associated with limited outbreaks of disease. *Vibrio cholerae* is a gram-negative, slightly curved rod with polar flagella. It is divided into six serogroups, 0:1 through 0:6, and four biotypes. Two of the biotypes, classic and El Tor, which belong to serogroup 0:1, are responsible for the devastating epidemic disease known as cholera. Serogroup 0:1 is further divided into three serotypes called Ogawa (containing A and B antigens), Inaba (containing A and C antigens), and Hikojima (containing A, B, and C antigens). The organisms are quite tolerant of alkaline conditions and are therefore capable of multiplying in medium adjusted to pH 8.5.

Pathogenicity

Vibrio cholerae, which is ingested in contaminated food or water, becomes attached to the epithelial cells of the small bowel. There is no evidence of penetration or morphologic alteration of intestinal epithelium. The organisms excrete an enterotoxin (choleragen) that is a protein with a molecular weight of 84,000 consisting of two major regions designated A and B. Region A consists of two polypeptides, designated A_1 and A_2, that are linked by a single disulfide bond. Region B (choleragenoid), which consists of five associated peptides, is responsible for attachment of

the toxin molecule to the glycolipid $G_{M}1$ ganglioside receptor located on small-intestinal epithelial cell membranes. The A_1 peptide has the effect of stabilizing the membrane-bound enzyme, adenylate cyclase, in an active conformation. The enzyme is complexed with a regulatory protein and guanosine triphosphate (GTP). Limitation of enzymatic activity occurs naturally by hydrolysis of GTP, which inactivates the complex. The A_1 peptide produces its toxic effect by ribosylating the complex, which prevents hydrolysis of GTP and locks the enzyme in an active state leading to excessive production of cyclic AMP.

Clinical Manifestations

High concentrations of cyclic AMP cause a derangement of the cellular ion transport processes and a hypersecretion of chloride and bicarbonate ions and water into the lumen of the small intestine. The feces of cholera patients are nearly isotonic with their plasma. Accumulation of fluid in the intestine is responsible for the voluminous stool and the diarrhea that develop. Fluid loss can exceed 1 liter per hour. Accompanying the diarrhea is demineralization, acidosis, and extreme dehydration. The watery stools produced by the patients usually contain small bits of mucus, which give them a characteristic rice-water appearance.

Treatment

The most important immediate treatment of cholera is replacement of lost body fluids and electrolytes. This is accomplished by infusing a solution of NaCl, $NaHCO_3$, and KCl intravenously or by administering the solution orally and including glucose in the replacement fluid. Antimicrobials effectively eliminate *V. cholerae* from the feces of most patients but are not a substitute for adequate fluid and electrolyte replacement.

Epidemiology

Cholera is endemic in southeast Asia and from this focus spreads to other areas of the world from time to time. In 1991, cholera appeared in several coastal cities in Peru and spread rapidly because of poor sanitation and unsafe water supplies. Hundreds of thousands of cases have been reported in Central and South America and Mexico, but the mortality has been less than 1 percent because of the effective response of the medical community. Sporadic cases of cholera are reported in Europe and the United States, although a cholera epidemic has not occurred in the United States in more than 100 years.

Enterotoxigenic Escherichia coli

Some strains of *E. coli* are capable of producing enteric infections, although most strains are nonpathogenic commensals in the intestinal tract. Predominant among the intestinal pathogens is enterotoxigenic *E. coli* (ETEC), which causes diarrhea, which is usually less severe than in cholera, in all age groups. Infection is acquired by ingesting food or water contaminated with the organisms. Colonization of the surface of small-intestinal epithelial cells occurs as a result of the presence of fibriae on the bacteria. The fibriae have been given antigenic designations. Colonization factor antigens (CFA/I, CFA/II, and CFA/IV) are associated with strains responsible for human infections, K88 with strains specific for swine, and K99 with strain specific for lambs and calves. The organisms produce heat-labile and heat-stable enterotoxins, both of which produce diarrhea in the host. Heat-labile enterotoxin (LT) functions in the same way as cholera toxin, increasing adenylate cyclase activity with the resultant elevation of cellular cyclic AMP. Interestingly, LT shares antigenic determinants with cholera toxin. Heat-stable enterotoxin (ST), which is a low-molecular-weight, nonantigenic molecule, stimulates guanylate cyclase activity by increasing cellular levels of cyclic guanosine monophosphate (cyclic GMP).

Enterotoxin production by *E coli* is controlled by a transmissible plasmid that, theoretically, can infect any *E. coli* serotype and confer on it the ability to produce enterotoxin. A single plasmid can carry genes for both LT and ST production or for either alone.

Enteropathogenic Escherichia coli

E. coli strains that cause diarrheal disease in infants but do not produce LT and ST are designated enteropathogenic *E. coli* (EPEC). Their mechanism of disease production is not clearly understood, although examination of small-intestinal biopsies from infected infants revealed that the organisms adhere intimately to enterocytes, causing dissolution of microvilli and the cupping of enterocytes around the bacteria. EPEC are known to produce a cytotoxin that also has enterotoxic activity and there is some recent evidence that the organisms may invade enterocytes. Certain *E. coli* O serotypes, such as O55 and O111, are commonly associated with these infections.

Invasive Enteric Pathogens Capable of Systemic Spread

Salmonellae

Organisms of the genus *Salmonella* are capable of invading intestinal tissue and spreading to the other areas of the body. They are gram-negative, motile rods that fail to ferment lactose but do ferment glucose, with the production of acid and gas. They are H_2S positive. An important exception is *Salmonella typhi*, which produces acid but no gas from carbohydrate fermentation.

Because of its antigenic complexity, the genus *Salmonella* consists of more than 2000 serotypes, each of which is given a species designation by the traditional system of classification. A simplified system of classification, emphasizing ecologic features, designates only three species: *S. typhi*, *Salmonella choloraesuis*, and *Salmonella enteritidis*. By this system *S. typhi* and *S. choleraesuis* each consists of a single serotype, and all remaining serotypes are assigned to the species *S. enteritidis*. The most recent scheme, based on genetic studies, maintains that all salmonellae belong to a single species. The species, which is called *Salmonella enterica*, contains six subspecies that can be differentiated biochemically.

Salmonellae cause disease in a variety of animals as well as in humans. In humans, there are three clinically distinguishable types of infection: gastroenteritis, enteric fever, and septicemia. They all result from eating food or drinking water contaminated with large numbers of the organisms.

Gastroenteritis

By far, the most common type of disease produced by salmonellae in humans is gastroenteritis, which is a localized infection of the ileum and colon. Any salmonella can produce gastroenteritis, but in the United States it is most frequently caused by *Salmonella typhimurium*. Symptoms begin between 18 and 24 hours after eating contaminated food. Strains of salmonella are known to excrete an exotoxin that may function as an enterotoxin, but its role in the pathogenesis of enterocolitis has not been established. The organisms invade the intestinal epithelium and proliferate within the epithelial cells and lymphoid follicles. This leads to an acute inflammatory response that occasionally causes ulceration. The resulting enterocolitis is characterized by diarrhea, chills and fever, abdominal pain, and leukocytosis. As a rule, the infection is self-limiting, and spontaneous recovery occurs within 5 days.

Enteric Fever

Enteric fever is a far more severe type of infection than gastroenteritis because it features systemic as well as intestinal involvement. The prototype of enteric fever is typhoid fever caused by *S. typhi*. When the organisms are ingested in contaminated food or water, they penetrate the intestinal epithelium, spread to the mesenteric lymph nodes, and are disseminated throughout the body in the blood. Although they are removed by the reticuloendothelial system, they are capable of multiplying in macrophages, are released into the bloodstream, and frequently produce infections in various body organs, including the liver, spleen, bone marrow, and gallbladder. The organisms reinfect the intestinal tract from the gallbladder, localize in

Peyer's patches, and cause necrosis. Ulcerations in Peyer's patches frequently lead to intestinal hemorrhaging and sometimes bowel perforation. Spiking fever, enlarged spleen, leukopenia, and hemorrhages of the skin, "rose spots," are common symptoms. Although diarrhea is usually absent, abdominal tenderness and distention are common. The incubation period for the disease varies between 1 and 2 weeks.

Paratyphoid Fever

Enteric fever caused by salmonellae other than *S. typhi* is referred to as paratyphoid fever. The incubation period is shorter than for typhoid fever (1–10 days), and the disease is less severe. Organisms commonly responsible for paratyphoid fever in the United States include *Salmonella paratyphi B* and *S. typhimurium*.

Septicemia

Salmonella septicemia is similar to enteric fever in that it is a generalized infection involving the bloodstream and various body organs. However, the organisms do not affect the gastrointestinal tract and therefore are not isolated from the feces. *Salmonella choleraesuis* is most often responsible for this type of disease.

Transmission

Typhoid and other enteric fevers are exclusively human diseases and human carriers who have recovered from the infection and have contaminated food or water are the primary sources of infection. Other salmonellae are associated with animals. Because farm animals, such as cattle, swine, and poultry, frequently harbor the organisms, contaminated meat is the main vehicle of infection. Household pets may also be carriers, and eggs may contain salmonellae.

Prevention

Prevention of salmonellosis requires sanitary control during food preparation, rigid exclusion of salmonella carriers from occupations in which they handle food, and proper disposal of sewage so that it does not contaminate drinking water supplies. Thorough cooking of meat, pasteurization of milk, and water treatment are additional measures used to prevent transmission of salmonellae and other enteric pathogens. Two vaccine types are currently available for protection against typhoid fever. One consists of a suspension of heat-phenol inactivated *S. typhi* that is administered subcutaneously and the other a suspension of live attenuated *S. typhi* strain Ty 2/a, that is given orally.

Diagnosis

Diagnosis of salmonellosis is made by isolating the organisms from the patient's blood, feces, urine, or pus. The organisms are identified using biochemical tests, and identification is frequently confirmed by antigenic analysis with typing sera.

Treatment

Antimicrobials are not recommended for treatment of uncomplicated gastroenteritis because they do not shorten the duration of illness. However, enteric fevers and septicemia require antibiotic therapy. Chloramphenicol, ampicillin, and trimethoprim-sulfamethoxazole are effective.

Campylobacter jejuni

C. jejuni, a gram-negative microaerophilic curved rod, frequently causes diarrheal disease in humans. The organism resides naturally in the intestinal and reproductive tracts of mammals and birds. Excreta from these animals, contaminating soil, water, and food, are responsible for transmission of the organisms to humans. When the organisms are ingested, infection is produced in both the small and large intestines. Invasion of intestinal tissue occurs, resulting in an acute exudative and hemorrhagic inflammation. The major symptoms are fever; diarrhea, which may be liquid or bloody; and abdominal pain. In severe cases, colonic involvement, including infiltration of the lamina propria with white blood cells and crypt abscess formation, may occur. Bacteremia also develops in a few individuals, indicating that the infection is capable of spreading systemically. Some strains produce a cytotoxin and others an enterotoxin that is similar to *E. coli* LT and cholera toxin.

Definitive diagnosis is made by isolating the organisms from the feces. Fecal material is streaked on selective agar medium containing antibiotics to which *C. jejuni* is resistant, but most flora components are susceptible. Because *C. jejuni* is microaerophilic, cultures are incubated in an atmosphere of 5% oxygen, often at 42°C to provide greater selectivity.

Helicobacter pylori

H. pylori is a recently recognized pathogen that resembles *Campylobacter* species morphologically. It is responsible for chronic gastritis in humans and there is evidence that the organism also causes gastric and duodenal ulceration. *Helicobacter pylori* is actively motile, penetrates gastric mucus, and colonizes gastric epithelium, especially the intercellular junctions. It produces the enzyme urease, which is particularly important because it raises the pH of the immediate environment to approximately 6.5 and allows the organism to survive in a normally acidic ecosystem. The urea present in the stomach is converted to ammonia and carbon dioxide by this enzyme and the ammonia produced is cytotoxic to gastric epithelial cells.

The organism also causes a depletion of gastric mucus, allowing gastric acid to erode denuded mucosa. A combination of antibiotics and bismuth-containing preparations are prescribed to treat ulcers caused by this organism.

Yersinia enterocolitica

Y. enterocolitica produces an enteric disease in humans that is similar in most respects to the disease produced by *C. jejuni*. This tiny, gram-negative rod produces enteritis in animals. Upon recovery, the animals frequently remain healthy carriers, excreting the organisms in their feces, and humans become infected by consuming contaminated food or water. The organisms invade the mucosa of the ileum to produce fever, diarrhea, and abdominal pain. From here they may spread, involving regional lymph nodes and other organs of the body.

Enteric Pathogens that Produce Infections Confined to Intestinal Tissue

Shigella

Organisms of the genus *Shigella* are nonmotile, gram-negative rods that ferment glucose, with the production of acid but not gas, and fail to ferment lactose. They are H_2S negative. There are four species within the genus—*Shigella boydii, S. dysenteriae, S. flexneri,* and *S. sonnei*—that are subdivided into serotypes on the basis of O-antigenic differences.

Disease

All of the species are capable of producing bacillary dysentery in humans and other primates. Infection occurs as a result of consuming food or water contaminated with the organisms. Studies show that ingestion of fewer than 200 organisms can result in infection, and on this basis, they are considered to be the most effective of the enteric pathogens in causing human disease. This has been attributed to resistance to stomach acidity. *Shigella* species produce an exotoxin that has cytotoxic, neurotoxic, and enterotoxic properties, and is undoubtedly responsible for much of the pathology that occurs with the disease. *Shigella dysenteriae,* serotype 1, also known as Shiga's bacillus, produces greater quantities than other *Shigella* strains (hence the term *Shiga toxin*). Enterotoxic activity is manifest early in the course of the disease in the small bowel, causing diarrhea, whereas cytotoxic activity is manifest later in the course of the disease in the colon. Cytotoxicity is a consequence of inactivation, by the toxin, of the 60S ribosomal subunit in eucaryotic cells, thus interfering with peptide elongation and protein synthesis. *Shigella* penetrates mucosal epithelial cells of the colon and kills them. Organisms that reach the lamina propria are readily phagocytized and destroyed, so that lymph node involvement and bacteremia are rare. Colonic epithelial cell death results in superficial ulceration, bleeding, and an inflammatory response. The infected individual develops fever, experiences severe abdominal cramps and tenesmus, and has frequent stools. Dysenteric stools are scant and contain blood, mucus, and inflammatory cells.

Epidemiology

The most common source of *Shigella* infection is the human carrier who continues to excrete the organisms in the feces long after clinical recovery and who contaminates food and water. There are no important animal reservoirs. This disease is prevalent among closed population groups, especially if hygienic conditions are substandard. In the United States, outbreaks occur most often in prisons, mental hospitals, children's institutions, and Indian reservations. *Shigella sonnei* is isolated with greatest frequency from cases of dysentery in the developed countries of the world. Prevention includes sanitary procedures, which effectively exclude or eliminate the pathogens from food or drinking water.

Diagnosis

Blood, mucus, and clumps of neutrophils and macrophages are observed in the stools of infected individuals. Definitive diagnosis depends, however, on the isolation of the organisms from fecal material.

Treatment

Oral rehydration therapy is used to treat chronic diarrhea. When dysentery is severe, patients are treated with ampicillin or trimethoprim-sulfamethoxazole.

Invasive Escherichia coli

A disease that resembles bacillary dysentery in every respect is caused by *E. coli* strains belonging to *Shigella*-like serogroups. These strains do not produce enterotoxin but invade colonic epithelial cells, with resulting tissue destruction and dysentery. The disease is limited to impoverished populations living under unsanitary conditions and, therefore, rarely occurs in the United States.

Enterohemorrhagic Escherichia coli

E. coli strains responsible for hemorrhagic colitis and hemolytic-uremic syndrome (HUS), most notably 0157:H7, adhere to colonic mucosa, producing histopathologic lesions similar to those produced by EPEC in the small bowel. In the colon, the bacteria produce relatively large amounts of Shiga-like toxins (SLT), which are also called verotoxins (VT) because of their cytotoxic effect on Vero tissue culture cells that are derived from African green monkey kidney cells. The *E. coli* strains that produce the toxins are sometimes referred to as verotoxin-producing *E.*

Pathogenic Bacteriology

coli (VTEC) and sometimes as enterohemorrhagic *E. coli* (EHEC). One of the verotoxins, VT1 or SLT I, is almost identical with Shiga toxin and the other, VT2 or SLT II, has similar biologic properties to VT1, but is not neutralized by Shiga toxin antibody. The toxins cause hemorrhages in the colon, resulting in bloody diarrhea and low-grade fever. Infected individuals, particularly young children, may also develop HUS manifested by hemolytic anemia, thrombocytopenia, and acute renal failure. Outbreaks of hemorrhagic colitis have been traced to contaminated food, primarily hamburger meat, indicating that cattle are a common reservoir for EHEC.

Information about the types of enteric infections produced by *E. coli* strains is summarized in Table 4-8.

Table 4-8 *Escherichia coli* Strains that Produce Enteric Infections

Strain	Pathogenic mechanism	Site of infection	Disease
Enterotoxigenic *E. coli* (ETEC)	Enterotoxin production	Small bowel	Diarrhea
Enteropathogenic *E. coli* (EPEC)	Cytotoxin production	Small bowel	Diarrhea
Enteroinvasive *E. coli* (EIEC)	Enterocyte invasion	Colon	Dysentery
Enterohemorrhagic *E. coli* (EHEC or VTEC)	Cytotoxin (verotoxin) production	Colon	Hemorrhagic colitis; HUS

Vibrio Parahaemolyticus

V. parahaemolyticus causes two types of disease in humans. The most common is watery diarrhea, but dysentery involving the colon also occurs. There is evidence that some organisms invade intestinal tissue and others produce a cytotoxin. Additionally, a hemolysin is produced (Kanagawa phenomenon) but its role in the pathology of the disease has not yet been determined. *Vibrio parahaemolyticus* is a halophilic marine organism that inhabits saltwater estuaries around the world. Gastroenteritis usually follows ingestion of contaminated seafood that is insufficiently cooked. In Japan, the organism accounts for roughly one quarter of the reported cases of "food poisoning," although *V. parahaemolyticus* is also occasionally responsible for enteric infection in the United States, especially on the West Coast.

Mycobacteria

David C. Straus

General Properties

The genus *Mycobacterium* contains numerous species that can cause a wide variety of chronic infections in humans. The two most important diseases caused by the *Mycobacterium* are the chronic lung infections seen in tuberculosis and the disseminated infections seen in leprosy. The *Mycobacterium* causes these long-term (chronic) infections by virtue of its ability to survive inside normal macrophages. The hallmark of the members of this genus is the capacity to retain such dyes as carbol-fuchsin following decolorization with acidic alcohol. The cells of the genus are said to be "acid-fast." The term *acid-fastness* refers to the fact that when the carbol-fuchsin stain is fixed in the cell by heat or chemical reaction, it cannot be eluted by acidic ethanol (95% ethanol and 3% HCl).

Mycobacteria are acid-fast because they contain large amounts of lipid in their cell walls. In fact, the most striking chemical feature of mycobacteria is their extraordinarily high cell-wall lipid content, which comprises 60 percent of the cell-wall dry weight. This lipid-rich cell wall accounts for their relative impermeability to stains, their acid fastness, their unusual resistance to killing by alkali and acid, and their resistance to the bactericidal activity of antibody and complement. Mycobacteria cannot be Gram stained but are considered gram-positive because of their cell-envelope structure. They are obligate aerobes that grow extremely slowly. For example, *M. tuberculosis* has a generation time of 6 to 12 hours. Slow growth has been attributed to the time required to synthesize the lipids present in their cell wall.

Because mycobacteria are obligate aerobes, they form a surface pellicle when growing in vitro that resembles a mold and accounts for their name.

Tuberculosis (TB)

The causative agent of TB is *Mycobacterium tuberculosis*. The tubercle bacilli are slightly bent or curved slender rods (2–4 μm long and 0.2–0.5 μm wide). *Mycobacterium tuberculosis* strains either grow as discrete rods or as aggregating, long arrangements, called serpentine cords. Virulent strains tend to grow on the surface of liquid or on solid media as intertwining serpentine cords in which the bacilli aggregate with their long axes parallel.

The Disease

There are an estimated 8 to 10 million new cases of tuberculosis in the world each year with about 3 million deaths. The annual incidence in the United States is 9.4 cases per 100,000. This, unfortunately, is increasing (Table 4-9), with no end in sight. The consequences of inhaling or ingesting tubercle bacilli depend on the size of the inoc-

Table 4-9 Factors Responsible for
the Increasing Incidence of TB in the United States

Acquired immunodeficiency syndrome

Increased immigration from countries where TB is common

An increase in the homeless population

An increased population in long-term-care facilities (prisons, nursing homes)

An increase in indigent populations

Occurrence of antibiotic-resistant strains of *Mycobacterium tuberculosis*

ulum, the virulence of the organism, and the resistance of the host. Humans exhibit a wide range of responses. Initial exposure in a tuberculin-negative individual most often results in a self-limiting lesion. However, in some cases (presumably because of low host resistance or a large inoculum) the disease progresses rapidly. After inhalation of tubercle bacilli, the initial lesion appears as an area of nonspecific pneumonitis, usually located in a well-aerated peripheral zone. It is only after delayed-type hypersensitivity (DTH) develops (2–4 weeks) that granulomatous inflammation intervenes and the characteristic tubercles (small lumps containing phagocytic cells) are formed. Tubercle bacilli are also carried to the draining lymph nodes and then (by way of the blood and lymph) throughout the body. The next stage consists of a caseous lesion that heals by fibrosis and calcification, which may result in extensive scar formation. The healed and frequently calcified primary complex lesions are referred to as the Ghon complex. Most TB in adults is due to reactivation of long-dormant foci remaining from the primary infection. Disseminated (miliary) TB may develop after the rupture of a caseous lesion into a pulmonary vein. Although most cases of tuberculosis are caused by *M. tuberculosis*, two additional species, *M. bovis* and *M. africanum*, can cause tuberculosis in humans.

Mycobacterium tuberculosis
Virulence Factors

M. tuberculosis does not produce exotoxins or endotoxins. The three most important virulence factors possessed by the organism are (1) ability to survive inside normal macrophages, (2) cord factor formation, and (3) sulfatide production. Cord factor is a mycoside (trehalose-6, 6'-dimycolate). The tendency to grow in cords is a function of the amount of cord factor the organism contains. Cord factor itself is toxic. Sulfatides are sulfur-containing glycolipids. Although not toxic in themselves, they enhance the survival of *M. tuberculosis* in normal macrophages by preventing phagolysosome formation, so that the organisms avoid enzymatic destruction.

Immune Response to Infection

Serum antibodies do not play a role in immunity against *M. tuberculosis*. Though macrophages of normal animals permit ingested tubercle bacilli to survive, macrophages from tuberculous animals destroy them. This is due to an increased number of lysosomes. While the enhanced activity of the altered (activated) macrophages is nonspecific, its induction is immunologically specific. These macrophages will kill all other bacteria at an accelerated rate, but only *M. tuberculosis* antigens will activate them.

Laboratory Diagnosis

A provisional diagnosis of TB is usually made by demonstrating acid-fast bacilli in stained sputum smears or gastric washings that contain swallowed sputum. Whether or not the smear is positive, the material is cultured on Löwenstein-Jensen media because cultivation can detect fewer organisms than staining and culture characteristics distinguish human tubercle bacilli from other acid-fast bacilli. A DTH test for *M. tuberculosis* antigens is also used in diagnosis. It is called the tuberculin test. DTH to tuberculin is highly specific for the tubercle bacillus. Purified protein derivative (PPD) from *M. tuberculosis* is injected intradermally into the superficial layers of the forearm (Mantoux test). The average diameter of induration at the injected site is measured at 48 hours. Reactivity occurs about one month after infection and usually persists for life. Thus, a positive test reveals previous mycobacterial infection but it does not establish the presence of an active infection.

Therapy

In 1945, streptomycin was first used to treat tuberculosis. The value of this antibiotic is restricted by its toxicity to the eighth cranial nerve on prolonged administration as well as by the frequent emergence of streptomycin-resistant tubercle bacilli during therapy. In an effort to circumvent the emergence of drug-resistant strains, rifampin and isoniazid are used in combination, but, unfortunately, drug-resistant *M. tuberculosis* strains continue to appear. A vaccine, consisting of a living, attenuated bovine strain called the bacillus of Calmette and Guérin (BCG), is currently available for protection against TB. The vaccine is about 60 to 80 percent effective and is commonly used in Europe. In the United States, where the general populace is at relatively low risk, BCG vaccination is not performed.

Mycobacteria Associated with Nontuberculosis Infections

A wide variety of diseases are caused by the nontuberculosis *Mycobacterium*. The diseases produced by this organism have pathologic and clinical similarities to TB, but important differences exist. The most common manifestation is pulmonary disease, which is seen primarily in elderly white men with emphysema and bronchitis. *Mycobacterium kansasii* and organisms of the *M. avium, intracellulare,* and *fortuitum* groups are frequently responsible for this type of infection.

Leprosy

Leprosy is caused by *Mycobacterium leprae* and is also called Hansen's disease after its discoverer. There are currently 12 million cases in the world, with about 4000 cases in the United States. *Mycobacterium leprae* is virtually indistinguishable in morphology and staining properties from *M. tuberculosis.* Similar to *M. tuberculosis,* it can also survive inside normal macrophages. *Mycobacterium leprae* has never been cultivated in vitro, whereas *M. tuberculosis* is easily grown in the laboratory.

Pathogenesis

Mycobacterium leprae causes chronic granulomatous lesions that closely resemble those of TB. The organisms are primarily intracellular and can evidently proliferate inside macrophages. Leprosy is distinguished by its chronic slow progress and by its mutilating and disfiguring lesions. The organism has a predilection for skin and nerve. In the cutaneous form of the disease, large firm nodules (lepromas) are widely distributed. In the neural form, segments of peripheral nerves are involved, leading to localized patches of anesthesia. The loss of sensation in fingers and toes increases the frequency of minor trauma, leading to secondary infections and mutilating injury. Leprosy occurs as either lepromatous or tuberculoid leprosy. Lepromatous leprosy is progressive and the prognosis is poor. Tuberculoid leprosy is the healing phase and the prognosis is better.

Diagnosis, Treatment, and Epidemiology

Diagnosis is accomplished by demonstrating acid-fast bacilli in scrapings from ulcerated lesions. Therapy with dapsone (diaminodiphenylsulfone) usually produces a gradual improvement over several years. However, resistance to dapsone may occur. Rifampin and clofazimine are promising new agents. Genetic factors have been shown to contribute considerably to the striking individual differences in susceptibility and type of response to infection with *M. leprae.* There is evidence for the existence of a gene that predisposes one to tuberculoid leprosy that is linked to the HLA complex. Finally, contrary to popular belief, leprosy is not highly contagious. It is transmitted only when exudates of mucous membrane lesions and

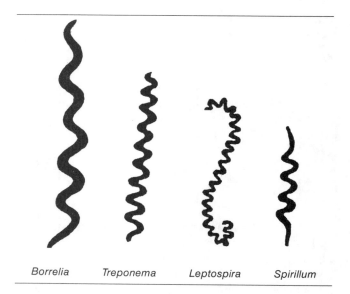

Fig. 4-7 Comparative morphology of spirochetes.

skin ulcers contaminate skin abrasions in uninfected individuals.

Spirochetes

Rial D. Rolfe

The spirochetes are heterogeneous group of actively motile, *spiral-shaped* organisms (Fig. 4-7). Four genera of spirochetes are pathogenic for humans: (1) *Treponema,* which causes syphilis and the nonvenereal treponematoses; (2) *Borrelia,* which causes epidemic relapsing fever, Lyme disease, and fusospirochetosis; (3) *Leptospira,* which causes leptospirosis; and (4) *Spirillum,* which is one cause of rat-bite fever.

Treponema

The genus *Treponema* includes species that are pathogenic for humans as well as nonpathogenic species that are components of the normal intestinal flora. The pathogenic treponemas include the human pathogens that cause syphilis (*Treponema pallidum* subspecies *pallidum*), yaws (*Treponema pallidum* subspecies *pertenue*), pinta (*Treponema pallidum* subspecies *carateum*), and bejel (*Treponema pallidum* subspecies *endemicum*). Naturally occurring infection by pathogenic treponema is limited to humans. The pathogenic treponemas are morphologically and immunologically indistinguishable. However, the disease manifestations they produce in humans are clinically distinct (Table 4-10). None of the pathogenic treponemas have been cultured on artificial media.

Table 4-10 Differentiation of the Treponematoses

	Venereal Syphilis	Yaws	Pinta	Bejel
Causative organism	*Treponema pallidum* subspecies *pallidum*	*Treponema pallidum* subspecies *pertenue*	*Treponema pallidum* subspecies *carateum*	*Treponema pallidum* subspecies *endemicum*
Mode of transmission	Sexual Congenital	Skin to skin	Skin to skin	Skin to skin Mouth to mouth
Usual age of onset	Adolescent Adult	Childhood	Childhood	Childhood
Primary lesion	Genital chancre	Skin lesion	Skin lesion	Skin lesion Oral lesion
Secondary lesion	Skin lesion	Skin lesion Bone lesion	Skin lesion	Mucous membrane lesion
Tertiary lesion	Gumma	Skin lesion Gumma	Skin lesion	Gumma

Treponema pallidum Subspecies *pallidum* (Syphilis)

Epidemiology

Treponema pallidum subspecies *pallidum* is distributed worldwide and occurs in epidemic proportion in virtually every country. The majority of cases of syphilis are transmitted *venereally,* and the primary lesion is usually found on the skin or mucous membranes of the genitalia.

In addition to transmission by venereal contact, *T. pallidum* subspecies *pallidum* can be acquired in utero, following passage of treponemas through the placenta, or the neonate may become infected as it passes through the birth canal. This is known as *congenital syphilis.* Neonatal infection can result in premature birth, stillbirth, neonatal death, neonatal disease, or latent infection.

Clinical Manifestations

Treponema pallidum subspecies *pallidum* infects almost every tissue of the body, resulting in a wide variety of clinical manifestations. The natural course of syphilis is complex and is arbitrarily divided into the following stages.

Incubation and Primary Stage. *Treponema pallidum* subspecies *pallidum* multiplies at the site of entry into the host and after about 3 weeks produces an inflammatory *chancre* at the site of inoculation. In men, the initial chancre is usually present on the penis, where it is readily detected. In women, the chancre is most commonly located in the perineal region or on the labia, vaginal wall, or cervix. Therefore, the chancre frequently goes unnoticed in women. The chancre causes little pain or discharge unless secondarily infected. Approximately 10 percent of chancres are extragenital, usually in or around the mouth. Soon after *T. pallidum* gains entrance into the host, the

spirochetes migrate through the lymphatics to the regional lymph nodes and then enter the bloodstream.

Primary Latent Period. The chancre heals spontaneously in 3 to 6 weeks, and the patient does not display any symptoms of disease for the next 4 to 8 weeks.

Secondary Stage (Stage of Systemic Involvement). *Secondary syphilis* is the most florid stage of the disease and occurs 2 to 10 weeks after the chancre heals. The most common manifestation of secondary syphilis is a generalized *skin rash,* which usually occurs on the trunk and proximal extremities, although any surface of the body may be involved, including the palms and soles. Both the primary chancre and secondary lesions contain large numbers of spirochetes and are highly infectious when located on exposed surfaces. The secondary lesions of syphilis subside spontaneously. Approximately one third of patients will progress to cure without treatment. In the remaining patients an asymptomatic stage called latent syphilis develops.

Latent Syphilis. During this stage of *subclinical* infection, the disease can only be detected serologically. Approximately one half of syphilitic patients never develop more severe clinical manifestations, and the latent stage either lasts a lifetime or progresses spontaneously to complete cure. The remaining patients develop clinical manifestations of tertiary syphilis, a slowly progressive inflammatory disease that can affect virtually any organ of the body.

Tertiary Syphilis. *Tertiary syphilis* can occur years after the primary infection. The most characteristic lesion of tertiary syphilis is the destructive *gumma* that most frequently involves the skin, liver, bones, and spleen. The gumma is a nonspecific granulomatous lesion. *Treponema pallidum* subspecies *pallidum* also has a predilection for infecting the *cardiovascular* and *central nervous systems.* Aortitis and aortic valve insufficiency are the most frequent clinical manifestations of syphilitic cardiovascular disease. *Treponema pallidum* subspecies *pallidum* infection of the central nervous system can be either asymptomatic or symptomatic. Symptomatic neurosyphilis encompasses three different clinical manifestations: (1) *meningovascular syphilis* (syphilitic meningitis); (2) *tabes dorsalis,* which is characterized by muscular incoordination and sensory disturbances; and (3) *general paresis,* which is characterized by progressive mental deterioration, insanity, and generalized paralysis, terminating in death.

Diagnosis

None of the pathogenic treponemas can be cultured in vitro. However, there are two important approaches to the diagnosis of syphilis. The first is direct *microscopic* demonstration of *T. pallidum* subspecies *pallidum* in exudate of chancres or secondary lesions, and the second diagnostic approach is the detection of antibody. The transverse diameter of all pathogenic treponemas is below the resolution of ordinary light microscopy, but can be visualized by *dark-field* microscopy or by staining with special reagents that are deposited on the cell's surface.

There are two types of serologic tests for syphilis: the *nonspecific nontreponemal reaginic antibody tests* and the *specific antitreponemal antibody tests.*

Nonspecific Nontreponemal Reaginic Antibody Tests.

Treponema pallidum subspecies *pallidum* infection results in the development of distinct antibodies (IgG and IgM) called *reagin.* Syphilitic reagin is different from the reagin antibody *(IgE)* involved in allergy. Reagin can be detected using complement fixation and flocculation tests with aqueous suspensions of lipids extracted from normal mammalian tissues (e.g., *cardiolipin* extracted from the heart muscle of an ox). Examples of nontreponemal tests include the Venereal Disease Research Laboratory *(VDRL)* test and the rapid plasma reagin *(RPR)* card test. Biologic *false-positive* reactions occur in nonsyphilitic individuals with a variety of diseases, including malaria, infectious mononucleosis, lupus erythematosus, and other spirochetal illnesses, such as yaws, pinta, bejel, leptospirosis, and rat-bite fever. The reaginic antibody tests are used for *screening* large numbers of sera and for following the *course of treatment.* Reagin usually disappears following adequate treatment.

Specific Antitreponemal Antibody Tests.

The other group of serologic tests detect antibody to *T. pallidum* subspecies *pallidum* antigens. The fluorescent treponemal-antibody absorption *(FTA-ABS)* test is an indirect immunofluorescent antibody test using *T. pallidum* subspecies *pallidum* harvested from rabbit testes as the antigen. The *T. pallidum* subspecies *pallidum* immobilization *(TPI)* test determines the ability of syphilitic serum to block or interfere with the motility of *T. pallidum* subspecies *pallidum*. *Treponema pallidum* subspecies *pallidum* agglutination has been used extensively to demonstrate antibody against specific antigens. Specific antitreponemal antibody tests are used to *confirm* a positive reagin test since false-positive reactions occur less commonly with these specific tests. Specific antitreponemal antibody also appears faster in serum following onset of infection as compared to reaginic antibody and remains *positive* after adequate treatment.

Treatment

Penicillin is the antibody of choice in the treatment of syphilis. Erythromycin or tetracycline can be used therapeutically in patients who are allergic to penicillin. Some patients will develop a systemic reaction consisting of headache, malaise, and fever following initial treatment. This is called the *Jarisch-Herxheimer* reaction, is self-limited, and does not affect the course of recovery.

A certain degree of immunity develops during or after infection with *T. pallidum* subspecies *pallidum*. However, protection is only relative and unreliable.

Nonvenereal Treponematoses

Epidemiology

The nonvenereal treponematoses are a group of contagious diseases endemic among rural populations of tropical and subtropical countries. The etiologic agents of these diseases are *T. pallidum* subspecies *pertenue* (yaws), *T. pallidum* subspecies *carateum* (pinta), and *T. pallidum* subspecies *endemicum* (bejel). There are no immunologic differences between the spirochetes of venereal syphilis and the spirochetes of the nonvenereal treponematoses; all four diseases give positive nonspecific and specific serologic tests for syphilis. Differences in *geographic* locations and *clinical manifestations* permit separation of the species (Table 4-10). The nonvenereal treponematoses are commonly transmitted when traumatized skin comes in contact with infectious exudate from primary or secondary lesions. Bejel may also be transmitted by inanimate objects (e.g., eating utensils, toothpicks, tobacco pipes) that come in contact with infectious mucosal lesions. All three diseases occur primarily in *children* and *adolescents.*

Clinical Manifestations

These three diseases are characterized by self-limiting primary and secondary lesions that are followed by tertiary lesions. An inflammatory superficial lesion develops at the site of inoculation and the bloodstream is invaded shortly after the initial infection. Superficial satellite lesions frequently develop as a result of bacteremia. In pinta, the initial lesion may also spread peripherally to form a squamous, erythematous patch. Yaws and bejel may pass through a latent phase before the appearance of tertiary lesions. The usual sites of tertiary lesions are the skin in pinta, the skin and bones in yaws, and the skin, bones, and mucous membranes in bejel.

Diagnosis

The methods used in the diagnosis of nonvenereal treponematoses are similar to the methods used in the diagnosis of syphilis. All the serologic tests for venereal syphilis become positive in the nonvenereal treponematoses.

Treatment

All the nonvenereal treponemas can be successfully treated with *penicillin,* tetracycline, or chloramphenicol.

Borrelia

Relapsing Fever

Epidemiology

Relapsing fever is an acute infectious disease caused by several species in the genus *Borrelia.* This disease is characterized clinically by an initial period of febrile illness followed by apparent recovery and successive relapses of fever. *Borrelia hermsii* and several other borreliae produce a natural infection of rodents and small animals (e.g., ground squirrels and prairie dogs) and this constitutes the natural reservoir of infection for humans. Humans usually acquire infection by the bite of an infected *insect vector.* *Tick-borne relapsing fever* is transmitted to humans by ticks that feed on the blood of infected animals. The *Borrelia* organisms rapidly multiply and invade all tissues of the tick. *Borrelia* persists for long periods in the tick and may be transmitted transovarially from generation to generation. Humans are infected when *Borrelia* organisms are released from the tick upon biting a human host. The tickborne disease occurs *endemically. Louse-borne relapsing fever* usually occurs in epidemics and is transmitted from person to person by the *human body louse. Borrelia recurrentis* is the causative agent of louse-borne relapsing fever. The spirochetes multiply in the hemolymph of a louse after ingestion of infected human blood. Transmission of louseborne fever occurs when the louse is crushed on a susceptible host, resulting in the release of infective organisms capable of penetrating intact skin or mucous membranes.

Clinical Manifestations

After *Borrelia* is introduced into the bloodstream, there is an incubation period of 3 to 10 days, followed by a sudden onset of fever, chills, headaches, and multiple organ dys-

function. The fever then declines, and an *afebrile period* lasting from 4 to 10 days is then followed by another attack of chills and fever. Successive *febrile relapses* occur at intervals of 2 to 14 days and are usually shorter in duration and less severe. During the febrile stages of the disease, the organisms are present in the blood, whereas they are absent during the afebrile periods.

Borrelia displays a high degree of *antigenic variation,* which is responsible for the relapsing course of the disease. During afebrile periods, the spirochetes are sequestered in internal organs and reemerge antigenically modified during the subsequent febrile period. The host must elaborate new circulating antibodies during each interval, and the appearance of these antibodies corresponds with clinical improvement and disappearance of the spirochetes from the blood.

Diagnosis

Borrelia cannot be readily cultured on artificial media. Therefore, the diagnosis of relapsing fever is usually made by microscopic examination of blood samples obtained during febrile periods. *Borrelia* is the *largest* of the pathogenic spirochetes and is easily identified in Giemsa's or Wright's stained smears of peripheral blood or by darkfield examination (Fig. 4-7).

Serologic tests are of little value in the diagnosis of this disease because of the antigenic variation of *Borrelia.* Approximately 10 percent of patients with relapsing fever display positive serologic tests for syphilis.

Treatment

Relapsing fever responds well to treatment with *penicillin* or tetracycline.

Lyme Disease

Epidemiology and Clinical Manifestations

Borrelia burgdorferi, a newly recognized species of *Borrelia,* is the causative agent of Lyme disease. In the United States mice and deer are the major reservoirs for this microorganism, which is transmitted by a *tick bite.*

The clinical disease commonly presents as three consecutive stages of illness. In the initial stage there is fever, severe headache, myalgia, stiff neck, and a typical skin lesion. The skin lesion *(erythema chronicum migrans)* gradually expands, usually shows a papule at the site of the tick bite, and has sharply demarcated borders. If left untreated, approximately 5 to 15 percent of patients develop the next stage of the disease, which is characterized by the onset of neurologic and cardiac involvement. The third stage of the disease primarily involves migrating episodes of arthritis.

Diagnosis

Lyme disease can be diagnosed serologically by indirect immunofluorescence or enzyme-linked immunosorbent assay (ELISA) tests for antibody.

Treatment

The treatment of choice is either penicillin or tetracycline. However, patients with the later stages of the disease frequently continue to have signs and symptoms despite antimicrobial therapy.

Fusospirochetosis

Epidemiology and Clinical Manifestations

Fusospirochetosis is a disease of the oral cavity that occurs when a normal spirochete of the mouth, *Borrelia vincentii*, and a gram-negative anaerobic bacillus, *Fusobacterium fusiforme*, find suitable conditions to increase in numbers. Conditions that predispose an individual to fusospirochetosis include injury to the mouth and decreased resistance, as with malnutrition, viral infection, or poor oral hygiene. These two organisms act *synergistically* in the production of oral suppurative infections.

Ulcerative gingivostomatitis ("trench mouth") is one form of fusospirochetal disease. Another form is *Vincent's angina,* an acute ulcerating disease of the oropharynx.

Diagnosis

Fusospirochetal organisms can be readily identified in a stained smear of exudate from suppurative lesions.

Treatment

Treatment of fusospirochetosis is twofold. First, antimicrobial agents are administered to inhibit the fusospirochetal flora. Second, the initial cause of tissue breakdown (e.g., malnutrition) is eliminated.

Leptospira

Epidemiology

Leptospirosis is an acute febrile disease caused by spirochetes in the genus *Leptospira*. The leptospiras are the smallest of the pathogenic spirochetes, and one or both ends of the cell are typically bent to form a *hook* (Fig. 4-7). There are only two species of *Leptospira: L. interrogans,* the pathogenic leptospira, and *L. biflexa,* the nonpathogenic leptospira. Antigenically distinct strains of *L. interrogans* are further classified into numerous serogroups and serotypes. Leptospiras are primarily animal pathogens and humans are infected through direct or indirect contact with

these animals. Person-to-person transmission is rare. In most of the world, infected rats are the common source of human infection, but in the United States, dogs are the important reservoir. Leptospira infection in animals is chronic and the microorganisms localize in the tissues and organs, especially the *kidneys,* where they are excreted profusely in the urine. Human infection is acquired by direct contact with infectious urine, with water and soil contaminated with infectious urine, or with infectious tissues. Leptospiras enter the body through abrasions in the skin or through the mucosal surfaces of the gastrointestinal tract. Especially vulnerable to disease are workers in rat-infested slaughterhouses, miners, farmers, veterinarians and sewage-disposal workers. Commonly used terms for leptospirosis include swineherd's disease, Fort Bragg fever, pretibial fever, Weil's disease, canicola fever, and autumnal fever.

Clinical Manifestations

After leptospiras penetrate the skin or mucous membranes, there is an incubation period of 1 to 2 weeks before onset of symptoms. A local lesion at the site of entry does not develop. During the incubation period, the organisms enter the bloodstream and are rapidly disseminated to all parts of the body. Leptospiras usually infect the kidneys. *Anicteric leptospirosis,* the most common and mild form of disease, is characterized by an abrupt onset of high fever, muscular pain, conjunctivitis, nausea, and aseptic meningitis. The most severe form of disease, referred to as *icteric leptospirosis* (also *Weil's disease* or *infectious jaundice*), is characterized by impaired renal and hepatic function, hemorrhage and necrosis of tissue, vascular collapse, and high mortality.

Recovery from leptospirosis is slow but is followed by lasting serotype-specific immunity.

Diagnosis

The laboratory diagnosis of leptospirosis is based on demonstration of the organism in clinical specimens and on the immune response to infection. Dark-field microscopic examination can be used to observe the distinctive morphology of leptospiras in blood, urine, or spinal fluid. However, direct demonstration of leptospira is successful in only a small portion of cases. Unlike other pathogenic spirochetes, leptospiras can be readily grown on a variety of *artificial media*. During the first week of the disease, *Leptospira* can be readily cultured from the blood or cerebrospinal fluid. Thereafter, it is shed intermittently in the urine. The immune response to infection can be assayed by agglutination, complement-dependent lysis, or complement-fixation tests.

Table 4-11   Incidence of Anaerobes as Normal Flora in Humans

| Location | *Clostridium* | Nonsporulating Bacilli | | Cocci | |
		Gram-Positive	Gram-Negative	Gram-Positive	Gram-Negative
Skin	−	+ +	−	+	−
Upper respiratory tract	−	+	+	+	+
Mouth	+ / −	+	+ +	+ +	+ +
Intestine	+ +	+ +	+ +	+ +	+
External genitalia	−	+ / −	+	+	−
Urethra	+ / −	+ / −	+	+	−
Vagina	+ / −	+ +	+	+	+

Key: − not found or rare; + usually present; + + usually present in large numbers; + / − irregularly present.

Treatment

In general, antimicrobial therapy of leptospirosis is disappointing unless initiated during the first 2 days after onset. Penicillin, streptomycin, tetracycline, and the macrolide antibiotics are active against *Leptospira*.

Spirillum

There are two completely different etiologic agents of rat-bite fever: *Spirillum minus*, a gram-negative, spiral-shaped organism, and *Streptobacillus moniliformis*, a gram-negative filamentous bacillus (see section on misc. gram-negative bacilli). *Rat-bite fever* due to *S. minus* is worldwide in distribution. The microorganism is transmitted to humans by the bite of a rat or other rodent. *Spirillum minus* is part of the normal oropharyngeal flora of rodents. After an incubation period of 5 to 14 days, an inflamed lesion develops at the site of the bite. This is accompanied by lymphadenopathy, erythematous skin rash radiating from the wound, and fever. In untreated cases the fever may be relapsing and persist for weeks or months. The most serious complication is subacute bacterial endocarditis.

Spirillum minus has not been cultured on artificial media, and diagnosis depends on microscopic demonstration of the organism in lesions, lymph nodes, or blood with phase contrast microscopy or with Giemsa's or Wright's stains.

Penicillin and streptomycin are both effective therapeutically in treating rat-bite fever due to *S. minus*.

Anaerobic Bacteria

Rial D. Rolfe

Obligate anaerobes are bacteria that require a very low oxygen tension for growth; they do not grow in the presence of atmospheric oxygen or in air that has been enriched with carbon dioxide. The reduction of oxygen by aerobic and anaerobic bacteria results in the production of several toxic compounds (e.g., hydrogen peroxide, superoxide radical, hydroxyl radical). Anaerobic bacteria do not contain or contain only low concentrations of enzymes (e.g., *superoxide dismutase, catalase, peroxidase*) that are present in aerobic or facultative bacteria to eliminate these toxic compounds. Anaerobic bacteria differ dramatically in their susceptibility to oxygen toxicity; some anaerobic bacteria can grow slowly in 20% oxygen while others can only grow in an atmosphere with less than 0.02% oxygen.

Epidemiology

Anaerobic bacteria are prevalent as *normal flora* components throughout the human body, particularly in such sites as the intestinal and genitourinary tracts, oropharynx, and skin (Table 4-11). In the large intestine, anaerobic bacteria outnumber facultative bacteria by a factor of 1000 : 1. Most anaerobic bacteria are not primary pathogens but are normal flora components that have managed, when they produce infections, to breach the barrier of the mucous membranes. Therefore, most anaerobic infections arise in proximity to the mucosal surfaces the bacteria normally colonize. Certain conditions, which lower *oxygen concentration*, favor the proliferation of anaerobic bacteria in tissue. These conditions include compromised blood supply, tissue necrosis, or antecedent infection by aerobic or facultative bacteria. Another characteristic of infections involving anaerobic bacteria is that the flora at the infected site is frequently *polymicrobial*, containing multiple mixed species of anaerobic and/or anaerobic plus aerobic bacteria.

Anaerobic bacteria may participate in all types of infections and may involve any organ or tissue of the body. In many types of infections, such as intraabdominal abscess, aspiration pneumonia, and brain abscess, anaerobes are the

Pathogenic Bacteriology

main etiologic agents. Anaerobes account for approximately 15 percent of all clinically significant blood culture isolates. Other infections, such as septic arthritis, meningitis, and endocarditis, are seldom caused by anaerobic bacteria.

Pathogenic Mechanisms

A number of factors determine the pathogenicity of anaerobic bacteria. The *exotoxins* produced by clostridia are largely responsible for the nature of the local lesions and the systemic manifestations caused by these bacteria. Several anaerobic bacteria produce extracellular and membrane-associated *enzymes* that contribute to their pathogenicity. These enzymes include lecithinases, collagenases, proteases, hyaluronidases, deoxyribonucleases, neuraminidases, and lipases. The gram-negative anaerobic bacilli also possess *endotoxin* that varies in potency from species to species. Some gram-negative anaerobic bacteria elaborate a polysaccharide *capsule* external to the outer membrane. This capsule functions as a virulence factor by promoting abscess formation and resistance to killing by polymorphonuclear leukocytes.

Characteristics of Anaerobic Bacteria

Anaerobic bacteria are represented by all morphologic types. However, of the hundreds of species that inhabit the mucosal surfaces of humans, only a relatively small number are actually involved in infection (Table 4-12).

Table 4-12   Major Genera of
Clinically Important Anaerobic Bacteria

Gram-negative bacilli
   Bacteroides
   Porphyromonas
   Prevotella
   Fusobacterium
Gram-positive, sporeforming bacilli
   Clostridium
Gram-positive, nonsporeforming bacilli
   Actinomyces
   Bifidobacterium
   Propionibacterium
   Eubacterium
   Morbiluncus
   Lactobacillus
Gram-positive cocci
   Peptostreptococcus
   Gemella
Gram-negative cocci
   Veillonella

Gram-Negative Bacilli

The gram-negative anaerobic bacilli of medical importance are included in the genera *Bacteroides*, *Porphyromonas*, *Prevotella*, and *Fusobacterium*. The genus *Bacteroides* comprises a heterogenous group of pleomorphic bacilli that are normal inhabitants of the respiratory, genital, and intestinal tracts. *Bacteroides fragilis* is the anaerobic microorganism most often isolated from infections and is more *resistant* to antimicrobial agents than any other anaerobe. Strains of *B. fragilis* that produce an *enterotoxin* have recently been described and may cause diarrheal disease in humans. *Porphyromonas* and *Prevotella* are isolated from a variety of infectious processes, usually in association with other bacteria. A characteristic of most species in these two genera is a *brown-to-black* colony pigment that develops on blood agar. *Prevotella bivia* is prevalent in the vaginal flora and may play a pathogenic role in bacterial *vaginosis* and other female genital tract infections.

Members of the genus *Fusobacterium* characteristically appear as thin, gram-negative bacilli with tapered ends. *Fusobacterium* are regular constituents of the normal flora of the oral cavity, gastrointestinal tract, and genital tract. The species of *Fusobacterium* most often encountered in clinical infections are *Fusobacterium nucleatum* and *Fusobacterium necrophorum*. These species are commonly isolated from infections of the upper and lower respiratory tracts or infections that occur as a consequence of distal spread from a respiratory focus.

Gram-Positive, Sporeforming Bacilli

All pathogenic anaerobic, sporeforming bacilli belong to the genus *Clostridium*. Although many different species of *Clostridium* have been described, a relatively small number play a significant role in clinical infections. *Clostridium perfringens* is the most common clostridial species isolated from infection and is responsible for *gas gangrene* as well as a variety of other infections (see next section, Clostridia). *Clostridium ramosum* is the second most frequently isolated clostridial species and is resistant to a number of commonly used antimicrobial agents. *Clostridium septicum* is most often recovered from patients with underlying malignancies, particularly colon carcinoma. *Clostridium botulinum*, *Clostridium tetani*, and *Clostridium difficile* cause disease by toxin production (see next section, Clostridia).

Gram-Positive, Nonsporeforming Bacilli

The nonsporeforming, gram-positive, anaerobic bacilli are a heterogeneous group of bacteria in the genera *Actinomyces*, *Bifidobacterium*, *Propionibacterium*, *Eubacterium*, *Morbiluncus*, and *Lactobacillus*. These anaerobic bacteria are normal flora components of the oral cavity, gastrointestinal tract, vagina, and skin.

Members of the genus *Actinomyces* are the major etiologic agents of human *actinomycosis* (see section entitled Pathogenic Actinomycetes). These microorganisms can also be recovered from pulmonary infections and brain abscesses.

The bifidobacteria are filamentous, pleomorphic bacilli that are part of the normal intestinal, mouth, and vaginal flora. They are principally isolated from mixed pulmonary infections. *Bifidobacterium dentium* is the species most frequently isolated from clinical infections.

Species in the genus *Propionibacterium* are the anaerobes most frequently found on normal skin and are common contaminants of blood and other specimens. The two most common species, *Propionibacterium acnes* and *Propionibacterium granulosum,* may be associated with infections involving implanted *prosthetic* devices, such as heart valves and orthopedic prostheses.

Eubacterium lentum is the most common of the eubacteria isolated from clinical specimens. Eubacteria are isolated from wound and other infections and are most always associated with other anaerobes or facultative bacteria.

Morbiluncus is a newly designated genus that consists of curved, gram-positive bacilli. *Morbiluncus mulieris* and *M. curtisii* are commonly isolated from patients with bacterial *vaginosis*.

Lactobacillus species are essentially nonpathogenic, although rare instances of endocarditis and pleuropulmonary disease associated with *L. catenaforme* have been reported.

Gram-Positive Cocci

The pathogenic, anaerobic, gram-positive cocci belong to the genera *Peptostreptococcus* and *Gemella*. They are prominent members of the indigenous flora, especially in the mouth, upper respiratory tract, and large intestine. Next to the anaerobic gram-negative bacilli, the anaerobic gram-positive cocci are the anaerobes most commonly encountered in clinically significant infections. They have been isolated from virtually all types of infections, usually in combination with other anaerobes or facultative bacteria. The species most commonly isolated from human infections are *Peptostreptococcus magnus, P. asaccharolyticus, P. prevotii, P. anaerobius,* and *P. tetradius.*

Gram-Negative Cocci

Veillonella is occasionally isolated from clinical specimens although usually in combination with other bacteria.

Isolation and Identification of Anaerobic Bacteria

The proper methods for collecting and transporting clinical specimens for the isolation of anaerobic bacteria are important considerations. Since anaerobes are prevalent as normal flora on virtually all mucous membranes, it is imperative to avoid contamination of the specimen with normal flora components. Specimens that are unacceptable for anaerobic culture because the collection sites are colonized or because contamination with indigenous flora often occurs include expectorated sputum, throat swabs, nasotracheal or bronchoscope aspirates, gastrointestinal contents, feces (except for *Clostridium difficile*), vaginal or endocervical secretions, midstream urine, and skin or superficial wound swabs. Whenever possible, a needle and syringe are used to obtain a specimen, and all bubbles of air and gas should be expelled from both the syringe and needle. The contents of the syringe are then injected into an oxygen-free sterile tube. Properly collected specimens need to be rapidly transported to the laboratory to minimize exposure of the microorganisms to oxygen.

A *Gram's stain* of the specimen is prepared and examined immediately after the specimen arrives in the laboratory. Many anaerobic bacteria assume a characteristic morphology that can be presumptively identified microscopically.

Basically there are two techniques for the cultivation of anaerobic bacteria in the clinical laboratory: the anaerobic jar and the anaerobic chamber, often called a "glove box." The *anaerobic jar* consists of a tightly sealed container from which oxygen is removed using a variety of different techniques. The *anaerobic chamber* consists of a plastic box with attached and sealed gloves, filled with oxygen-free gas, into which specimens are introduced through an entry lock. Since anaerobic infections are frequently polymicrobic, all clinical specimens are cultured aerobically as well as anaerobically.

Definitive identification of anaerobic bacteria is based on morphology, susceptibility to antibiotics, fermentation of carbohydrates, and other physiologic characteristics. Gas-liquid chromatographic analysis of volatile fatty acids and nonvolatile organic acids produced during carbohydrate fermentation is also used to aid in the identification of anaerobic bacteria.

Treatment

Successful therapy of anaerobic infections often involves both rational antibiotic selection and *surgical drainage* of pus and debridement of necrotic tissue. In general, *antimicrobial therapy* of most serious anaerobic infections requires high dosages and prolonged treatment to minimize the possibility of relapses. Antimicrobial agents commonly used to treat anaerobic infections are beta-lactam agents and beta-lactamase inhibitors, cefoxitin, imipenem, chloramphenicol, clindamycin, and metronidazole. Because many anaerobic infections tend to be polymicrobial, with aerobic or facultative organisms, or both, antimicrobial agents that are effective against all infective components must be used.

Clostridia

Rial D. Rolfe

The clostridia are gram-positive, *sporeforming* bacilli that are involved in a variety of human diseases. They are widely distributed and are present in soil and in the intestinal tracts of humans and animals.

Clostridium perfringens

C. perfringens is divided into five types, A through E, on the basis of their ability to produce four major lethal toxins: alpha, beta, epsilon, and iota. Only types A, C, and D are pathogenic for humans. Type A is an etiologic agent of clostridial myonecrosis (gas gangrene) and a common form of food poisoning. Type C is the etiologic agent of enteritis necroticans.

Clostridial Myonecrosis

Epidemiology

Clostridial myonecrosis, or gas gangrene, is a rapidly progressive and life-threatening illness caused by pathogenic clostridia. This disease is characterized by extensive *necrosis* of muscle and connective tissue, and is a consequence of compromised blood supply, either through direct injury or underlying vascular disease, and contamination with clostridia. Clostridia are unable to initiate infection in healthy tissue in which the oxidation-reduction potential is normal. Most cases of clostridial myonecrosis occur following serious injuries or surgical procedures. Several clostridial species are able to cause invasive infection in humans. Most cases of clostridial myonecrosis are caused by *C. perfringens*. Other clostridial species that can be involved in gas gangrene are *C. novyi, C. septicum, C. fallax, C. histolyticum,* and *C. sordellii*. All these clostridia produce a variety of toxins of different potencies. These clostridial species are widely distributed in nature and can be found in soil, sewage, water, and the intestinal tracts of humans and animals. Therefore, contamination of wounds with these bacteria is very common. Gas gangrene is usually a *mixed infection,* and both aerobic and anaerobic bacteria may be isolated from a single gangrenous lesion.

Occasionally, more than one pathogenic species of *Clostridium* may be isolated from a wound.

Clinical Manifestations

Once pathogenic clostridia are established in damaged tissue, they rapidly invade the surrounding healthy tissue by elaborating toxins that produce ischemia in adjacent muscle. The most important is *alpha toxin* (lecithinase C or phospholipase C), which damages cell membranes. Other exotoxins include neuraminidases, proteases, deoxyribonucleases, hyaluronidases, lecithinases, and collagenases. The involved muscle and overlying soft tissue undergo necrosis and autolysis with little inflammatory cell reaction.

Diagnosis

There are no specific tests for the early detection of clostridial myonecrosis and diagnosis is made on the basis of *clinical manifestations*. Direct visualization of muscle to determine the characteristic appearance of the disease is required to make a definitive diagnosis in early cases. A Gram's stain smear of the wound exudate may support the diagnosis by revealing the presence of clostridia and the absence of inflammatory cells.

Treatment

Without prompt effective therapy, refractory septic shock, circulatory failure, CNS depression, and death may soon follow the onset of symptoms. Total *excision* of all diseased muscle is a necessity for survival of the patient. Adjunctive measures such as therapy with *penicillin* to halt further spread of infection and *hyperbaric oxygen* to raise the oxygen concentration in tissues may also be useful in treatment. The therapeutic use of polyvalent equine gas gangrene *antitoxin* is controversial because of the high incidence of adverse side effects.

Food Poisoning

Epidemiology

Clostridium perfringens type A is a common cause of *food poisoning* throughout the world. This type of food poisoning is caused by ingestion of improperly cooked food, particularly *meat* products (e.g., beef and gravy), that are contaminated with an enterotoxin-producing strain of *C. perfringens* type A.

Clinical Manifestations

The ingested bacterial cells reach the intestine and undergo sporulation. The heat-labile *enterotoxin* of *C. perfringens* is released during sporulation. Usual onset of symptoms is 8 to 12 hours following ingestion of contaminated food.

The disease is rather mild, and symptoms include abdominal pain and acute diarrhea lasting 12 to 24 hours. Fever and vomiting are uncommon.

Diagnosis

Diagnosis of *C. perfringens* food poisoning is made on the basis of clinical features, incubation period, and attack rate. Recovery of enterotoxin-producing strains of *C. perfringens* from the implicated food and the patient's feces helps establish the diagnosis. Immunologic assays can be used to detect enterotoxin in food.

Treatment

Clostridium perfringens food poisoning is self-limiting, is typically mild, and usually requires only *supportive therapy*. There are no known agents to counteract the effects of the enterotoxin.

Enteritis necroticans

Enteritis necroticans (pigbel) is a severe, necrotizing disease of the small intestine caused by *C. perfringens* type C. This disease occurs primarily in the highlands of Papua, *New Guinea,* and is associated with the ingestion of undercooked *pork* contaminated with *C. perfringens* type C. This clostridial species proliferates in the human intestine and elaborates large quantities of *beta toxin*. The toxin causes widespread necrosis of the intestine since there is inadequate intestinal proteolytic activity to inactivate the toxin. The natives are deficient in *intestinal proteases* due to a normal low-protein diet and the presence of a heat-stable *trypsin inhibitor* in sweet potatoes, the staple diet of these people. The disease ensues within 24 hours of ingestion of the contaminated pork and is characterized by acute abdominal pain, bloody diarrhea, and vomiting. Death due to shock and peritonitis occurs in approximately 40 percent of patients. There is no effective therapy for enteritis necroticans. However, this disease can be prevented by active immunization with *beta toxoid*.

Clostridium tetani

Epidemiology

Tetanus is a severe infection produced by the action of a potent *neurotoxin* elaborated by *C. tetani*. The spores of *C. tetani* that are widely distributed in soil and in the intestinal tracts of humans and animals contaminate a wound. Germination of spores is favored by necrotic tissue and poor blood supply in the wound. The cause of infection with *C. tetani* varies from accidental injuries to surgical procedures.

Pathogenic Mechanisms

The clinical manifestation of tetanus is due to the elaboration of an exotoxin, called *tetanospasmin,* by *C. tetani.* Tetanospasmin is a neurotoxin that has an affinity for cells of the central nervous system. Although the tetanus bacilli are antigenically heterogeneous, the neurotoxin produced by all strains is immunologically *identical.*

Under appropriate in vivo environmental conditions, spores of *C. tetani* germinate and produce tetanospasmin. The presence of other organisms and necrotic tissue enhances the reversion of *C. tetani* spores to vegetative cells. The tetanus bacilli *do not invade* healthy tissue but remain at the site of infection. Tetanospasmin travels from the site of infection to the central nervous system along the axis cylinders of motor nerves, where it is fixed by cerebral gangliosides. The neurotoxin interferes with neuromuscular transmission by inhibiting the release of *inhibitory transmitters* (e.g., glycine) at spinal synapses. This results in excess motor activity and the typical muscle spasms of tetanus. All symptoms of tetanus are attributable to this neurotoxin.

Clinical Manifestations

The incubation period for tetanus may range from a few days to several weeks. The first symptom of generalized tetanus is *trismus* (lockjaw). This may be accompanied by stiffness of the neck, difficulty in swallowing, and rigidity of abdominal muscles. Eventually, generalized tonic convulsions develop and the ultimate cause of death is asphyxia from spasms of respiratory muscles.

Local tetanus is a rare form of the disease. It is characterized by persistent contraction of muscles near the site of injury. Local tetanus may progress to the generalized form of disease, but it is generally milder and much less likely to be fatal.

Cephalic tetanus is another rare form of tetanus that may follow injuries to the head or otitis media when *C. tetani* is part of the infecting flora. Cephalic tetanus is characterized by isolated or combined dysfunction of any of the cranial nerves. This form of tetanus may progress to generalized tetanus.

Tetanus neonatorum results from postnatal infection of the umbilicus. This is a serious and frequently fatal form of tetanus seen most often in developing countries.

Clinical tetanus does not induce immunity because the disease is produced by amounts of neurotoxin that are too small for immunization.

Diagnosis

The diagnosis of tetanus is usually based on clinical findings. However, bacteriologic studies can confirm the diagnosis. Attempts should be made to culture *C. tetani* from all suspicious lesions. A Gram's stain smear of wound exudate may reveal typical clostridia that have a "drumstick" or "tennis racket" appearance because of the presence of *terminal spores* that are larger in diameter than the vegetative cells.

Treatment and Prevention

Tetanus *antitoxin* (human immunoglobulin) is administered in all cases of suspected tetanus. Antitoxin neutralizes circulating toxin but is ineffective against toxin already fixed in the central nervous system. Tissue debridement of the wound and administration of penicillin to prevent further toxin formation are also indicated.

The only effective means to prevent tetanus is by prophylactic active *immunization. Tetanus toxoid,* in combination with diphtheria toxoid and pertussis vaccine, is usually given during the first year of life. Toxoid given to women before and during the first 6 months of pregnancy prevents tetanus neonatorum. A booster injection of toxoid can induce protective levels of amnestic antibody within 1 to 2 weeks and is frequently administered at the time of injury.

Clostridium botulinum

Epidemiology

Botulism is a life-threatening, paralytic illness produced by a powerful neurotoxin elaborated by *C. botulinum.* This microorganism is ubiquitous in soil and frequently contaminates fruits, vegetables, fish, and other foods.

Clostridium botulinum is subdivided into eight toxicologic types (A, B, C1, C2, D, E, F, and G), which differ from one another in the production of *immunologically distinct neurotoxins.* However, the pharmacologic action of these toxins is identical. Types A, B, and E most commonly produce disease in humans.

Pathogenic Mechanisms

The polypeptide neurotoxins elaborated by *C. botulinum* are the most potent exotoxins known. These toxins produce paralysis by preventing the release of the neurotransmitter *acetylcholine* from the nerve terminals of neuromuscular junctions. The neurotoxins are heat labile but resistant to the acid and proteolytic enzymes present in the intestinal tract. The production of botulinum toxin is governed by specific *bacteriophages.*

Clinical Manifestations

Clostridium botulinum produces three forms of botulism in humans: food-borne, wound, and infant.

Food-Borne Botulism

Human botulism is ordinarily not an infectious disease but rather an intoxication resulting from the ingestion of food containing preformed neurotoxin. The foods most often responsible for botulism are sausage, pork, and home-canned vegetables, such as beans, peas, and asparagus. Food items contaminated by toxin have a completely normal appearance and taste. The spores of *C. botulinum* are highly resistant to heat and can withstand boiling for several hours. Under appropriate environmental conditions, the spores of *C. botulinum* germinate, and the multiplying vegetative cells elaborate neurotoxin. After ingestion, the toxin is absorbed from the stomach and upper small bowel and reaches susceptible neurons by way of the bloodstream. Symptoms of botulism usually begin 12 to 36 hours after the ingestion of contaminated food. The cranial nerves are generally affected first, followed by a descending pattern of weakness or paralysis. The early involvement of cranial nerves causes problems with eyesight, hearing, and speech. Respiratory failure is the most common cause of death.

Wound Botulism

Wound botulism is a rare disorder that occurs when neurotoxin is produced by *C. botulinum* contaminating traumatic wounds. *Clostridium botulinum* does not invade healthy tissue. The clinical symptoms are like those of food-borne botulism.

Infant Botulism

Infant botulism is due to neurotoxin production by *C. botulinum* within the gastrointestinal tracts of infants between 3 and 26 weeks of age. *Honey* has been implicated as a source of *C. botulinum* for infants. Constipation and weak sucking are often the first symptoms of infant botulism. Cranial nerve deficits then appear, usually manifested by a flaccid facial expression, ptosis, and paralysis of eye muscles. Intensive supportive care enables the vast majority of infected infants to recover completely. However, infant botulism accounts for some cases of sudden infant death syndrome.

There are no long-term sequelae in patients who survive any form of botulism. Clinical botulism does not induce natural immunity because the amount of toxin required to elicit an antibody response is lethal.

Diagnosis

The diagnosis of botulism should be considered in a patient with symmetric descending weakness or paralysis of the cranial nerves, extremities, and trunk. The clinical diagnosis of botulism can be confirmed by demonstrating either botulinum toxin in the blood or gastric contents of a patient or toxin and *C. botulinum* in the suspected food. Toxin is detected by bioassay in mice, whereas isolation of *C. botulinum* requires special anaerobic culture techniques.

Treatment and Prevention

Administration of polyvalent *antitoxin* is the principal means of treating botulism. This antitoxin is prepared in horses and contains antibodies for the three most common types of neurotoxins encountered in humans (types A, B, and E). Desensitization may be necessary if the patient is allergic to horse serum. This antitoxin only neutralizes circulating toxin and has no effect on toxin bound to susceptible nerve cells. Recovery from botulism is very gradual, occurring over weeks to months.

A pentavalent *toxoid* is available for administration to laboratory workers. Immunization of the public is not recommended because of the low incidence of botulism.

Clostridium difficile

Epidemiology

Clostridium difficile is the major cause of *pseudomembranous colitis* associated with antimicrobial therapy in humans. Pseudomembranous colitis is a severe, necrotizing process of the large intestine. Essentially all antimicrobial agents are capable of inducing pseudomembranous colitis, but it is seen most often following the administration of clindamycin, ampicillin, or the cephalosporins.

Pathogenic Mechanisms

Antimicrobial agents may sufficiently suppress the normal colonic flora to permit intestinal overgrowth by *C. difficile*. This microorganism produces two antigenically distinct, heat-labile protein toxins, referred to as *enterotoxin* (toxin A) and *cytotoxin* (toxin B), which are responsible for the clinical manifestations of this disease. Intestinal diseases due to *C. difficile* vary from a relatively mild, self-limiting diarrhea to a severe, fulminating pseudomembranous colitis.

Diagnosis

Diagnosis of *C. difficile*–associated diarrhea is based initially on the clinical setting of diarrhea that is related temporally to antibiotic therapy. *Colonoscopy* and *sigmoidoscopy* examination may reveal the presence of a pseudomembrane on the colonic mucosa. The cytotoxin of *C. difficile* can be detected in feces by demonstrating a histotoxic effect in tissue culture cells. In addition, immunoassays for detection of toxins A or B, or both, are commer-

cially available. A selective agar medium significantly aids in the isolation of *C. difficile* from feces. However, culture of *C. difficile* is less specific than toxin detection.

Treatment

Oral *vancomycin, metronidazole,* or *bacitracin* is used in the treatment of pseudomembranous colitis. In addition, the implicated antimicrobial agent should be discontinued.

Pathogenic Actinomycetes

W. LaJean Chaffin

Actinomycetous Bacteria

The actinomycetes are a large, diverse group of gram-positive bacilli that differ in some characteristics, such as tolerance for oxygen and ability to form spores, but share a tendency to form filaments. These bacteria also have related pathogenicities and are responsible for three major infections—actinomycosis, nocardiosis, and actinomycetoma. Filamentation is quite pronounced in some species, and at one time these organisms were thought to form an intermediate stage between bacteria and fungi. As a consequence, historically they have been more studied by mycologists as agents of infection than by bacteriologists but they are true bacteria. They lack a nucleus and have a bacterial cell-wall structure. In addition to the basic components of the cell wall, the walls also contain components that are useful in speciation and classification. Several genera are associated with human infection, including *Actinomyces, Arachnia, Nocardia, Actinomadura,* and *Streptomyces*. Members of the genus *Streptomyces* are probably more important to medical science as sources of antibiotics than as agents of infection.

Actinomycosis

The three major species that have been implicated in actinomycosis are *Actinomyces israelii, Arachnia propionica,* and *Actinomyces naeslundii*, in decreasing frequency of isolation (Table 4-13). Actinomycosis is a chronic, suppurative disease that spreads to contiguous tissue and is subdivided into disease types based on site of infection. In cervicofacial disease, infection may be initiated following dental caries or gingival disease or by trauma that introduces the organism to a potential site of infection. A swollen area develops, producing discomfort but rarely pain. If unattended, pyogenic abscesses occur that will eventually develop draining sinus tracts. The infection often spreads to adjacent areas including bone. This type of infection is known in cattle as lumpy jaw. A

Table 4-13 Actinomycetous Infections

Infection	Lesions	Frequent etiology	Usual habitat	Exposure	Granules	Direct examination of positive patient specimens
Actinomycosis	Abcess formation Sinus tracts	*Actinomyces israelii* *Actinomyces naeslundii* *Arachnia propionica*	Normal flora	Displacement from normal oral, gastrointestinal tract/site	+ Rare +	Gram-positive filaments ≤1 μm in diameter
Nocardiosis	Abscess formation Sinus tracts rare	*Nocardia asteroides* *Nocardia brasiliensis*	Soil	Inhalation	− +	Gram-positive filaments ≤1 μm in diameter Partially acid-fast
Actinomycetoma	Abscess formation Sinus tracts	*Actinomadura madurae* *Actinomadura pelletieri* *Nocardia brasiliensis* *Streptomyces somaliensis*	Soil	Trauma to subcutaneous tissue followed by contamination with soil containing microbe	+ + + +	Gram-positive filaments ≤1 μm in diameter

thoracic form of the disease may be initiated by extension from above or by aspiration of organisms. Respiratory symptoms develop, and eventually lung tissue may be destroyed and draining sinus tracts develop. The third major manifestation is abdominal infection, which is usually initiated by perforation of the intestinal wall (e.g., ruptured appendix), and the organisms are introduced to a potential site of infection. The infection develops very slowly with symptoms dependent on the infected site. Eventually, if untreated, the draining sinus tracts often erupt through the abdominal wall. In addition a genital infection has been described in women, generally those who use intrauterine contraceptive devices that have been in place for months to years. The symptoms are generally those of pelvic inflammatory disease. Occasionally, primary lesions have been noted in other tissues, and rare cases of hematogenous spread have been reported.

Epidemiology

The agents of actinomycosis are components of the normal flora of the oral cavity and intestinal mucosa. Two additional normal flora species of *Actinomyces* are not associated with disease but may contribute to dental caries. Infections occur in men about twice as often as in women and generally in the 15- to 35-year-old age group. During infection, most of the organisms grow as discrete colonies, producing granules that may be recovered from the sinus tract exudate. The frequently yellowish color of these granules probably results from lipid in the macrophages.

The granules are up to 2.5 mm in size and have tissue cells adhering to them.

Laboratory Diagnosis

The granule size and color assist in identification of the organisms. When crushed, the granules reveal gram-positive bacterial forms of about 1 μm in diameter that are present as delicate intertwined filaments and diphtheroids. Most isolates of these genera are described as facultative anaerobes that grow best in the presence of carbon dioxide (*A. propionica* growth is not enhanced by carbon dioxide). On rich solid medium or in thioglycolate broth, they initially produce microcolonies of short, branching filaments. With time, the filaments fragment into diphtheroids, short chains, or coccobacillary forms. They are not acid-fast. Colony morphology and biochemical tests are used to distinguish species.

Treatment

As bacteria, these organisms are susceptible to a variety of antibacterial antibiotics. Penicillin is frequently the drug of choice. Other antimicrobials that have been used are clindamycin and sulfa drugs. Surgical excision and cleaning may also be recommended for treatment of infection.

Nocardiosis

Nocardiosis is initiated as a primary pulmonary infection that may range from subclinical to pneumonic (see Table

4-13). The infection may be transitory, chronic, or an acute necrotizing pneumonia. The development of draining sinuses is rare. Infection is sometimes disseminated by hematogenous spread to other sites, with the central nervous system being the most common. Other disseminated sites include the kidney and heart. Multiple or large abscesses develop. The majority of cases (80–90%) are caused by *Nocardia asteroides*. Occasionally, *Nocardia brasiliensis* and *Nocardia otitidiscaviarum* are involved.

Epidemiology

In the United States, the number of cases of nocardiosis is estimated at 500 to 1000 a year. About 50 percent of the patients are compromised by conditions such as leukemia or treatment with corticosteroids or immunosuppressive drugs. In another 25 percent, some defect in cellular immune defense is suspected. However, about 25 percent of the cases occur in apparently normal individuals. Individuals of all ages can be infected, but the greatest incidence is in the 30- to 50-year-old age group. About 75 percent of the patients are men. Opportunistic infection also occurs in a small percentage of patients with acquired immunodeficiency syndrome (AIDS). *Nocardia* species occur worldwide as soil inhabitants, but infections are more frequent in rural than in urban environments.

Laboratory Diagnosis

For diagnosis, pus, sputum, or biopsy material is examined for gram-positive, partially acid-fast bacteria. In positive smears, delicate, multiple branched and beaded filaments appear. *Nocardia* species are aerobic and will grow on most laboratory media. The colonial morphology, filamentous pattern, and partial acid-fastness coupled with characteristic biochemical tests are used in species identification. The partial acid-fastness is associated with short-chain mycolic acids present in the cell wall.

Treatment

The prognosis in nocardiosis is grave, with high mortality for both pulmonary and disseminated infections. The organisms respond to a number of antibacterial antibiotics. The sulfonamides are generally the drugs of choice. For chronic infections, treatment is continued for 6 to 12 months. Surgery can be used to drain and clean abscesses.

Actinomycetoma

Several genera of actinomycetes are implicated as bacterial etiologic agents of mycetoma (Table 4-13). Mycetoma is a chronic, suppurative, and granulomatous infection of subcutaneous tissue. The organisms are present as a granule that may be recovered from sinus tracts that drain the abscesses. The infection results from traumatic implantation of the organism into subcutaneous tissue. The infection can be caused by a variety of dematiacious and non-dematiacious fungi (eumycetoma) or bacteria (actinomycetoma). The fungal agents of mycetoma are discussed in Chap. 6 in the section on subcutaneous mycoses. Although generally slow-developing infections, mycetomas of bacterial etiology progress somewhat more rapidly than those of fungal etiology. Among the implicated bacteria are *Actinomadura madurae*, *Actinomadura pelletieri*, *Actinomyces israelii* (rarely), *Nocardia asteroides*, *Nocardia brasiliensis*, *Nocardia otitidiscaviarum*, *Nocardiopsis dassonvillei*, and *Streptomyces somaliensis*.

Epidemiology

The agents of actinomycetoma are ubiquitous soil inhabitants that occur with greatest frequency in subtropical and tropical soils. The infecting organism is introduced into tissue by implantation such as caused by a puncture wound. Lesions often are found on the feet, initiated from a wound obtained while walking barefoot. The frequency of isolation of a species in a geographic location is similar to the prevalence of the agent in the soil.

Laboratory Diagnosis

Diagnosis of a bacterial etiology for this infection is based on direct examination of material removed from lesions and by culture identification. The size and color of granules are noted, along with the size of the microbial elements and gram-positive character of the organism. The colonial morphology and color, biochemical tests, and cell-wall composition are used in species identification.

Treatment

Long-term antibiotic treatment is generally required. The treatment of infections caused by species of *Actinomyces* and *Nocardia* was discussed under treatment of actinomycosis and nocardiosis. Penicillin and sulfa drugs have been used in medical management of infections associated with these organisms. Streptomycin has been recommended for use with infections attributed to *Actinomadura* and *Streptomyces*. Surgical intervention may also be recommended, and in advanced cases, amputation may be considered.

Mycoplasma, L-Forms, Legionella

David C. Straus

Mycoplasma
Morphology and History

Mycoplasma species are the smallest known free-living organisms. They are extremely pleomorphic because they lack a cell wall. They stain poorly and are not gram-stainable. On solid media, *Mycoplasma* forms minute, transparent colonies. Typical colonies range from 10 to 600 μm in diameter and show a "fried egg" appearance. Many human strains show complete or incomplete hemolysis. The *Mycoplasma* species were originally referred to as pleuropneumonia organisms (PPO) or pleuropneumonia-like organisms (PPLO). The first human disease known to be associated with *Mycoplasma* was primary atypical pneumonia (PAP). PAP is thus named because the word "atypical" implies that the disease does not resemble that produced by *Streptococcus pneumoniae,* which causes a "typical" lobar pneumonia. The causative agent of PAP is *Mycoplasma pneumoniae.*

Growth Requirement

Strains of *Mycoplasma* vary widely in their growth rates. Most strains require a rich medium (serum protein and a sterol) for growth. They incorporate the sterol into their cell membrane to strengthen it and help them tolerate the differences between the internal and external osmotic pressures. Approximately 15 percent of the dry weight of the parasitic human *Mycoplasma* strains is composed of lipid, and a very great percentage (65%) of this is sterol. *Mycoplasma* are generally susceptible to kanamycin and tetracylines but are resistant to sulfonamides and penicillin.

Primary Atypical Pneumonia

Only one human disease (PAP) has been definitely shown to be caused by *Mycoplasma. M. pneumoniae,* which is responsible for PAP, is also referred to as Eaton's agent and differs antigenically from all other mycoplasmas. Cold agglutinins, agglutinins to *Streptococcus MG,* and *Mycoplasma* growth-inhibiting antibody can be found in the sera of those individuals recovering from PAP. This disease is usually diagnosed employing a complement-fixation test for a lipid antigen complex in the organism. The development of a DTH reaction to *M. pneumoniae* appears to correlate with the severity of disease and explain the observed differences between infections in young children and adults. PAP caused by *M. pneumoniae* is more severe in adults than it is in children.

Epidemiologic studies show that this disease is most commonly found in children and young adults. It has an incubation period of 9 to 12 days. Treatment involves administration of tetracylines or kanamycin.

Other Mycoplasmas

Mycoplasma hominus has been implicated as one of the causative agents of pelvic inflammatory disease. A form of *Mycoplasma,* once called t-strains (for tiny colony strains), is now called *Ureaplasma urealyticus. Ureaplasma* differs from the true *Mycoplasma* in that it requires urea for growth. It produces urease, which splits urea into ammonia and carbon dioxide. *Ureaplasma* is implicated in some cases of nongonococcal urethritis.

L-Forms

L-forms are bacteria without cell walls. They can be obtained from almost every bacterial species. L-forms are capable of reversion to the parent form by generating cell-wall material. They differ from *Mycoplasma* in this respect, because *Mycoplasma* never produces a cell wall. Agents that are capable of converting bacteria to L-forms include antibiotics, lithium chloride, caffeine, lysozyme, and specific antibody plus complement. L-forms are highly susceptible to osmotic pressure gradients and need such stabilizing agents as salts, sugars, polypeptides, and spermines to survive. Their role in human infection is unknown.

Legionella pneumophila

Morphology, Characteristics, and Virulence Factors

Legionella pneumophila is the cause of "Legionnaires' disease," a respiratory illness that may be severe and is often associated with a common-source air-borne infection. The organism is a short rod (0.5 mm × 3 mm). It stains poorly with Gram's stain but is gram-negative. *Legionella pneumophila* is an intracellular parasite that produces a cytotoxin that selectively inhibits the activation of polymorphonuclear leukocyte oxidative metabolism. There are at least 11 serotypes as defined by direct immunofluorescence staining of whole bacteria cells. Most clinical diseases seen to date have been caused by *Legionella pneumophila* serotype 1.

Epidemiology

Legionnaires' disease first came under close scrutiny in 1976, when 182 persons attending the annual convention of the American Legion became ill (49 deaths; 27% mortality). Subsequent outbreaks have occurred in the United States and elsewhere in the world. The infection can occasionally be dust-borne, but in most cases it has been traced to water-cooling towers connected to air-conditioning plants (aerosols). This is particularly important in hospitals because immunologically compromised patients appear to be especially susceptible to infection with this pathogen. Person-to-person spread is rare. There are two distinct clinical diseases caused by *L. pneumophila.* These are pneumonia (Legionnaires' disease) and Pontiac fever (a self-limiting illness characterized by the abrupt onset of fever, chills, headache, and myalgia).

Table 4-14 *Rickettsia:* Classification per Common Complement-Fixing Antigens

Group	*Rickettsia*	Disease	Reservoir	Vector
Typhus fever	*R. prowazekii*	Epidemic louse-borne typhus	Humans	Human head and body louse
		Brill's disease or Brill-Zinsser disease	Humans	Recrudescence
	R. typhi	Endemic flea-borne typhus	Rodents	Rat flea
Spotted fever	*R. rickettsii*	Rocky Mountain Spotted fever	Rodents, ticks	Tick
	R. conorii	Boutonneuse fever; Mediterranean fever; South African tick-bite fever; Kenya tick typhus	Dogs, ticks, rodents	Tick
	R. sibirica	North Asian tick typhus	Wild rodents	Tick
	R. australis	Queensland tick typhus	Wild rodents, marsupials	Tick
	R. akari	Rickettsialpox	House mice	Mite
Scrub typhus	*R. tsutsugamushi*	Scrub typhus	Wild rodents	Mite
Q fever	*Coxiella burnetii*	Q fever	Sheep, goats, and cattle	Milk ingestion Tick Dust inhalation
Trench fever	*Rochalimaea quintana*	Trench fever	Humans	Body louse

Clinical Findings, Diagnosis, and Treatment

Pathologic examinations have failed to demonstrate the organism in any tissue other than the lung. A sudden onset of fever, chills, myalgia, and dry cough, which may progress to a severe pneumonia, is commonly observed. Diagnosis is usually achieved by direct fluorescent antibody staining or culture of the organism from lung tissue. Culture of *Legionella* species has been greatly enhanced by the development of charcoal yeast extract (CYE) media. The addition of antibiotics to this medium allows for the isolation of the organism from sputum samples, which contain other microorganisms. Erythromycin is the drug of choice, and rifampin is also very effective. It should be kept in mind that the organism produces a beta lactamase.

Obligate Intracellular Parasites

David C. Straus

General Characteristics

In previous chapters we have referred to certain bacteria as intracellular pathogens. Examples are *Mycobacterium tuberculosis, Mycobacterium leprae, Salmonella typhi, Listeria monocytogenes, Legionella pneumophila,* and *Brucella abortus.* These organisms can all survive in normal macrophages but are killed by activated macrophages. However, they can also survive outside of cells and are considered, therefore, to be "optional" intracellular parasites. The *Rickettsia* and *Chlamydia,* on the other hand, cannot (with one exception) multiply outside of cells. They therefore are considered to be "obligate" intracellular parasites. In addition to this difference, another important distinction exists. The intracellular life of the *Rickettsia* and *Chlamydia* is not confined to professional phagocytes, but occurs primarily in other cell types. Other than this one common trait, the *Chlamydia* and *Rickettsia* do not appear to be related.

Rickettsiae

Classification

The rickettsiae are small, pleomorphic coccobacilli, approximately 0.3 to 1.0 μm. They possess the typical gram-negative bacterial structure; that is, they possess an outer membrane. As mentioned above, all of the rickettsiae are obligate intracellular parasites. Their intracellular location allows them access to many preformed materials required for their survival. The rickettsiae obtain energy by coupling the production of adenosine triphosphate (ATP) with the oxidation of glutamate via the tricarboxylic acid cycle. The cells that the rickettsiae infect are normally nonphagocytic. There are four medically important genera: *Rickettsia* (several species), *Rochalimaea* (only one species), *Coxiella* (only one species), and *Ehrlichia* (several species). The only *Ehrlichia* species to cause infections in humans is *E. sennetsu.* This organism has no known arthropod vector. Its reservoir is man and it is found only in western Japan. The *rickettsiae* can be grouped according to common complement-fixing antigens (Table 4-14).

Pathogenesis

Most rickettsiae are transmitted to humans by arthropod vectors. In general, they multiply in vascular endothelial cells, causing local pathology, but they can also be distributed throughout the body, causing characteristic rash. Fever and intense headaches occur. Death is the result of toxin build-up in the blood.

Rickettsioses

Typhus Fever Group

Epidemic Louse-borne Typhus (R. prowazekii). This disease is fortunately rare in the United States, but it occurs in countries where human body and head lice are common (Africa, Central and South America). Humans are the only reservoir, and the louse, which is the vector, dies of the infection. The louse feeds on the blood of the infected person and the organism multiplies in the gut of the louse. The infected louse defecates as it feeds on another individual and as the bite itches a great deal, the person scratches and inoculates the louse feces into the skin (autoinoculation). The onset of epidemic typhus occurs with fever, headache, and muscle pain. A rash appears on about the fourth day. The illness is quite severe and the fatality rates range from 10 to 40 percent, increasing with increasing age. A recrudescence of long-standing infection can occur. This is referred to as Brill's or Brill-Zinsser disease. Recurrence of symptoms is usually the result of lowered immunity, stress, or some other unknown factor.

Endemic Flea-borne Murine Typhus (R. typhi). This disease has worldwide distribution but only a few cases occur in the United States each year. Rat lice and fleas maintain a natural cycle in rats and the human is an accidental host, becoming infected when bitten by a rat flea. The illness resembles that of louse-borne typhus but is less severe, with only a 5 percent fatality rate.

Spotted Fever Group

Rocky Mountain Spotted Fever (RMSF) (R. rickettsii). This disease accounts for greater than 95 percent of all rickettsial diseases that occur in the U.S. It has a wide distribution in the United States, especially in the eastern states. The first cases of RMSF occurred in the Rocky Mountains (hence the name), but the disease is now rare in this region. Wild rodents and dogs are reservoirs of infection and humans become infected when bitten by ticks harbored by infected animals. The incubation period of the disease is about 6 days, after which a characteristic rickettsial onset (fever, headache, myalgia, rash) occurs. The fatality rate is 10 to 50 percent if the disease is untreated. Death is due to a rickettsial toxin.

Boutonneuse Fever, South African Tick-Bite Fever, Mediterranean Fever, Kenya Tick Typhus (R. conorii). There are a number of different names for this disease entity, which occurs primarily in Africa and India. It is transmitted by ticks. Other tick-borne typhus fevers are caused by *R. sibirica* (North Asian tick typhus), *R. australis* (Queensland tick typhus), and *R. japonica* (Japanese spotted fever). All of these diseases have symptoms that resemble RMSF but are usually milder.

Rickettsialpox (R. akari). This disease is occasionally seen in the United States. The illness is mild and is transmitted to humans from mice by the bite of a mite.

Scrub Typhus Group *(R. tsutsugamushi)*

"Tsutsugamushi" is Japanese for small, dangerous creature. This is indeed an excellent description of the rickettsial agent that causes scrub typhus. The disease is seen primarily in India, southeastern Asia, and Australia. It is transmitted to humans by the bite of the trombiculide mite (chigger) that parasitizes rodents. The human is usually an accidental host. The illness greatly resembles epidemic typhus and may result in a 30 percent fatality rate in untreated cases.

Trench Fever Group *(Rochalimaea quintana)*

Trench fever is transmitted by the body louse, with the human as its only reservoir. The illness is moderately severe, with only rare fatalities. The course of the disease may be short or it may be protracted with relapses. *Rochalimaea quintana* can be cultivated on blood agar under 10% carbon dioxide. It differs from all other rickettsiae in this property.

Q Fever *(Coxiella burnetii; Q stands for "query")*

Q fever occurs in many countries including the U.S. The natural cycle is maintained in various mammals (rodents, cattle, sheep, goats) by ticks. The organism is excreted by these animals in milk, urine feces, and so forth. It is inhaled by man or ingested in unpasteurized milk. The organism is usually stable outside host cells, but does not multiply. No rash occurs, but there is an atypical pneumonitis.

Diagnosis of Rickettsial Disease

Patient history (possible exposure to lice, fleas, ticks, or aerosols that might contain *C. burnetii*) is very important in diagnosing rickettsial diseases. Laboratory diagnosis is usually based on cultivation of the organism by inoculation of acute-phase blood from patients into chick embryo yoke sacs, chick embryo cell cultures, and the peritoneal cavity of guinea pigs. *Rochalimaea quintana* can be cultivated on blood agar under 10% CO_2. The Weil-Felix test, involving the agglutination of *Proteus vulgaris* strains OX19, OX2, and OXK by antibody against rickettsiae with which *Proteus* has antigens in common, used to be widely used. However, it is nonspecific and is no longer performed. The laboratory diagnosis is usually confirmed by demonstration of antibody in the patient's serum. Serologic tests for this purpose, using known rickettsial antigens, include the indirect fluorescent antibody test and complement-fixation tests.

Treatment

Tetracycline is the drug of choice. Chloramphenicol is also effective but usually avoided because of the danger of aplastic anemia.

Chlamydiae
Classification

The chlamydiae are classified as bacteria, but they differ from most bacteria in several important ways. They are obligate intracellular parasites that multiply only in living host cells since they lack energy-producing enzyme systems. They have a predilection for columnar epithelial cells that line mucous membranes. These organisms are also differentiated from other bacteria by their morphology and by a common group antigen. They are the only bacteria to have a unique development cycle involving two morphogenic forms—one adapted to intracellular survival (reticulate body) and one adapted to extracellular multiplication (elementary body). The intracellular form contains cytoplasmic vesicles called inclusions. *Chlamydia* consist of three species, *C. trachomatis*, *C. psittaci*, and *C. pneumoniae*.

Chlamydial Properties

The infectious particle (elementary body) outside the cell is a coccoid form about 0.3 μm in diameter. This enlarges inside cells to form a reticulate body, which is also called an initial body (0.5–1.0 μm in diameter) and which divides by binary fission to form additional reticulate bodies. From these, numerous elementary bodies develop. Multiplication takes place with the chlamydia being embedded in a matrix to comprise a colony that is the pathognomonic inclusion. The matrix of inclusion of *C. trachomatis* stains with iodine; those of *C. psittaci* and *C. pneumoniae* do not.

Diseases Caused by Chlamydia trachomatis

The species *C. trachomatis* consists of a number of distinct serotypes (A–L). The strains that cause trachoma and inclusion conjunctivitis are collectively referred to as TRIC (*TR*achoma, *I*nclusion, *C*onjunctivitis) agents.

Trachoma

This is a disease of the conjunctiva and cornea that constitutes a major cause of blindness in many parts of the world. Transmission is from eye to eye by fingers and contaminated washcloths. The organism causes inflammation of the conjunctiva of the upper part of the eye. There is infiltration by lymphocytes and plasma cells, and lymphoid follicles and germ centers develop in the conjunctiva of the upper lid. The upper part of the cornea is infiltrated by blood vessels and fibroblasts forming a structure referred to as a pannus. Scarring results in eyelid inversion (entropion), with damage to the cornea by eyelashes (trichiasis). Corneal inflammation also leads to scarring and results in blindness. Trachoma can be treated successfully with tetracycline and the sulfonamides.

Inclusion Conjunctivitis

Inclusion conjunctivitis is a genital disease transmitted from an infected mother to her infant during the process of birth. An eye infection called inclusion blennorrhea (mucous discharge) develops in the newborn. A severe purulent conjunctivitis occurs during the first 2 weeks of life. Adults and older children contract the disease from genital secretions in poorly chlorinated swimming pools.

Genital Infections

As a genital infection transmitted venereally, *C. trachomatis* is responsible for many cases of nonspecific urethritis. In the female the organism can cause cervicitis and salpingitis (inflammation of the fallopian tubes).

Pneumonitis of Infants

This disease usually occurs in the first months of life. Fever is absent, but there are marked respiratory signs and symptoms and prolonged cough.

Lymphogranuloma Venereum (LGV)

LGV is caused by serotypes L1, L2, and L3 of *C. trachomatis* and is venereally transmitted. A small herpetiform vesicle first appears on the genitals, followed by inflammation of regional lymph nodes and bubo formation.

Disease Caused by Chlamydia psittaci
Psittacosis

Psittacosis, also called ornithosis, is a zoonosis acquired by humans from psittacine, parrot-like birds and poultry. Birds develop a chronic carrier state that can be aggregated to a frank illness by the stress of shipping. The organism is excreted in the feces and may be present in various tissues of the birds, presenting a possible source of infection for poultry workers. Birds are treated with tetracycline. In humans, the infection is primarily manifest as primary atypical pneumonia. Tetracycline is the antibiotic of choice.

Disease Caused by Chlamydia pneumoniae

Acute Respiratory Illness

In 1986, a series of isolations of a new strain of *C. psittaci* from acute respiratory infections was reported. It was later identified as a separate species now called *C. pneumoniae*. This organism can cause a relatively mild upper respiratory tract infection that can occasionally develop into pneumonia. Symptoms include chronic cough, mild fever, and a raspy throat. Pneumonia caused by *C. pneumoniae* can be transferred from person to person with no intervening host. Patients infected with *C. pneumoniae* can be treated with tetracycline and erythromycin.

Questions

1. Which of the following refers to the ability of bacteria to produce pathologic changes or disease in the host?
   A. Virulence
   B. Pathogenicity
   C. Attenuation
   D. In vitro growth rates
   E. In vivo growth rates
2. The two *major* components of virulence include:
   A. Invasiveness and toxigenicity
   B. Intracellular and extracellular survival
   C. Adherence factors and antiphagocytic mechanisms
   D. Capsules and spreading factors
   E. Cell walls and nucleic acids
3. All of the following are examples of aggressins **except**:
   A. The pili of *Pseudomonas aeruginosa*
   B. The carbohydrate capsule of *Streptococcus pneumoniae*
   C. The Panton-Valentine leukocidin of *Staphylococcus aureus*
   D. The cell wall of *Streptococcus sanguis*
   E. The M protein of *Streptococcus pyogenes*
4. The organism that is known to be an intracellular bacterial parasite is:
   A. *Streptococcus pyogenes*
   B. *Klebsiella pneumoniae*

C. *Clostridium perfringens*
D. *Mycobacterium tuberculosis*
E. *Streptococcus agalactiae*

5. The bacterial toxin that attaches to presynaptic terminals of cholinergic nerves (where it blocks release of acetylcholine) is produced by:
   A. *Bacillus anthracis*
   B. *Clostridium botulinum*
   C. *Clostridium tetani*
   D. *Corynebacterium diphtheriae*
   E. *Pseudomonas aeruginosa*
6. The bacterial toxin that causes cessation of mammalian protein synthesis by inactivating EF-2 of eucaryotic cells is produced by:
   A. *Bacillus anthracis*
   B. *Clostridium botulinum*
   C. *Clostridium tetani*
   D. *Corynebacterium diphtheriae*
   E. *Vibrio cholerae*
7. The bacterium that produces a toxin with the same molecular mechanism as the diphtheria toxin is:
   A. *Bacillus anthracis*
   B. *Pseudomonas aeruginosa*
   C. *Streptococcus pneumoniae*
   D. *Staphylococcus aureus*
   E. *Vibrio cholerae*
8. The bacterium that produces a toxin that activates adenylate cyclase, resulting in an accumulation of cyclic AMP in the epithelial cells of the mucosal lining, is:
   A. *Escherichia coli*
   B. *Pseudomonas aeruginosa*
   C. *Streptococcus pneumoniae*
   D. *Staphylococcus aureus*
   E. *Streptococcus pyogenes*
9. All of the following statements about endotoxins are true **except** that:
   A. They are also referred to as lipopolysaccharides
   B. They are an integral part of the cell walls of gram-negative bacteria
   C. They are normally not as toxic as bacterial exotoxins
   D. Their toxicity can be destroyed by autoclaving
   E. They contain ketodeoxyoctonate
10. Which of the following pairs of bacteria produce toxins with the same mechanism of action?
    A. *Streptococcus pyogenes* and *Shigella dysenteriae*
    B. *Escherichia coli* and *Vibrio cholerae*
    C. *Bacillus anthracis* and *Clostridium perfringens*
    D. *Legionella pneumophila* and *Salmonella typhi*
    E. *Klebsiella pneumoniae* and *Mycobacterium tuberculosis*
11. Which of the following statements correctly describes superantigens (toxins)?

A. They are more toxic than most bacterial toxins
B. They are produced only by highly virulent bacteria
C. They cannot be neutralized by host antibody
D. They stimulate T-cell proliferation at very low concentrations
E. They are produced only by bacteria that are highly resistant to antibiotics

12. Which of the following refers to the mechanism by which diphtheria toxin kills cells?
    A. Cessation of protein synthesis by inactivation of EF-2
    B. Activation of adenylate cyclase
    C. Interaction with cell membranes, causing lysis of cells
    D. Activation of guanylate cyclase
    E. Direct inactivation of DNA

13. The pseudomembrane seen in clinical diphtheria is composed primarily of:
    A. Fibrin
    B. DNA
    C. RNA
    D. Lipid
    E. Carbohydrate

14. The DTP vaccine is composed of which of the following?
    A. Diphtheria toxin, tetanus toxin, heat-killed *Bordetella pertussis*
    B. Diphtheria toxoid, tetanus toxoid, heat-killed *Pseudomonas aeruginosa*
    C. Diphtheria toxoid, tetanus toxoid, heat-killed *Bordetella pertussis*
    D. Diphtheria toxin, tetanus toxin, heat-killed *Pseudomonas aeruginosa*
    E. Diphtheria toxoid, tetanus toxin, heat-killed *Pseudomonas aeruginosa*

15. The capsule of *Bacillus anthracis* is composed of:
    A. L-Glutamic acid
    B. D-Glutamic acid
    C. Polysaccharide
    D. Nucleic acid
    E. Lipid

16. *Bacillus anthracis* possesses all of the following characteristics **except** that:
    A. It is a large, gram-positive rod
    B. It is a sporeformer
    C. It produces a potent exotoxin composed of three antigenically distinct thermolabile proteins
    D. It can live inside phagocytic cells
    E. It can be killed by antibiotics

17. *Listeria monocytogenes* has all of the following characteristics **except** that:
    A. It is a sporeformer
    B. It is a short, gram-positive rod
    C. It can live inside phagocytic cells

D. It is actively motile
E. It can be killed by antibiotics

18. *Bacillus cereus* is most commonly associated with human
    A. Intrauterine infections
    B. Food poisoning
    C. Venereal disease
    D. Respiratory infections
    E. Urinary tract infections

19. The staphylococci differ from the streptococci in:
    A. Gram reactivity
    B. Cell diameter
    C. Cell morphology
    D. Catalase production
    E. Acid-fast staining

20. The most important antiphagocytic structure of the group A streptococci is the:
    A. M protein
    B. Group A carbohydrate
    C. Hyaluronic acid capsule
    D. Protein A
    E. Mycolic acids

21. *Staphylococcus aureus* can best be differentiated from *Staphylococcus epidermidis* by:
    A. Gram's stain
    B. Colonial morphology
    C. Coagulase production
    D. Catalase production
    E. Cell diameter

22. The toxin produced by *Staphylococcus aureus* that is responsible for the staphylococcal scalded skin syndrome is:
    A. The Panton-Valentine leukocidin
    B. Exfoliatin
    C. Protein A
    D. Alpha toxin
    E. Beta toxin

23. *Staphylococcus epidermidis:*
    A. Produces protein A
    B. Produces alpha toxin
    C. Produces enterotoxins
    D. Has been shown to cause subacute endocarditis
    E. Produces beta toxin

24. The genus-species name for the group A streptococci is:
    A. *Streptococcus pneumoniae*
    B. *Streptococcus mutans*
    C. *Streptococcus pyogenes*
    D. *Streptococcus agalactiae*
    E. *Streptococcus sanguis*

25. The streptococci most commonly involved in serious neonatal infections are:
    A. *Streptococcus pneumoniae*
    B. *Streptococcus mutans*

C. *Streptococcus pyogenes*
D. *Streptococcus agalactiae*
E. *Streptococcus sanguis*

26. The group A streptococcus serotype most commonly associated with acute glomerulonephritis (AGN) after pharyngitis is:
    A. 2
    B. 7
    C. 12
    D. 19
    E. 20

27. The streptococci most commonly associated with subacute bacterial endocarditis are:
    A. *Streptococcus pyogenes*
    B. *Streptococcus agalactiae*
    C. Viridans streptococci
    D. *Streptococcus pneumoniae*
    E. *Streptococcus bovis*

28. The member of the genus *Staphylococcus* most commonly associated with urinary tract infections in young, sexually active females is:
    A. *Staphylococcus aureus*
    B. *Staphylococcus epidermidis*
    C. *Staphylococcus saprophyticus*
    D. *Staphylococcus hominus*
    E. *Staphylococcus capitis*

29. The smallest known free-living organisms are:
    A. Viruses
    B. *Mycoplasma* species
    C. *Rickettsiae*
    D. *Chlamydiae*
    E. Fungi

30. L-forms:
    A. Are bacteria without a cell wall
    B. Can be obtained only from *Mycoplasma*
    C. Will never revert to the parent form
    D. Are more similar to viruses than to bacteria
    E. Are highly virulent forms of fungi

31. *Legionella pneumophila:*
    A. Is a gram-positive rod
    B. Is an intracellular parasite
    C. Produces no known toxins
    D. Can spread from person to person
    E. Can infect any tissue in the human body

32. Clinically, Legionnaires' disease:
    A. Is a respiratory illness that may be severe
    B. Is highly resistant to antibiotics
    C. Is best treated with penicillin
    D. Is a self-limiting disease
    E. Takes several years to develop

33. The material produced by *M. tuberculosis* that is responsible for serpentine formation is
    A. Sulfatide
    B. Mycolic acid

C. Cord factor
D. PPD
E. M protein

34. The material produced by *M. tuberculosis* that promotes the survival of the bacterium inside normal macrophages is:
    A. Sulfatide
    B. Mycolic acid
    C. Cord factor
    D. PPD
    E. M protein

35. Which of the following bacteria can cause tuberculosis in humans?
    A. *Mycobacterium marinum*
    B. *Mycobacterium bovis*
    C. *Mycobacterium kansasii*
    D. *Mycobacterium xenopi*
    E. *Mycobacterium simiae*

36. *Mycobacterium leprae* is similar to *Mycobacterium tuberculosis* **except** for its:
    A. Gram's stain reaction
    B. Acid-fast reaction
    C. In vitro cultivation
    D. Survival inside normal macrophages
    E. Cell morphology

37. Which of the following organisms has a unique development cycle with two morphogenic forms?
    A. *Rickettsia rickettsii*
    B. *Chlamydia trachomatis*
    C. *Coxiella burnetii*
    D. *Rochalimaea quintana*
    E. *Rickettsia typhi*

38. Epidemic louse-borne typhus is caused by:
    A. *Rickettsia prowazekii*
    B. *Rickettsia typhi*
    C. *Rickettsia rickettsii*
    D. *Rickettsia conorii*
    E. *Rickettsia akari*

39. The vector for Brill's disease is:
    A. The tick
    B. The louse
    C. The mite
    D. The mosquito
    E. No vector is involved

40. The most common rickettsial disease in the U.S. is:
    A. Rocky Mountain spotted fever
    B. Epidemic tick-borne typhus
    C. Scrub fever
    D. Q fever
    E. Epidemic louse-borne typhus

41. Which of the following bacteria can be grown in vitro?
    A. *Rickettsia prowazekii*
    B. *Chlamydia trachomatis*

C. *Rochalimaea quintana*
D. *Coxiella burnetii*
E. *Chlamydia psittaci*

42. *Chlamydia trachomatis* can cause which of the following diseases?
    A. Inclusion conjunctivitis
    B. Psittacosis
    C. Rocky Mountain spotted fever
    D. Q fever
    E. Scrub fever

43. Which of the following would be a TRIC agent?
    A. *Chlamydia trachomatis*
    B. *Chlamydia psittaci*
    C. *Chlamydia pneumoniae*
    D. *Rickettsia rickettsii*
    E. *Rickettsia prowazekii*

44. Anaerobic bacteria do not normally inhabit which region of the human body?
    A. Pharynx
    B. Mouth
    C. Skin
    D. Stomach
    E. Vagina

45. The indigenous flora interfere with the colonization of the human body by pathogens by which of the following mechanisms?
    A. Producing bacteriocins
    B. Competing for cellular attachment sites
    C. Generating toxic metabolites
    D. Maintaining an inhospitable environment
    E. All of the above may be involved

46. Dental caries are a *direct* consequence of:
    A. The production of organic acids by plaque bacteria
    B. The synthesis of glucan by *Streptococcus mutans*
    C. The colonization of plaque by anaerobes
    D. The presence of a salivary glycoprotein matrix on teeth
    E. The development of agglutinating IgA antibodies against oral flora components

47. The predominant anaerobic bacteria inhabiting the human skin belong to the genus:
    A. *Clostridium*
    B. *Propionibacterium*
    C. *Bacteroides*
    D. *Fusobacterium*
    E. *Bifidobacterium*

48. The single most important beneficial activity of the indigenous flora for the human host is:
    A. Enhancement of fluid absorption from the gut
    B. Interference with colonization by pathogenic organisms
    C. Stimulation of epithelial cell regeneration
    D. Vitamin production
    E. Stimulation of IgM antibody production

49. The region of the body with the largest population of indigenous anaerobic bacteria is the:
    A. Skin
    B. Vagina
    C. Urethra
    D. Colon
    E. Nose

50. Which of the following bodily structures contains no resident flora?
    A. Nose
    B. Teeth
    C. Bronchi
    D. Urethra
    E. Vagina

51. The O-specific side chains of gram-negative enteric bacteria are composed of:
    A. Repeating units of various monosaccharides
    B. Porins
    C. Eight carbon sugar acids
    D. Lipoteichoic acid
    E. Repeating units of D-glutamic acid

52. The toxic moiety of the outer membrane of gram-negative enteric bacteria consists of:
    A. Peptidoglycan
    B. Diaminopimelic acid
    C. Lipid A
    D. Ketodeoxyoctonate
    E. Glycoprotein

Use the following choices (A–D) to answer questions 53–57. Each lettered choice may be used once, more than once, or not at all.

    A. *Escherichia coli*
    B. *Klebsiella pneumoniae*
    C. *Proteus mirabilis*
    D. *Pseudomonas aeruginosa*

53. Produces characteristic blue-green pigments.

54. Characterized as being heavily encapsulated and producing pneumonia in debilitated individuals.

55. A lactose fermenting nosocomial pathogen that resides exclusively in the intestinal tract.

56. This organism is urease positive.

57. A ubiquitous, nonfermenting organism that frequently produces infections in compromised hospitalized patients.

58. Urease production by enteric bacteria involved with urinary tract infections is clinically significant because:
    A. The enzyme destroys the epithelial lining of the bladder
    B. Products of urease activity cause an alkalinization of the urine and precipitation of calcium and magnesium phosphates
    C. The enzyme facilitates migration of bacteria into the kidneys

D. Urease is the primary enzyme involved with digestion of mucus on epithelial cell surfaces

E. The enzyme is required for adherence of bacteria to uroepithelial cells

59. An individual experiences severe diarrhea after eating sushi (raw fish) in a West Coast restaurant. The most probable cause of the problem is:
   A. *Salmonella enteritidis*
   B. *Campylobacter jejuni*
   C. *Shigella sonnei*
   D. *Vibrio parahaemolyticus*
   E. *Yersinia enterocolitica*

60. *Salmonella* species can be differentiated from *Shigella* species in the diagnostic laboratory on the basis of:
   A. Motility
   B. Lactose fermentation
   C. Gram's stain
   D. Glucose fermentation
   E. Tolerance to anaerobic conditions

61. An outbreak of gastroenteritis occurred after a dinner party in New York. Twenty-eight of 33 persons who attended the party developed symptoms of diarrhea, headache, abdominal pain, nausea, fever, and vomiting within 24 hours after the dinner was consumed. The food implicated in the outbreak was caesar salad, which was prepared with raw eggs. The most likely cause of the outbreak was:
   A. Enterotoxigenic *E. coli*
   B. *Salmonella enteritidis*
   C. *Vibrio cholerae*
   D. *Shigella dysenteriae*
   E. *Vibrio parahaemolyticus*

62. There is no animal reservoir for:
   A. *Campylobacter jejuni*
   B. *Salmonella typhimurium*
   C. *Vibrio cholerae*
   D. *Yersinia enterocolitica*
   E. Enterohemorrhagic *E. coli*

63. One would **not** expect to find erythrocytes and neutrophils in the stools of patients with:
   A. Bacillary dysentery
   B. Cholera
   C. *Salmonella* gastroenteritis
   D. Colitis caused by enteroinvasive *E. coli*
   E. *Campylobacter* enteritis

64. Systemic infections in humans are caused by:
   A. *Vibrio cholerae*
   B. Enterotoxigenic *E. coli*
   C. *Vibrio parahaemolyticus*
   D. *Salmonella typhi*
   E. *Shigella sonnei*

Match the principal mechanism of toxin action given below (A–E) with the toxins listed in questions 65–69. Each choice may be used once, more than once, or not at all.

A. Ribosylates elongation factor 2
B. Inactivates the 60S ribosomal subunit
C. Locks the enzyme adenylate cyclase into active conformation
D. Blocks glucose dehydrogenase activity
E. Locks the enzyme guanylate cyclase into active conformation

65. *E. coli* LT enterotoxin
66. Shiga cytotoxin
67. *E. coli* ST enterotoxin
68. Cholera toxin
69. *Pseudomonas aeruginosa* exotoxin A

70. When symptoms of typhoid fever first become apparent, *Salmonella typhi* is most frequently isolated from:
   A. The sputum
   B. The feces
   C. Purulent exudates
   D. The blood
   E. The urine

71. The enzyme produced by *Helicobacter pylori* that appears to be important for survival of the organism in the stomach is:
   A. Urease
   B. Protease
   C. Adenylate cyclase
   D. Lipase
   E. Alkaline phosphatase

72. This microaerophilic curved rod, which frequently causes enteritis in humans, resides in the intestinal and reproductive tracts of animals.
   A. *Vibrio cholerae*
   B. *Salmonella choleraesuis*
   C. *Shigella flexneri*
   D. *Vibrio parahaemolyticus*
   E. *Campylobacter jejuni*

73. The virulence factor primarily responsible for the systemic aspects of salmonella infection is:
   A. Antiphagocytic activity
   B. Motility
   C. Exotoxin A production
   D. Ability to survive in phagocytes
   E. Resistant to lysis

74. Which of the following was most likely responsible for an outbreak of bacillary dysentery that occurred in a nursery school?
   A. A pet dog belonging to one of the children
   B. The school gardener
   C. Turtles in the school aquarium
   D. The school cook
   E. A parakeet brought in by one of the children

Select the method that is most appropriate for each sterilization or disinfection situation.
   A. Autoclaving

B. Ethylene oxide application
C. Tincture of iodine application
D. Filtration
E. Use of dry heat

75. A serum sample
76. The surface of the skin
77. Bacteriologic medium
78. Capped, empty test tubes
79. A plastic catheter

Match the following techniques or substances to the means by which they sterilize or disinfect.

A. Autoclave
B. Zephiran
C. Glutaraldehyde
D. Chlorine
E. Mercurochrome

80. Acts as an alkylating agent
81. Causes mercaptide production
82. Produces moist heat
83. Causes cell membrane disruption
84. Acts as an oxidizing agent

85. Penicillinases mediate bacterial resistance to penicillins by hydrolyzing:
A. The transpeptidases on the bacterial cell membrane
B. The beta-lactam ring
C. The dihydrothiazine ring
D. The thiazolidine ring
E. The side-chain radicals

86. Clavulanic acid is characterized by its:
A. Broad spectrum of antimicrobial activity
B. Inhibition of transpeptidases and carboxypeptidases
C. Reversible inhibition of bacterial protein synthesis
D. Irreversible inhibition of folic acid synthesis
E. Inactivation of beta lactamases

87. Metronidazole is **most** effective against:
A. Aerobic bacteria
B. Facultative aerobic bacteria
C. Obligate anaerobic bacteria
D. *Neisseria meningitidis*
E. *Staphylococcus aureus*

88. Trimethoprim:
A. Is an analogue of PABA (*P*-aminobenzoic acid)
B. Competitvely inhibits dihydrofolate reductase activity and blocks folic acid synthesis
C. Antagonizes the action of sulfonamides
D. Has limited use because mammalian enzymes have as high an affinity for the antibiotic as do bacterial enzymes
E. Is effective against bacteria that require preformed folic acid as a growth factor

89. Which one of the following agents is used in the treatment of leprosy?

A. Trimethoprim
B. Nitrofurantoin
C. Diaminodiphenylsulfone (DDS)
D. Co-trimoxazole
E. Polymyxin

90. Which of the following antibiotics binds to the 50S ribosomal subunit?
A. Polymyxin
B. Streptomycin
C. Penicillin
D. Chloramphenicol
E. Cephalothin

91. Erythromycin:
A. Blocks cross-linking of the peptidoglycan chain
B. Causes direct damage to the cell membrane by a detergent-like action
C. Damages the cytoplasmic membrane by attaching to sterols
D. Inhibits synthesis of protein
E. Inhibits RNA polymerase

92. Against which microorganism would metronidazole be most active?
A. *Haemophilus influenzae*
B. *Bordetella pertussis*
C. *Bacteroides fragilis*
D. *Neisseria meningitidis*
E. *Staphylococcus aureus*

Match each lettered antimicrobial agent with one of the numbered characteristics listed in items 93–95. Each antimicrobial agent may be used once, more than once, or not at all.

A. Cephalosporins
B. Erythromycin
C. Nalidixic acid
D. Polymyxins
E. Rifampin
F. Neomycin
G. Metronidazole

93. Inactivation of DNA-dependent RNA polymerase
94. Interferes with replication of DNA
95. Ototoxic and nephrotoxic

96. Clindamycin:
A. Is not active against anaerobic bacteria
B. Is always bactericidal against actively multiplying bacteria
C. Binds to the 50S ribosomal subunit, preventing peptide-chain elongation
D. Causes single- and double-strand breaks in DNA
E. All of the above answers are correct

97. Sulfonamides:
A. Are structural analogues of tetrahydropteroic acid synthetase
B. Interfere with microbial folic acid synthesis

C. Are structural analogues of dihydrofolate reductase

D. Are inactivated by beta lactamases

E. Are not absorbed from the gastrointestinal tract

98. All of the following are bacteriostatic chemotherapeutic agents **except:**
    A. Chloramphenicol
    B. Bacitracin
    C. Novobiocin
    D. Tetracycline
    E. Sulfonamides

99. The highest incidence of meningococcal infection occurs in which age group?
    A. 0 to 6 months of age
    B. 6 to 24 months of age
    C. 2 years to 5 years of age
    D. 5 years to 21 years of age
    E. Over 21 years of age

100. Animals other than humans constitute the primary reservoir for each of the following **except:**
    A. *Brucella abortus*
    B. *Leptospira pomona*
    C. *Neisseria gonorrhoeae*
    D. *Borrelia hermsii*
    E. *Yersinia pestis*

101. Effective vaccines presently in use against meningococcal disease contain which of the following as the primary immunizing agent?
    A. Heat-killed bacilli
    B. Lipopolysaccharide
    C. Pili (fimbriae)
    D. Capsular polysaccharide
    E. Major outer-membrane protein

102. Serogroup classification of *Neisseria meningitidis* is based on:
    A. The protein pili
    B. The polysaccharide capsule
    C. The outer-membrane proteins
    D. The lipopolysaccharide
    E. The IgA protease

103. The two most common complications of meningococcemia are:
    A. Brain abscess, endocarditis
    B. Urinary tract infection, pneumonia
    C. Myocarditis, arthritis
    D. Arthritis, meningitis
    E. Meningitis, pneumonia

104. There are six capsular types of this bacterium and type b seems to confer the potential for increased virulence:
    A. *Bordetella pertussis*
    B. *Haemophilus influenzae*
    C. *Brucella abortus*
    D. *Gardnerella vaginalis*
    E. *Haemophilus aegyptius*

105. A Gram's stain of spinal fluid from a 2-year-old child revealed gram-negative, small coccobacillary organisms. The most probable etiologic agent is:
    A. *Staphylococcus aureus*
    B. *Neisseria meningitidis*
    C. *Streptococcus pneumoniae*
    D. *Haemophilus influenzae*
    E. *Bordetella pertussis*

106. This disease is most commonly a result of occupational exposure (e.g., slaughterhouse workers, veterinarians, farmers) to diseased animals:
    A. Plague
    B. Tularemia
    C. Granuloma inguinale
    D. Brucellosis
    E. Fusospirochetosis

107. The most common clinical manifestation of *Yersinia pestis* infection is:
    A. Septicemic plague
    B. Meningitic plague
    C. Bubonic plague
    D. Pneumonic plague
    E. All of the above occur with about the same incidence

108. The vaccine used in the prevention of tularemia contains:
    A. Formalin-killed *Francisella tularensis*
    B. Formalin-inactivated endotoxin
    C. Live attenuated *Francisella tularensis*
    D. Live attenuated *Yersinia pestis*
    E. Formalin-inactivated murine toxin

109. A patient presents to the emergency room with a cellulitis that developed 24 hours following a cat bite. The **most likely** etiologic agent of the cellulitis is:
    A. *Pasteurella multocida*
    B. *Yersinia pestis*
    C. *Brucella abortus*
    D. *Francisella tularensis*
    E. *Bordetella pertussis*

110. In the diagnosis of pertussis, *Bordetella pertussis* is most likely isolated from:
    A. Blood culture during bacteremic phase of disease
    B. Joint fluid
    C. A nasopharyngeal swab cultured on Bordet-Gengou medium
    D. Abscess on the skin
    E. Spinal fluid

111. Patients with whooping cough are most infectious (contagious) during what stage of the illness?
    A. Incubation
    B. Catarrhal
    C. Paroxysmal
    D. Convalescent
    E. Spasmodic

112. This microorganism causes a sexually transmitted disease that can be diagnosed by demonstrating "Donovan bodies" in skin biopsies:
    A. *Plesiomonas shigelloides*
    B. *Calymmatobacterium granulomatis*
    C. *Cardiobacterium hominis*
    D. *Chromobacterium violaceum*
    E. *Bartonella bacilliformis*

113. Which microorganism may preferentially utilize erythritol as a nutrient source?
    A. *Pasteurella*
    B. *Brucella*
    C. *Yersinia*
    D. *Haemophilus*
    E. *Francisella*

114. Plague is transmitted by the:
    A. Louse
    B. Chigger
    C. Flea
    D. Mosquito
    E. Tick

115. Which spirochete(s) can be seen under ordinary light microscopy after staining with Giemsa or Wright stains?
    A. *Treponema pallidum*
    B. *Borrelia recurrentis*
    C. *Leptospira interrogans*
    D. Two of the above are correct
    E. All of the above are correct

116. Which spirochete(s) can be grown in vitro on artificial media and this growth used in the diagnosis of infection?
    A. *Treponema pallidum*
    B. *Spirillum minus*
    C. *Leptospira interrogans*
    D. *Treponema pertenue*
    E. *Borrelia recurrentis*

117. All of the following statements regarding the secondary stage of syphilis are true **except:**
    A. Skin and mucous membrane lesions are usually present
    B. Some individuals can pass through this stage with no symptoms
    C. *Treponema pallidum* is not present in the mucous membrane lesions
    D. Some patients will experience one or more relapses of the secondary stage of syphilis
    E. Serologic tests for syphilis are positive

118. The nonvenereal treponematoses can be differentiated from syphilis by:
    A. Microscopically examining skin lesions for morphologically distinct spirochetes
    B. Serologic detection of reaginic antibody
    C. Isolating and identifying the causative microorganisms

    D. Antimicrobial susceptibility testing
    E. None of the above are correct

119. The body louse is the vector for:
    A. Leptospirosis:
    B. Pinta
    C. Epidemic relapsing fever
    D. Lyme disease
    E. Meningitis

120. Leptospirosis:
    A. Is caused by a small, gram-negative coccobacillus
    B. Is frequently transmitted from human to human by inanimate objects
    C. Can result in a severe form of jaundice
    D. Is a sexually transmitted disease
    E. All of the above are correct

121. *Specific* treponemal tests for syphilis include:
    A. *Treponema pallidum* immobilization (TPI) test
    B. Fluorescent treponema antibody-absorption (FTA-ABS) test
    C. Both of the above
    D. Neither of the above

122. An individual with symptoms typical of secondary syphilis and high antibody titers in the VDRL (Venereal Disease Research Laboratory) and FTA-ABS (fluorescent treponema antibody-absorption) tests for syphilis is given the recommended treatment for syphilis. Which of the following would most likely occur if treatment were successful?
    A. Both the VDRL and FTA-ABS tests would remain positive
    B. The VDRL would remain positive and the FTA-ABS would become negative
    C. Both the VDRL and FTA-ABS tests would become negative
    D. The VDRL would become negative and the FTA-ABS would remain positive

Match each lettered microorganism with one of the numbered characteristics listed in items 123–128. Each microorganism may be selected once, more than once, or not at all.

    A. *Veillonella*
    B. *Bacteroides fragilis*
    C. *Bifidobacterium adolescentis*
    D. *Propionibacterium acnes*
    E. *Clostridium perfringens*
    F. *Porphyromonas*

123. Gram-positive nonsporeforming bacillus frequently found in the gastrointestinal tract

124. Gram-negative bacillus that produces black to brown pigmented colonies on blood agar medium

125. Gram-negative coccus

126. Anaerobic bacterium most frequently isolated from human infections

127. Common inhabitant of normal skin
128. Produces an enterotoxin as well as numerous toxic enzymes that contribute to its pathogenic potential as a causative agent of disease
129. Antibiotic-associated pseudomembranous colitis is caused by an exotoxin elaborated by:
    A. *Bacteroides fragilis*
    B. Toxigenic strains of *Escherichia coli*
    C. *Vibrio cholerae*
    D. *Clostridium difficile*
    E. *Clostridium perfringens*
130. "Tetanus neonatorum":
    A. Is caused by placental passage of *Clostridium tetani* into the neonate's circulatory system
    B. Is caused by failure of protective antibodies to cross the placenta
    C. Usually results from infection of the umbilicus by *Clostridium tetani*
    D. Is caused by placental passage of tetanospasmin into the neonate's circulatory system
    E. All of the above are correct
131. Which microorganism(s) produce(s) enzymes or toxins that cause tissue necrosis?
    A. *Clostridium botulinum*
    B. *Clostridium perfringens*
    C. Both of the above microorganisms
    D. Neither of the above microorganisms
132. The eitiologic agent of which of the following diseases produces several antigenically distinct neurotoxins that require a polyvalent antitoxin preparation for neutralization?
    A. Tetanus
    B. Botulism
    C. Gas gangrene
    D. Pseudomembranous colitis
    E. Enteritis necroticans
133. Tetanus toxin:
    A. Blocks release of acetylcholine at the neuromuscular junction
    B. Is directly toxic to contractile proteins of cardiac muscle
    C. Blocks inhibitory impulses of neurons causing muscular spasms
    D. Functions as a lecithinase
    E. Stimulates the level of adenylate cyclase in mammalian cells
134. Enterotoxin plays a role in producing clinical manifestations of disease produced by:
    A. *Clostridium perfringens*
    B. *Clostridium difficile*
    C. Both are correct
    D. Neither is correct
135. Gas gangrene can be caused by:
    A. *Clostridium perfringens*

B. *Clostridium novyi*
    C. *Clostridium septicum*
    D. *Clostridium fallax*
    E. All of the above
136. The agent for artificial immunization against *Clostridium tetani* consists of:
    A. Purified capsular antigen
    B. Purified cell-wall protein
    C. A toxic protein treated with formaldehyde
    D. An attenuated live organism
    E. O and Vi antigens
137. In which infection does an organism considered to be part of the normal flora become pathogenic?
    A. Nocardiosis
    B. Mycoplasmal pneumonia
    C. Actinomycosis
    D. Histoplasmosis
    E. Tuberculosis
138. Actinomycetous bacteria are:
    A. Gram-negative bacilli
    B. Gram-positive bacilli
    C. Gram-negative cocci
    D. Gram-positive cocci
    E. Gram-negative curved rods
139. Which organism has a predilection for brain tissue in disseminated disease?
    A. *Nocardia asteroides*
    B. *Chlamydia psittaci*
    C. Toxigenic strains of *Escherichia coli*
    D. *Actinomyces israelii*
    E. *Clostridium botulinum*
140. Which infection, in a large number of cases (about 75%), may be considered opportunistic in compromised hosts?
    A. Actinomycosis
    B. Eumycetoma
    C. Nocardiosis
    D. Actinomycetoma
    E. Coccidioidomycosis
141. The formation of sinus tracts from infected areas is a characteristic of which of the following infections?
    A. Nocardiosis
    B. Actinomycosis
    C. Pelvic inflammatory disease
    D. Erythrasma
    E. Listeriosis
142. Which of the following is **not** true about pathogenic species of *Nocardia?*
    A. Normal soil inhabitants
    B. Partially acid-fast
    C. Gram-positive
    D. Carry a lysogenic phage responsible for virulence
    E. May be implicated in more than one disease

Answers

1. B The pathogenicity of a microorganism is directly related to its ability to cause pathologic changes. The virulence of a bacterium is what allows it to be pathogenic.

2. A Bacteria cause disease by being able to invade and/or produce toxins.

3. D Answers A, B, C, and E refer to bacterial virulence factors. Answer D is a cell-wall structure, not a virulence factor.

4. D *Mycobacterium tuberculosis* can survive inside normal macrophages because it produces sulfatides that stop phagosomes from fusing with lysosomes. The other organisms listed cannot do this.

5. B The botulism toxin produces a flaccid paralysis in patients. It does this by virtue of preventing the release of the neurotransmitter, acetylcholine.

6. D *Corynebacterium diphtheriae* is the only bacterium listed in this question that produces a toxin that inactivates EF-2.

7. B *Pseudomonas aeruginosa* produces exotoxin A, a toxin that also inactivates EF-2.

8. A Much of the diarrhea caused by *E. coli* is a result of the production of the toxin that causes cyclic AMP accumulation in the epithelial cells of the mucosal lining. This causes fluids to diffuse into the gut.

9. D The toxicity of endotoxin cannot be destroyed by autoclaving. The endotoxin of gram-negative bacteria is the only place in nature where ketodeoxyoctonate is found.

10. B *Vibrio cholerae* and *E. coli* produce toxins that activate adenylate cyclase, resulting in an accumulation of cyclic AMP in the epithelial cells of the mucosal lining.

11. D Certain bacterial toxins are called "superantigens" because they induce an immune response (T-cell proliferation) in doses far lower than the "typical" antigen.

12. A Diphtheria toxin kills cells by inactivating EF-2, which causes protein synthesis to stop.

13. A The pseudomembrane seen in clinical diphtheria is composed of dead host cells (killed by the diphtheria toxin), fibrin, and bacteria (most notably *C. diphtheriae*).

14. C Only toxoids would be included in a vaccine. Toxins cause adverse reactions. The third portion of the DTP vaccine is against *Bordetella pertussis* (whooping cough).

15. B The capsule of *Bacillus anthracis* is the only bacterial capsule composed of amino acids (D-glutamic acid).

16. D *Bacillus anthracis* is unlike *Mycobacterium tuberculosis* in that it cannot live inside normal macrophages.

17. A *Listeria monocytogenes* does not produce spores. The only important genera that produce spores are *Bacillus* and *Clostridia*.

18. B *Bacillus cereus* is not associated with intrauterine or respiratory tract infection, or venereal disease. It is an infrequently recognized cause of food poisoning in the U.S.

19. D The staphylococci produce catalase, while the streptococci do not.

20. A The most important antiphagocytic structure of the group A streptococci is the M protein. The group A carbohydrate has no antiphagocytic capability. The hyaluronic acid capsule is an antiphagocytic structure but is clearly of less importance than the M protein. The group A streptococci do not produce protein A or mycolic acids.

21. C *Staphylococcus aureus* produces coagulase; *Staph. epidermidis* does not.

22. B The exfoliation toxin is so named because it causes the shedding of skin.

23. D *Staphylococcus epidermidis* does not produce the same virulence factors as *Staph. aureus*.

24. C Pyogenes means pus formation. Among the streptococci, the group A streptococci cause the largest number of streptococcal diseases and are thus the most important. For this reason, they were assigned the first letter of the alphabet.

25. D *Agalactiae* means cessation of milk production. The group B streptococci were first observed to cause mastitis in dairy cattle, resulting in a decrease in milk production. The GBS were first observed to cause bacterial neonatal meningitis in humans in the 1970s.

26. C Type 12 has been most frequently associated with AGN after pharyngitis, with the majority of the other strains being associated with pyoderma.

27. C The viridans streptococci are commonly found in the nasopharynx and mouth. From these sites the organisms may invade the bloodstream after chewing or dental manipulation. Once in the bloodstream they can reach defective heart valves.

28. C *Staphylococcus saprophyticus* occurs on normal skin and in the periurethral and urethral flora. It is second only to *E. coli* as a cause of urinary tract infections in young, sexually active females.

29. B Viruses, rickettsia, and chlamydia are not free-living.

30. A The term *L-forms* comes from the fact that they were discovered at the Lister Institute in the early 1900s. They are bacteria without cell walls.

31. B *Legionella pneumophila* can survive inside normal macrophages but the mechanism by which it does this is presently unknown.

32. A Legionnaires' disease is normally an upper respiratory tract infection that can develop into pneumonia. Its usual source is the air-conditioning system.

33. C Cord factor is 6,6'-dimycolyl trehalose. Cord factor itself is toxic.

34. A Sulfatides produced by *M. tuberculosis* do not allow lysosomes and phagosomes to fuse, which means that inside normal macrophages, this organism is not exposed to the degradative enzymes that would normally kill it.

35. B *Mycobacterium tuberculosis, M. bovis,* and *M. africanum* can cause tuberculosis in humans.

36. C *Mycobacterium leprae* has never been cultivated in vitro, while *M. tuberculosis* is easily cultivated on Lowenstein-Jensen medium.

37. B The *Chlamydia* produce an intracellular life form (reticulate body) and an extracellular, infectious particle (elementary body).

38. A *Rickettsia prowazekii* can infect both the human body louse *(Pediculus humanus corporis)* and the head louse *(Pediculus humanus capitis),* the former being the more significant vector.

39. E Brill's disease is a recrudescence (reactivation) of epidemic louse-borne typhus. No vector is involved.

40. A Rocky Mountain spotted fever accounts for 95 percent of the rickettsial disease in the U.S.

41. C *Rochalimaea quintana* can be grown on blood agar in the presence of 10% CO_2.

42. A Diseases caused by *C. trachomatis* include trachoma, inclusion conjunctivitis, LGV, and so forth.

43. A All TRIC agents belong to the species *C. trachomatis,* which causes *tr*achoma and *i*nclusion conjunctivitis.

44. D The stomach contains no resident flora. All other regions harbor anaerobic bacteria.

45. E All of the activities listed (A–D) are thought to interfere with colonization by pathogenic bacteria.

46. A Although activities B through D are involved with plaque formation, only A is directly responsible for dental caries production.

47. B These organisms are present primarily in the hair follicles.

48. B Of the activities listed, B is considered to be most important.

49. D It is estimated that the colon contains a total of between 10^{13} and 10^{14} organisms. Most are anaerobes.

50. C Transient organisms are present in the bronchi but the region contains no resident flora.

51. A The monosaccharides are hexoses that occur in repeating units of three or four.

52. C Purified lipid A is toxic when injected into animals.

53. D

54. B

55. A

56. C

57. D

58. B *Proteus mirabilis* and *P. vulgaris* as well as *Morganella morganii* and *Providencia rettgeri* produce urease.

59. D *Vibrio parahaemolyticus,* which inhabits estuaries and contaminates seafood, most likely caused the diarrhea.

60. A *Salmonella* species are motile and *Shigella* species nonmotile. The two genera are the same regarding the other characteristics.

61. B Eggs sometimes harbor *Salmonella* species and when eaten raw are a source of gastroenteritis.

62. C This organism is found in humans only.

63. B *Vibrio cholerae,* the cause of cholera, is a noninvasive toxin producer. The other diseases listed are produced by invasive organisms that induce inflammation and often cause ulceration so that inflammatory cells are found in the stool.

64. D The other organisms produce diseases confined to the intestinal tract.

65. C

66. B

67. E

68. C

69. A

70. D In the course of this systemic disease, the organisms quickly pass from the intestinal tract to the bloodstream, after which they produce infections in various organs of the body and eventually reinfect the intestine.

71. A Urease breaks down the urea in the stomach, producing ammonia and causing an increase in pH. Thus, the organisms survive in a normally acidic environment.

72. E

73. D After traversing the intestinal tract, salmonella that are able to survive in phagocytic cells are disseminated throughout the body to produce infections in various organs.

74. D *Shigella* species, responsible for bacillary dysentery, infect only humans and other primates. The school cook, who handles food, was a more likely source of the disease than the school gardener.

75. D Serum, which is heat sensitive, can be filtered.

76. C Tincture of iodine is an effective skin antiseptic.

77. A As long as the medium is exposed to the steam

(gauze and cotton stopped flask) autoclaving is the best method.

78. E   Autoclaving is ineffective because the tubes are capped.

79. B   The plastic catheter, which could be damaged by heat, can be sterilized with ethylene oxide.

80. C

81. E

82. A

83. B   Zephiran is a cationic surface-active agent.

84. D   This is due to hypochlorous acid formation.

85. B   Structural integrity of the beta-lactam ring is essential for the antimicrobial activity of the penicillins. Penicillinases (also called beta lactamases) hydrolyze the beta-lactam ring.

86. E   Clavulanic acid is a beta-lactamase inhibitor that irreversibly binds to and inactivates beta lactamases. It has very little intrinsic antibacterial activity and it is administered simultaneously with a beta-lactam antimicrobial agent.

87. C   Metronidazole has selective antimicrobial activity against obligate anaerobic bacteria, some microaerophilic bacteria, and certain anaerobic protozoan pathogens.

88. B   Trimethoprim is a structural analogue of dihydrofolic acid that competitively inhibits bacterial dihydrofolic acid reductase, resulting in an inhibition of folic acid and ultimately purine and DNA synthesis. Mammalian cells and bacteria that use environmental preformed folic acid for growth are not inhibited by trimethoprim (or the sulfonamides).

89. C   Diaminodiphenylsulfone is used only in the treatment of leprosy.

90. D   Chloramphenicol binds reversibly to the 50S ribosomal subunit resulting in an inhibition of protein synthesis. Streptomycin, on the other hand, binds to the 30S ribosomal subunit. The other antimicrobial agents do not inhibit protein synthesis.

91. D   Erythromycin inhibits protein synthesis by binding to the 50S ribosomal subunit.

92. C   Metronidazole is selectively active against obligate anaerobic bacteria; *Bacteroides fragilis* is the only obligate anaerobe listed.

93. E   Rifampin selectively inhibits bacterial DNA-dependent RNA polymerase while having no effect on mammalian DNA-dependent RNA polymerase.

94. C   Nalidixic acid blocks DNA synthesis by inhibiting bacterial DNA gyrase.

95. F   Two of the most serious adverse reactions associated with aminoglycoside use are nephrotoxicity and ototoxicity.

96. C   Clindamycin is primarily used in the treatment of infections caused by anaerobic bacteria. It revers-

ibly binds to the 50S ribosomal subunit resulting in bacteriostatic inhibition of susceptible bacteria.

97. B   Sulfonamides are structural analogues of PABA that competitively inhibit tetrahydropteroic acid synthesis. This results in an inhibition of folic acid synthesis.

98. B   Bacitracin is the only antimicrobial agent listed that is bactericidal. All the other antimicrobial agents are bacteriostatic.

99. B   Passive transfer of maternal antibody protects the majority of infants less than 6 months of age against meningococcal infection. The incidence of natural immunity increases with age and this accounts for the greater prevalence of disease in children than in adults.

100. C   The only known reservoirs for *N. gonorrhoeae* are symptomatic and asymptomatic humans. All the other microorganisms listed in this question are zoonoses with animal reservoirs.

101. D   Vaccination with purified meningococcal capsular polysaccharide is an effective means of preventing epidemics of *N. meningitidis* infection and reducing the carrier state.

102. B   Nine serogroups of *N. meningitidis* have been identified on the basis of immunologic specificity of capsular polysaccharides.

103. D   The most frequent clinical manifestation of the meningococcemia is a petechial skin rash whereas the most frequent complications of meningococcemia are arthritis and meningitis.

104. B   Six antigenically distinct capsular types have been described for *H. influenzae*. Virtually all strains of *H. influenzae* isolated from invasive infections belong to serotype b.

105. D   Of the microorganisms listed, only *H. influenzae* and *B. pertussis* are gram-negative, small coccobacillary organisms. *Bordetella pertussis* is rarely a cause of meningitis while *H. influenzae* is the leading cause of meningitis in young children.

106. D   Brucellosis in humans is a zoonosis. Within the U.S., infection in humans is primarily from occupational exposure either through inhalation of infected droplets or handling of infected tissue.

107. C   In bubonic plague the microorganism enters the host through the skin and is carried by the lymphatics to the lymph nodes. In some individuals *Y. pestis* will enter the bloodstream and be carried to the lungs or meninges.

108. C   A live, attenuated strain of *F. tularensis* is available to immunize both animals and humans against tularemia.

109. A   *Pasteurella multocida* is a normal inhabitant of the upper respiratory tract of cats and other lower

animals. Approximately 25 percent of cat bites become infected with this microorganism and acute onset of cellulitis is the primary clinical manifestation.

110. C The bacteriologic diagnosis of pertussis is made by recovering the organism from respiratory secretions. *Bordetella pertussis* rarely penetrates the mucous membranes of the respiratory tract. Bordet-Gengou medium is an enriched medium for isolation of *B. pertussis.*

111. B Communicability of *B. pertussis* is greatest during the catarrhal stage of the disease when the patient is displaying symptoms of a minor upper respiratory tract infection.

112. B *Calymmatobacterium granulomatis* causes a venereal disease known as granuloma inguinale. Diagnosis of granuloma inguinale depends on the demonstration of encapsulated, oval bodies (Donovan bodies) in the cytoplasma of large histiocytic endothelial cells.

113. B The predilection of brucellae for placental tissue of animals is due to the presence of a growth stimulant, erythritol.

114. C The flea can transmit *Y. pestis* from infected rodents to humans or from person to person. There are no other arthropod vectors for *Y. pestis.*

115. B *Borrelia recurrentis* is the largest of the spirochetes and can be seen under ordinary light microscopy. *Treponema* species and *L. interrogans* are too small to be visualized by ordinary light microscopy and require special techniques (e.g., dark-field microscopy) to be observed in the laboratory.

116. C *Leptospira* species are the only pathogenic spirochetes that can be readily grown on a variety of artificial media.

117. C Both the primary chancre and secondary lesions of syphilis contain large numbers of treponemes and are highly infectious when located on exposed surfaces.

118. E All the pathogenic treponemes are morphologically and immunologically indistinguishable. Differences in geographic locations, where the diseases occur, and clinical manifestations permit separation of the species.

119. C *Borrelia recurrentis,* the causative agent of epidemic relapsing fever, is transmitted from person to person by the human body louse.

120. C The most severe form of leptospirosis, referred to as icteric leptospirosis, is characterized by impaired renal and hepatic function.

121. C Both tests detect antibody to *T. pallidum* subspecies *pallidum* antigens rather than to reagin.

122. D Following successful treatment, the nonspecific,

nontreponemal reaginic antibody tests (e.g., VDRL) become negative while the specific antitreponemal antibody tests (e.g., FTA-ABS) remain positive.

123. C *Bifidobacterium adolescentis* is the only grampositive nonsporeforming bacillus listed. Others include *Lactobacillus, Actinomyces, Arachnia, Eubacterium,* and *Propionibacterium.*

124. F Most species in both *Porphyromonas* and *Prevotella* produce brown to black colony pigment on blood agar.

125. A *Veillonella* is the only obligately anaerobic gramnegative coccus of clinical importance.

126. B *Bacteroides fragilis* is also more resistant to antimicrobials than any other anaerobe.

127. D *P. acnes* is a gram-positive bacillus that is a common contaminant of blood and other specimens. However, it may be associated with infections involving implanted prosthetic devices, such as heart valves, and orthopedic prostheses.

128. E *C. perfringens* is the most common clostridial species isolated from infection. The exotoxins it produces are responsible for the symptoms of gas gangrene and the enterotoxin it produces is responsible for the symptoms of food poisoning.

129. D Although all the bacteria listed produce enterotoxins, only *C. difficile* causes pseudomembranous colitis associated with antibiotic administration.

130. C Tetanus neonatorum results from postnatal infection of the umbilicus of infants from inadequately immunized mothers. Proper immunization of mothers will transfer protective antibodies to the infants.

131. B *Clostridium perfringens* elaborates several exotoxins that destroy healthy tissue. *Clostridium botulinum,* on the other hand, is not invasive in tissue.

132. B *Clostridium botulinum* produces eight antigenically distinct neurotoxins. However, the pharmacologic action of these toxins is identical. *Clostridium tetani,* on the other hand, produces only one antigenic type of neurotoxin.

133. C *Clostridium tetani* neurotoxin interferes with neuromuscular transmission by inhibiting the release of inhibitory transmitters (e.g., glycine) at spinal synapses. This results in excess motor activity and the typical muscle spasms of tetanus.

134. C The enterotoxin produced by *C. perfringens* is responsible for the clinical manifestations of food poisoning while the enterotoxin produced by *C. difficile* in partially responsible for the clinical manifestations of pseudomembranous colitis.

135. E Most cases of gas gangrene are caused by *C.*

perfringens. However, several other clostridial species that can be involved in gas gangrene include *C. novyi, C. septicum, C. fallax, C. histolyticum,* and *C. sordellii.*

136. C The only effective means to prevent tetanus is by prophylactic immunization. Tetanus toxoid consists of inactivated neurotoxin. In combination with diphtheria toxoid and pertussis vaccine, it is usually given during the first year of life.

137. C *Actinomyces israelii, Actinomyces naeslundii,* and *Arachnia propionica,* agents of actinomycosis, are components of normal oral and intestinal flora.

138. B Actinomycetes are gram-positive bacilli with varying tendencies to form filaments.

139. A *Clostridium botulinum* produces a neurotoxin but does not itself propagate in brain tissue. *Nocardia asteroides* may cause abscesses in the brain following dissemination.

140. C Nearly half of cases of nocardiosis occur in known compromised patients while another 25 percent occur in patients with a suspected defect in host defense.

141. B Abscess formation is characteristic of actinomycotic infections, and sinus tracts may form characteristically in actinomycosis and actinomycetoma but rarely in nocardiosis.

142. D Virulence of *Nocardia* species is not known to be attributable to a lysogenic phage.

Suggested Reading

Baron, S. (ed.). *Medical Microbiology* (3rd ed.). New York: Churchill Livingstone, 1991.

Boyd, R. F., and Hoerl, G. B. *Basic Medical Microbiology* (4th ed.). Boston: Little, Brown, 1991.

Davis, B. D., Dulbecco, R., Eisen, H. N., and Ginsberg, H. S. *Microbiology* (4th ed.). Philadelphia: Lippincott, 1990.

Joklik, W. K., Willett, H. P., Amos, D. B., and Wilfert, C. M. *Zinsser Microbiology* (20th ed.). Norwalk, CT: Appleton and Lange, 1992.

Schaechter, M., Medoff, G., and Eisenstein, B. I. (eds.). *Mechanisms of Microbial Disease* (2nd ed.). Baltimore: Williams & Wilkins, 1993.

Sherris, J. C. (ed.). *Medical Microbiology: An Introduction to Infectious Diseases* (2nd ed.). New York: Elsevier, 1990.

Volk, W. A., Benjamin, D. C., Kadner, R. J., and Parsons, J. T. *Essentials of Medical Microbiology* (4th ed.). Philadelphia: Lippincott, 1991.

Pathogenic Bacteriology

Virology

General Characteristics and Structure of Viruses

Earl M. Ritzi

Viruses are the smallest infectious agents, having a 20- to 300-nm diameter. This small size led viruses to be characterized in light-microscopy studies as submicroscopic infectious entities. Only poxviruses, which are the largest of the deoxyribonucleic acid (DNA) viruses, proved to be exceptions to this characterization. The term *filterable agents* has also been applied to viruses. Since viruses are smaller than bacteria, they pass through 0.22-μ filters that retain other microbes. Loeffler and Frosch discovered that a bacteria-free filtrate could transmit foot-and-mouth disease. This finding led to the discovery of the foot-and-mouth disease virus. Similarly, filtrates transmitted leukemia in mice, tobacco mosaic virus (TMV) disease in tobacco plants, and agents responsible for lysis of bacteria. These findings, which respectively led to the discovery of oncogenic murine retroviruses, tobacco mosaic virus, and the bacteriophages, contributed to the use of the term *filterable agent.*

Organismic Nature of Viruses

Viruses can be thought of as genetic parasites whose DNA or ribonucleic acid (RNA) genomes invade cells. These genomes replicate within cells, often utilizing a combination of preexisting or induced cellular enzymes and unique viral genome-encoded enzymes that may be present within viral particles (virion associated), or may be synthesized de novo in viral-infected cells. The nature of a virus is further revealed as progeny genomes, encoding unique viral structural proteins, become complete virus particles (virions) by utilizing cellular energy-producing systems and cellular protein-synthesizing systems to form protective protein shells. Rather than argue whether viruses are living or dead, viruses are best thought of as biologically active during intracellular replication and inactive as extracellu-

lar viral particles. The medical importance of virology has always been associated with acute, chronic, and fatal human diseases; however, in addition, the present-day study of virology views viral genomes containing 10 to 200 genes as relatively simple molecular models that permit new insights into complex biologic problems (such as cancer induction or immune deficiency) and further add to our basic knowledge of life at the cellular and molecular level.

Distinctive Characteristics of Viruses

While many properties of viruses are common or shared with bacteria, several characteristics distinguish viruses from other microorganisms. The following are distinctive characteristics of viruses:

1. Viruses contain only a single type of nucleic acid as their genome. The type of nucleic acid present may be either DNA or RNA but not both.
2. Viruses replicate from their own genetic material utilizing different replication strategies, not by the process of binary fission.
3. Viruses are obligate intracellular parasites that are dependent on cellular energy production and cellular machinery (e.g., ribosomes, transfer RNA) for protein synthesis.
4. Viruses synthesize their parts separately and then rely on spontaneous macromolecular interactions for their maturation.
5. Viruses are not sensitive to the usual antibiotics.

Host Range

Individual viruses may demonstrate a narrow species-specific host range for replication or even a tissue-specific tropism; however, as a group, viruses have a very broad host range, infecting humans, other vertebrates, insects, plants, and bacteria.

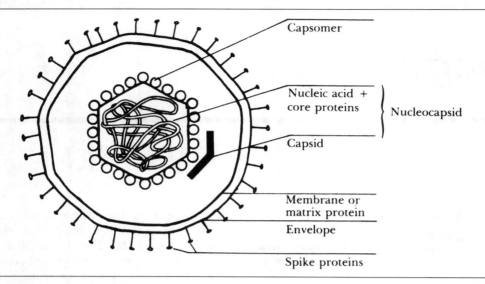

Capsomer

Nucleic acid +
core proteins   } Nucleocapsid

Capsid

Membrane or
matrix protein

Envelope

Spike proteins

Fig. 5-1   Components of a complete virus particle, or virion.

Theories of Viral Evolution

The origin of viruses, while still unknown, has been the subject of considerable speculation. The following are three widely discussed hypotheses:

1. Viruses evolved from some cellular component or structure that became autonomous or free of cellular control. These components may have been cellular regulatory genes or structures such as mitochondria. Smaller viruses and retroviruses are good candidates for evolution from cellular components.
2. Viruses may have evolved from primitive bacteria, by retrograde evolution. While there is some support for the evolution of chlamydiae and rickettsiae, there is little documentation to support viral evolution. This hypothesis has been suggested for evolution of the larger viruses.
3. Viruses, while parasites of ancestral cell types, evolved together with them, maintaining the host-parasite relationship. This theory is supported by the nonlethal persistent and latent infections caused by many viruses.

Structure

The electron microscope has permitted a detailed examination of both the size and morphology of DNA and RNA viruses that infect eucaryotic cells, as well as the bacteriophages that infect bacteria. There is a striking diversity in both size and morphology among members of the RNA and DNA virus families. To examine these structural differences and define similar or unifying aspects of structure,

virologists have generated a nomenclature for the various components of virus particles and a means for defining the symmetry of virus particles. The components of a complete virus particle, or virion, are presented in Fig. 5-1.

The following descriptions of viral nomenclature provide useful definitions of these terms and explain the basic functions of these viral structures.

Core

The innermost part of the viral particle, consisting of the viral nucleic acid and associated proteins, is the core. The viral nucleic acid, or genome, encodes viral-specific functions. The proteins associated with viral nucleic acids in the core may be specific enzymes such as DNA or RNA polymerase, reverse transcriptase, or histone-like proteins. In small viruses such as the papovaviruses, host-cell nuclear histones are incorporated as core proteins, whereas in larger viruses such as retroviruses, core proteins may be coded by the viral genome.

Capsid

The symmetric protein shell that surrounds the viral nucleic acid in the core is termed the capsid. The capsid protects the viral nucleic acid. In naked capsid viruses, it is important in adsorption to host-cell receptors, thereby determining the host range of virus infection.

Capsomers

The morphologic units that compose the capsid are capsomers. These are the morphologic units visualized with the electron microscope on the surface of naked capsid viruses. Capsomers are composed of clusters of polypeptides, or structural units.

Structural Units

The chemical units or single polypeptide chains that aggregate to form capsomers are referred to as structural units.

Nucleocapsid

The structure consisting of the nucleic acid protected by a protein capsid is the nucleocapsid.

Envelope

A membrane-like outer coat, or peplos, is termed the envelope. This structure is a membrane-like lipid bilayer with viral-coded glycoproteins and cell-derived lipids. While viral polypeptides are viral coded and lipids (with the exception of poxviruses) are of cellular origin, the carbohydrate portions of viral glycoproteins are influenced by both the viral-encoded primary protein structures and the particular host cell's complement of enzymes such as glycosyl transferases. The membrane may be obtained from host-cell membrane, nuclear membrane, or cytoplasmic membranes, or, in the case of poxviruses, it may be synthesized de novo in the cytoplasm. With enveloped viruses, the envelope antigens play decisive roles in determining the host range of infection and the specificity of host immune responses.

Tegument

Tegument is a term used exclusively in describing herpes viral particles. It is an amorphous asymmetric layer of material rich in viral-coded globular proteins that is found between the icosahedral nucleocapsid and the envelope of herpesviruses.

Membrane or Matrix Protein

A relatively hydrophobic protein located on the inside of the viral envelope of many enveloped RNA viruses is referred to as the matrix protein. This protein is located beneath the external spike proteins of the viral envelope and beneath the plasma membrane of RNA virus–producing cells. The viral nucleocapsid interacts with the matrix protein in budding through the host-cell membrane.

Spike Proteins

Viral-coded envelope glycoproteins that project from the envelope surface are spike proteins. These proteins may have specialized functions such as hemagglutination or neuraminidase activity, or they may promote cell-membrane fusion.

Virion

The complete or mature infectious virus particle is a virion. Depending on the virus in question, the virion may be a naked or enveloped capsid.

Pseudovirion

A virus particle that acquired host-cell genetic material during replication rather than viral nucleic acid is a pseudovirion. These particles have the potential to transduce cellular genes from one host cell to another.

Viroid

The viroid is a small infectious agent that causes disease in plants and possibly some slow-virus infections of animals. This agent is composed of nucleic acid (closed, circular RNA molecules of 70,000–120,000 molecular weight) without a structural protein coat.

Types of Symmetry

The architecture of a virion is strongly influenced by the symmetry of the viral capsid. Virus morphologies fall into one of the following three types of symmetry: helical, cubic, or complex.

Helical Symmetry

The nucleic acid of the virus with helical symmetry has a springlike or screwlike flexible configuration (helical), and the protein capsid is condensed on the helical nucleic acid. The prototype of helical symmetry is the plant virus, tobacco mosaic virus. Protein structure determines the diameter of the nucleocapsid, while length is determined by the nucleic acid. Medically important human viruses do not exist as naked helical nucleocapsids. These nucleocapsids are typically coiled within envelopes. Helical nucleocapsids are characteristic of virion structure in the orthomyxoviruses, paramyxoviruses, rhabdoviruses, bunyaviruses, filoviruses, arenaviruses, and coronaviruses. Helical nucleocapsids differ in length, width, periodicity, and flexibility.

Cubic Symmetry

All animal viruses that utilize cubic symmetry have capsids that form an icosahedron. An icosahedron is similar in structure to a geodesic dome. This structure has 20 faces or facets, each composed of an equilateral triangle, 12 vertices, and 30 edges. It is unique in possessing three types of rotational symmetry: fivefold, threefold, and twofold. The icosahedron can be assembled from a small number of repeating identical subunits (capsomers) to form a rigid protein structure. This means that only a small number of

Virology

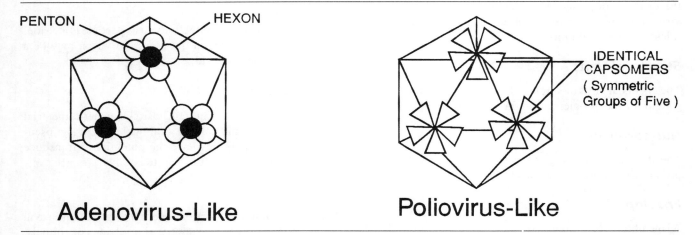

Fig. 5-2 Two different capsomer icosahedral patterns.

viral genes are required to specify capsid structure. In addition to genome economy, icosahedral symmetry provides a minimal energy design for a closed-shell capsid and a structure with a maximum volume and minimum surface area. As icosahedrons increase in size, the number of equilateral triangles on a face increases. This number of triangles is referred to as the triangulation number T. The total number of capsomers in a virion also increases with T, and the following equation can be used to determine the total number of capsomers if the triangulation number is known: capsomer number = 10T + 2. Two very different icosahedral patterns of capsomers utilize 5:3:2-fold rotational symmetry (Fig. 5-2). Adenovirus can be thought of as the prototype for one pattern shared by herpesvirus and iridovirus capsids. This pattern consists of 12 penton capsomers (each having 5 neighboring capsomers) that are situated at each of the 12 vertices and X number of hexon capsomers (each having 6 neighbors) situated on edges and faces. A second capsomer pattern (see Fig. 5-2) is exemplified by picornaviruses such as polio and is shared by papova-, parvo-, and birnavirus capsids. In this case, identical capsomers are spaced equidistantly from a common center to yield a more spherical structure; however, in poliovirus symmetric groups of 5 identical capsomers at each of the 12 vertices maintain the fivefold symmetry of icosahedral structure. The parvo-, papova-, adeno-, herpes-, picorna-, calici-, birna-, reo-, hepadna-, flavi-, and togaviruses are examples of viruses with icosahedral symmetry.

Complex Symmetry

Viruses that cannot be categorized as helical or cubic are complex. Viruses are considered complex if they have complex structures, such as poxviruses, or if they have two types of nucleocapsid symmetry (helical and cubic), such as retro-

viruses; however, some authorities emphasize the cubic capsid shell and place retroviruses in the icosahedral group.

Morphology

Symmetry is combined with presence or absence of an envelope to define viral morphology. Table 5-1 associates viral families and human viral representatives of each with their morphologic descriptions.

Classification

Earl M. Ritzi

Despite the diversity in morphology and striking differences in the size of both RNA and DNA viruses, shared characteristics have been utilized to classify human viruses into different genera and families. Over the years, many different taxonomic groupings have been created. The division of viruses into different families have shared features has relied on different sets of viral properties. The present-day classification scheme has, in large part, used morphology, physical composition of the virion, and replication strategies to achieve an orderly classification scheme.

Rationale for Classification

The following viral features have played important roles in classification, while symptomatology has assumed a secondary role.

Symmetry

The property of symmetry of viral structure has allowed both DNA and RNA viruses to be divided into three distinct groups: (1) helical, (2) cubic, and (3) complex.

Table 5-1 Morphology of Viral Agents and Families

Virus family	Representative virus	Morphology
DNA viruses		
Parvovirus	Parvovirus-like agent strain B-19	Naked icosahedral
Papovavirus	Human papilloma virus (HPV) 1-58	Naked icosahedral
Adenovirus	Human adenovirus (1-42 serotypes)	Naked icosahedral
Hepadnavirus	Hepatitis B virus	Enveloped icosahedral
Herpesvirus	Herpes simplex virus	Enveloped icosahedral
Poxvirus	Vaccinia	Complex
RNA viruses		
Picornavirus	Poliovirus 1-3	Naked icosahedral
Calicivirus	Hepatitis E virus	Naked icosahedral
Togavirus	Eastern equine encephalitis virus	Enveloped icosahedral
Flavivirus	St. Louis encephalitis virus	Enveloped icosahedral
Coronavirus	Human coronavirus HCV-229E	Enveloped helical
Reovirus	Mammalian reovirus (1-3)	Naked icosahedral
Rhabdovirus	Rabiesvirus	Enveloped helical
Filovirus	Marburg virus	Enveloped helical
Paramyxovirus	Parainfluenza viruses (types 1–4)	Enveloped helical
Orthomyxovirus	Influenza virus (type A)	Enveloped helical
Bunyavirus	LaCrosse virus (California encephalitis group)	Enveloped helical
Arenavirus	Lymphocytic choriomeningitis virus (LCM)	Enveloped helical
Retrovirus	Human immunodeficiency virus (type 1)	Enveloped icosahedral or complex (?)

Enveloped or Naked Virion

The presence or absence of a viral envelope has been a useful feature in classifying both DNA and RNA viruses. When this property is combined with symmetry, the following five different morphologic forms of viruses are delineated: (1) naked icosahedral, (2) enveloped icosahedral, (3) naked helical, (4) enveloped helical, and (5) complex. Each morphologic type is represented by one or more animal virus family, with the exception of the naked helical form. The following viral families are representatives of these four morphologic types: (1) Parvo-, Papova-, Adeno-, Picorna-, and Reoviridae are naked icosahedral forms; (2) Herpes-, Hepadna-, and Togaviridae are enveloped icosahedral forms; (3) Orthomyxo-, Paramyxo-, Rhabdo-, Corona-, Arena-, and Bunyaviridae are enveloped helical forms; and (4) Pox- and Retroviridae are complex forms.

Nucleic Acid

The nucleic acid of the virion has a number of distinct features that are useful in classification. The first basic point considered in classification is the type of nucleic acid. Viruses are of either the DNA type or RNA type. Secondly, the strandedness and physical nature of viral nucleic acids permit further distinctions to be made. The DNA viruses are nearly all double-stranded, with the exception of the parvoviridae family, which contains single-stranded DNA, and the hepadnaviridae, which contains two DNA strands of different length. The situation is reversed with the RNA viruses, which are predominantly single-stranded, with the exception of the reoviridae family, which contains double-stranded RNA. In addition, the RNA viruses may have segmented genomes, as found in Orthomyxo-, Reo-, Retro, Arena-, and Bunyaviridae families, or genomes may consist of a single RNA molecule, as seen in Picorna-, Toga-, Flavi-, Corona-, Rhabdo-, and Paramyxoviridae families. The presence of a closed, circular, double-stranded DNA genome in the Papovaviridae family distinguishes this group from Adeno-, Herpes-, and Poxviridae, which have linear, double-stranded DNA genomes. The members of the new DNA virus family termed the Hepadnaviridae (e.g., hepatitis virus B) all share a very unique double-stranded, circular-gapped DNA genome in which one strand has a constant length of 3182 bases and the other strand varies between 1700 and 2800 bases. In each case, the physical nature of the nucleic acid provides distinctions between classification groups. In addition, the size of the viral genome (molecular weight of the nucleic acid) has proved useful in distinguishing different families and genera. Lastly, the location of nucleic acid replication and capsid assembly (nuclear versus cytoplasmic) may distinguish one family, such as Poxviridae, from other nuclear DNA viruses, such as papova-, adeno-, and herpesviruses. Tables in the following replication section summarize unique structural differences in genomes, sites of nucleic acid replication, and functional aspects of replication strategy.

Virology

Replication Strategy

The molecular biology of genome replication and the methods for producing viral messenger RNA (mRNA; + sense) differ strikingly for viral families. Viral taxonomy has increasingly recognized that replication strategy is very fundamental to the nature of a virus and, therefore, has increasingly utilized similarities and distinct differences for grouping viruses. For example, the failure to detect subgenomic messages during flavivirus replication contrasted with existing knowledge of other alphaviruses of the togavirus family. This distinction, at least in part, led to the establishment of a separate family for the flaviviruses. These differences are detailed further in the following replication section.

Virion Diameter and Capsomer Number

The virion diameter and capsomer number are useful physical factors in current classification.

Site of Nucleocapsid Envelopment

The site of nucleocapsid envelopment has been useful in distinguishing members of the alphavirus genus of the togaviridae, which bud through the plasma membrane, from members of the flaviviridae family, which bud through intracytoplasmic membranes.

Enzymes

It is important in the study of virus-specific enzymes to distinguish between enzymes found within the virion (virion-associated enzymes) and virus-specific enzymes that are expressed by the viral genome during replication but that are not packaged within the viral particle. The presence of specific virion-associated transcriptases (RNA polymerases, DNA polymerases, and RNA-dependent DNA polymerases) and of specific functional spike proteins such as neuraminidase or membrane fusion protein have provided distinctions between genera and families. Tables following the replication section indicate the presence or absence of virion-associated enzymes and define those unique to each virus family.

Ether Sensitivity

Sensitivity to viral inactivation by ether is generally demonstrated in viral families that possess envelopes.

Antigenic Cross-Reactivity

In general, antigenic determinants of viral proteins are shared or cross-reactive within a genus or, in some cases, a family, while determinants are dissimilar or unreactive between different genera. This rule, however, is not universally held, and exceptions can be found.

Symptomatology

The use of symptoms has not been satisfactory in developing an international classification scheme because the same virus may be found in several disease groups and structurally dissimilar viruses may cause similar symptoms. However, this approach has proved useful to the clinician, and an alternative system of classification has utilized affected organs and systems as means for classification (e.g., dermatropic viruses, neurotropic viruses, viruses of the respiratory system).

Current Classification

The scheme presented in Figs. 5-3 through 5-7 is a current attempt to simplify and order the animal viruses. The five basic subgroups used to generate viral families have been derived by combining the important characteristics of nucleic acid type, symmetry, and naked versus enveloped morphology.

Fig. 5-3 Classification group I: DNA viruses with icosahedral symmetry and naked nucleocapsids.

Family
Parvoviridae
Parvoviruses:
B19 Virus: Erythema infectiosum
AAV: Adenoassociated Virus

Papovaviridae
Papovaviruses:
JC Virus: Progressive Multifocal Leukoencephalopathy
BK Virus
Human Papillomavirus: Warts and cervical cancer
Polyoma Virus: Tumors
Simian Vacuolating Virus (SV40)

Adenoviridae
Adenoviruses:
Pharyngitis–Respiratory tract infections
Eye infections
Gastroenteritis

Family
Hepadnaviridae
Hepadnaviruses:
Hepatitis B Virus: Acute and chronic hepatitis

Herpesviridae
Herpesviruses:
Herpes simplex: Fever blisters, genital herpes
Varicella-zoster: Chickenpox, shingles
Cytomegalovirus: Cytomegalic
inclusion disease
Epstein-Barr: Burkitt's lymphoma,
mononucleosis
B virus: Ascending myelitis
Human Herpesvirus 6: Roseola
(Exanthem Subitum)
Human Herpesvirus 7

Poxviridae
Poxviruses:
Variola: Smallpox
Vaccinia: Complications following vaccination
Molluscum contagiosum: Benign skin nodules
Orf: Milker's nodules
Cowpox virus: Vesicular lesions
Monkeypox virus: Smallpox-like

Fig. 5-4 Classification group II: DNA viruses with envelopes or complex coats.

Replication

Earl M. Ritzi

A lytic or productive viral infection will proceed if the cells or species of cells infected are permissive for the infecting virus. The term *permissive* when used to describe the host cell means that both a suitable cell receptor and intracellular requirements such as host-cell enzymes are sufficient for supporting the replication of a particular virus. The terms *nonpermissive* and *nonproductive infection* are utilized to describe the contrasting situation where cells are transformed in growth properties but viral replication is not supported. Synchronous viral infections of cells permitting a single replication cycle have given rise to one-step growth curves. When infectious units are assayed during synchronous infection, it is found that infectivity disappears rapidly after adsorption of virus to cells and that hours later there is a single rise in intracellular infectivity

Family
Picornaviridae
Enteroviruses:
Polioviruses: Poliomyelitis, meningitis
Coxsackieviruses: Aseptic meningitis,
herpangina, pleurodynia, myocarditis and
pericarditis, febrile illness
Echoviruses: Aseptic meningitis, febrile illness with or
without rash, common cold
Enterovirus 72: Hepatitis A virus
Rhinoviruses:
Common cold

Caliciviridae
Norwalk Agent
Hepatitis E Virus

Reoviridae
Reoviruses
Orbiviruses
Colorado Tick Fever Virus: Biphasic fever
Rotavirus: Nonbacterial infantile diarrhea.

Togaviridae
Alphaviruses:
Eastern and Western Encephalitis viruses
Rubivirus:
Rubella virus: German measles

Flaviviridae:
Flaviviruses:
Yellow Fever Virus: yellow fever
Dengue: Bone-Break fever
St. Louis encephalitis virus: Encephalitis
Hepatitis C virus: Posttransfusion hepatitis

Fig. 5-5 Classification group III: RNA viruses with cubic (icosahedral) symmetry.

followed by a subsequent rise in extracellular infectivity. The period from uncoating to the first appearance of intracellular virus is termed the eclipse period. A second period, from uncoating to the appearance of extracellular virus, is referred to as the latent period. For viruses that mature by budding through the cell membrane only extracellular virus is infective; therefore, only a latent period can be defined.

There are six basic steps in a viral replication cycle. In order of occurrence, these are (1) adsorption, (2) penetration, (3) uncoating, (4) biosynthesis, (5) maturation, and

Family

Orthomyxoviridae

Influenza viruses: Influenza

Paramyxoviridae

Pneumovirus:
Respiratory syncytial virus: Pneumonia and
severe bronchiolitis in infants, common cold
in adults.
Paramyxoviruses:
Parainfluenza viruses 1-4: Croup and
pneumonia in children.
Mumps virus: Mumps (epidemic parotitis)
Morbillivirus:
Measles virus: Measles (Rubeola)

Rhabdoviridae

Rabies virus: Rabies

Filoviridae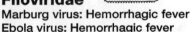

Marburg virus: Hemorrhagic fever
Ebola virus: Hemorrhagic fever

Arenaviridae

Arenaviruses:

Lymphocytic Choriomeningitis Virus (LCM):
Influenza-like disease with meningitis.
Lassa fever: Hemorrhagic fever

Coronaviridae

Human Coronaviruses: Upper Respiratory Tract
Infections:
Common colds

Bunyaviridae

Bunyaviruses: California Encephalitis Group,
La Crosse Virus: Encephalitis

Fig. 5-6 Classification group IV: RNA viruses with helical symmetry.

(6) release of progeny virus. These steps are common to both DNA and RNA viruses; however, the following discussion of these steps describes important differences.

Adsorption

The attachment of a virus to a cell involves specific cellular receptors and viral reacting sites termed the viral attachment protein(s). Often, well-defined host cell surface proteins with known cellular functions serve as virus recep-

Family

Retrovirdae

Retroviruses:
Oncoviruses: Endogenous leukemia/leukosis
viruses and defective sarcoma/ acute leukemia
viruses of many nonhuman species
Human T cell leukemia virus (HTLV-I):
Adult T cell leukemia; HTLV-II: Hairy cell
leukemia.

Lentiviruses:

Human immunodeficiency virus
(HIV-1and HIV-2): AIDS
Simian immunodeficiency virus (SIV):
A monkey disease virus.
Visna and Maedi virus of sheep.

Spumaviruses:

Human foamy virus: No symptoms
Simian foamy virus: Monkey kidney cells

Fig. 5-7 Classification group V: RNA viruses of mixed or complex symmetry.

tors; however, the cellular receptors may be virus specific, leading to specific viral cell and tissue tropisms, as well as species-specific host ranges. Poliovirus demonstrates this point by infecting receptor-positive human cells while failing to infect receptor-negative mouse cells. With enveloped viruses, the viral glycoproteins play a major role in adsorption, while naked capsid viruses may have a single viral attachment protein, such as the fiber of adenoviruses, or a mosaic of viral proteins forming a site on the capsid surface, such as the picornaviruses. Generally, adsorption involves electrostatic interactions and is influenced by pH; however, it shows little temperature dependence occurring in a similar manner at 4°C and 37°C.

Penetration

The process by which a virus enters a cell is termed penetration. Naked capsid viruses generally enter a cell by phagocytosis (viropexis) and are initially found in vacuoles. A second, important mechanism utilized by enveloped viruses such as paramyxoviruses entails a fusion of the viral envelope with the cellular membrane, resulting in the release of the nucleocapsid into the cytoplasm.

A modification of this mechanism is demonstrated by orthomyxoviruses, which undergo viropexis followed by vacuole fusion with a lysosome. This results in a lowered pH and a release of the nucleocapsid from the vacuole into the cytoplasm. More rarely, the nucleic acid may be directly injected into a cell (e.g., bacteriophage) or released into the cell upon a conformational change in the viral capsid (e.g., poliovirus). The process of penetration is a temperature-dependent one and proceeds much more rapidly at 37°C than at 4°C.

Uncoating

The removal of capsid and core proteins, liberating viral nucleic acid, is termed uncoating. With the exception of poxviruses, the process utilizes preexisting cellular proteases, negating the need for de novo synthesis of these enzymes. This cytoplasmic process may involve fusion of a lysosome with the viral vacuole (true for many naked capsid viruses), a conformational change in the viral capsid (picornaviruses like polio), only partial uncoating to leave a nucleic acid–protein core (reoviruses), or removal of proteins from nucleocapsids after envelopes have been removed by fusion with cellular membranes.

The uncoating of poxviruses is unique and involves a two-stage uncoating process. First, the outer coat and lateral bodies of poxviruses are removed, liberating a core structure. This is accomplished by preexisting cellular enzymes in a phagolysosome. The second stage of core uncoating is dependent on a unique viral enzyme in the poxvirus core, a DNA-dependent RNA polymerase. This virion-associated enzyme transcribes a message for a new uncoating protein while the poxvirus core is still intact. The new protein produced by translation of this message then uncoats the core structure, liberating the viral nucleic acid. Unlike most other viruses, complete poxvirus uncoating requires the synthesis of a new poxvirus-coded protease.

The viral uncoating process generally leads to a loss in infectivity and marks the true beginning of the viral eclipse period.

Biosynthesis of DNA-Containing Viruses

The biosyntheses of DNA viruses have generally been divided into two phases: an early phase, those events that occur before DNA replication, and a late phase, those events that follow the initiation of DNA replication. With the exception of poxviruses, which replicate in the cytoplasm, DNA viruses begin the biosynthesis phase when viral nucleic acid migrates into the nucleus through nuclear pores and host-cell DNA-dependent RNA polymerase transcribes selective early regions of the viral genome. Viral messenger RNA is then processed (polyadenylated, capped, and/or spliced) in a similar manner as cellular mRNA and transported to the cytoplasm where host-cell ribosomes and transfer RNA (tRNA) molecules synthesize viral proteins. The newly synthesized viral proteins move to the cell nucleus or cellular membranes. Many of the early viral proteins entering the nucleus are nonstructural proteins such as the T antigens (tumor antigens) of papova- or adenoviruses or the Epstein-Barr nuclear antigen (EBNA) of herpesviruses. During the early phase of replication, host-cell macromolecular processes such as DNA replication may be stimulated, as noted for papovaviruses, or inhibited, as noted for adeno- and herpesviruses.

In general, the replication of viral DNA proceeds on a double-stranded, linear DNA template and is characterized as both semiconservative and bidirectional. Adenovirus DNA appears to be an exception and is synthesized in a unidirectional, asymmetric fashion. The papovaviruses also present an exception to this rule by replicating viral DNA bidirectionally on a closed, circular DNA template. During and subsequent to nucleic acid replication, the late phase of protein synthesis, which is responsible for structural protein production, occurs. The capsid proteins produced migrate to the nucleus for capsid assembly.

The principal exception to the general DNA virus replication scheme is the poxvirus cycle of cytoplasmic replication. The presence of a DNA-dependent RNA polymerase in the poxvirus virion eliminates the requirement for nuclear host-cell transcription of the viral genome. The two-stage uncoating process provides for an extended period of early viral mRNA synthesis. Feulgen-staining cytoplasmic factories for DNA synthesis are detected in the cytoplasm, and a unique de novo synthesis of the poxvirus coat occurs in the cytoplasm. This coat is the only viral envelope that is not obtained by budding and is not an altered host-cell membrane.

Biosynthesis of RNA-Containing Viruses

The majority of RNA viruses replicate in the cytoplasm rather than in the nucleus. The two exceptions to this rule are the orthomyxoviruses and retroviruses, which have a nuclear phase in their replication cycles. Since transcription or replication of viral RNA relies on the presence of specific enzymes, the absence of RNA-dependent RNA polymerase activity in the host cell has imposed a need for different replication strategies to deal with this deficiency. If the unique retrovirus strategy is excluded, RNA viruses can be considered to be plus (encapsidating messenger-sense form), negative (encapsidating messenger-template form), or double-stranded (encapsidating the replicative form of their genomes). Four different types of viral RNA replication are recognized. The type of replication is determined by the physical nature of the viral genome and the presence or absence of virion-associated enzymes. The RNA virus families and representative agents are separated in Fig. 5-8 into four replication groups. Each group shares one of the following replication strategies:

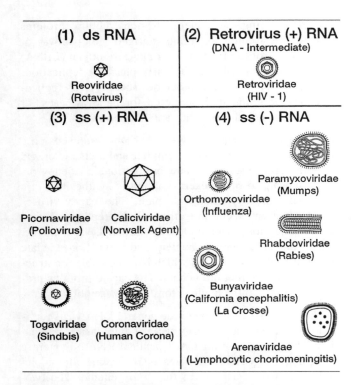

Fig. 5-8 Replication strategies of RNA viruses.

Double-Stranded RNA

The Reoviridae family, the only double-stranded RNA viruses, possesses a virion-associated transcriptase and exemplifies the first type of viral replication strategy. These viruses replicate their double-stranded RNA in a unique conservative and asymmetric manner. Since the viral core never completely uncoats, the segmented double-stranded genome remains protected against cellular nucleases during replication.

Retrovirus-RNA Replication Via a DNA Intermediate

A second replication strategy (repliation involving a DNA intermediate) is unique to the retrovirus family. Viruses contain an RNA-dependent DNA polymerase (reverse transcriptase) that catalyzes the synthesis of double-stranded DNA from the single-stranded RNA genome. The viral DNA circularizes and integrates into cellular nuclear DNA. The integrated DNA provirus is transcribed by host-cell DNA-dependent RNA polymerase to yield viral RNA genomes and polycistronic mRNAs. The extracted RNA genome of the retroviruses is not infective despite its positive polarity; however, the DNA provirus of transformed cells is infective.

Single-Stranded Plus (+) RNA

A third replication strategy is exhibited by the single-stranded RNA viruses that have genomes of positive polarity (similar to mRNA). The picorna-, toga-, flavi-, and coronaviruses are examples of single-stranded RNA viruses with positive (messenger) polarity. The entering genome of these viruses acts directly as genome-length polycistronic mRNA and is utilized to synthesize an RNA-dependent RNA polymerase and capsid proteins. The polymerase generates a complementary negative strand that can be released from the template and encapsidated as genomes in progeny virus particles or utilized as polycistronic messages for viral protein synthesis. The positive-stranded RNA viruses do not require virion-associated enzymes; therefore, nucleic acid alone, extracted from virions, acts as mRNA and is infective in permissive cells. The polycistronic mRNA of positive-stranded viruses is translated into a giant polypeptide that is subjected to posttranslational cleavage to obtain structural and nonstructural proteins.

Single-Stranded Minus (−) RNA

A fourth strategy employed by single-stranded RNA viruses of negative polarity differs significantly from that of positive-stranded viruses. The orthomyxo-, paramyxo-, and rhabdoviruses are examples of negative-stranded RNA viruses. These viruses have genomes that are complementary to mRNA and are characterized as negative-polarity genomes. Since the genome cannot act as mRNA, these viruses all must possess virion-associated transcriptases to synthesize monocistronic messages (smaller than genome size) upon entering the host cell. A polymerase and structural proteins are synthesized from monocistronic messages, and a replicative intermediate with growing negative RNA strands is formed to generate progeny viral genomes. The negative-strand viruses differ from positive-strand RNA viruses by utilizing monocistronic mRNAs, by having polymerase encapsidated in progeny virions, by packaging negative RNA strands, and by having viral nucleic acid that is noninfective when extracted from the virion.

Maturation

For naked capsid viruses, the process of maturation refers to the aggregation of viral polypeptides into capsomers and the subsequent self-assembly of the capsomers into a capsid. The maturation of naked capsid DNA viruses occurs in the nucleus, while all RNA virus maturation, with the exception of orthomyxoviruses, occurs in the cytoplasm. The enveloped viruses only complete their maturation during or after budding from an altered host-cell membrane.

Release of Progeny Virus

The release of naked capsid viruses such as papova-, adeno-, or picornaviruses occurs by a process of cell death and plasma membrane disintegration. The enveloped viruses are released from cells by budding through a cellular membrane. The herpesviruses bud through the inner layer of the nuclear membrane and are released either by passage through the endoplasmic reticulum or in vacuoles formed from the outer layer of the nuclear membrane. The most prevalent form of RNA virus budding occurs at the plasma membrane of the host cell. Release of progeny virus by budding through the surface membrane of infected cells is characteristic of the orthomyxo-, paramyxo-, rhabdo-, arena-, retro-, and togaviruses. A third type of viral budding is characteristic of corona-, bunya-, flaviviruses. Viruses of these families bud through intracytoplasmic membranes.

Unique Molecular Aspects of Genome Structure and Replication

Terminal Redundancy

The presence of terminal repeats in nucleotide sequence is noted at the ends of viral genomes. A terminally redundant base sequence such as A, B, C, D, . . . X, Y, A is revealed in DNA viruses by showing that endonuclease treatment followed by melting and reannealing produces DNA circles. Terminal redundancy (without sequence inversion) is associated with herpesvirus and retrovirus genomes.

Inverted Terminal Repeats (ITRs)

Reversed or inverted complementary sequences are found at the ends of adenovirus, poxvirus, parvovirus, rhabdovirus, bunyavirus, and arenavirus genomes. These ITRs are demonstrated by "panhandle" formation on melting and reannealing of adenovirus genomes.

Protein Linkage to Viral Genomes

Proteins are covalently coupled to genomes of selected viral families. Picornaviruses (like polio) have a Vpg protein. Adenovirus DNA has a 55 kD protein, and hepatitis B, caliciviruses, and parvoviruses have proteins attached as replication primers or packaging signals.

Cross-Linked Viral DNA

Vaccinia virus and other ds poxviruses are unique in being covalently cross-linked at genome ends.

Viral Enhancers

These are genome structures such as the 72bp repeats found in the SV40 genome that potentiate, activate, and may, in general, enhance transcription even when located thousands of bases away. Viral enhancers are usually located upstream of key viral promoter elements and play important roles in transcriptional control. While present in many viruses, enhancers of papovaviruses (such as simian virus 40) and retroviruses are well studied.

Transactivators of Transcription

Many viruses have important multifunctional proteins that serve as transactive transcriptional regulators. These proteins (e.g., simian virus 40 T antigens, adenovirus E1A and E1B proteins, herpes alpha-transinduction factor [alpha-TIF] and human immunodeficiency virus 1 [HIV-1] *tat* protein) turn on and regulate viral transcription programs.

mRNA Splicing

This phenomenon, which occurs in eucaryotic cells, was discovered in adenovirus transcription studies. In adenovirus one large late mRNA from the late promoter is spliced into different smaller-sized mRNAs to produce a complete assortment of adenovirus late proteins. Splicing of mRNA controls the abundance of each late protein. While mRNA splicing may occur during expression of other viruses, it is most noted in adenovirus replication.

Herpes Transcription Cascade

Rather than employing DNA replication as a simple division between early and late transcription programs, herpesviruses induce transcription of alpha genes with alpha-TIF (in the absence of protein synthesis). These alpha genes induce transcription of beta-1 and beta-2 genes. These beta genes allow DNA replication and the subsequent induction of gamma genes, thereby forming a transcription cascade of alpha, beta, and gamma genes where gene products induce subsequent steps and downregulate prior steps.

Summary of Viral Structure and Replication Relationships

Tables 5-2 and 5-3 associate genome structures of DNA and RNA viruses with pertinent replication concepts. Tables 5-4 and 5-5 describe enzyme activities that have been associated with virions of DNA and RNA viruses. Table 5-6 describes host-cell surface proteins that were found to serve as receptors for animal viruses.

Virology

Table 5-2   Nucleic Acid in DNA Virus Families

Family	Type of genome	Molecular wt. × 10^{-6}	Virion-associated transcriptase	Site of nucleic acid replication and capsid assembly
Parvoviridae	Single-stranded linear DNA, + or − polarity	1.2–1.8	No	N
Hepadnaviridae	Double-stranded circular DNA with a single-stranded region (linear dsDNA with cohesive ends)	1.6–2.1	Yes	N
Papovaviridae	Double-stranded circular DNA, supercoiled	3.0–3.5	No	N
Adenoviridae	Double-stranded linear DNA	23–26	No	N
Herpesviridae	Double-stranded linear DNA	100–150	No	N
Poxviridae	Double-stranded linear DNA, cross-linked	150–200	Yes	C

Key: N = nucleus; C = cytoplasm. *Yes* indicates the presence of a transcriptase, whereas *no* indicates the absence of one.

Table 5-3   Nucleic Acid in RNA Virus Families

Family	Structure of genome	No. of segments	Polarity (mRNA sense)	Transcriptase in virion	Genomic RNA infectious	Sub-genomic messages	Polyprotein precursors (posttranslational cleavage)	Site of N.A. replication
Picornaviridae	Single-stranded	1	+	No	Yes	No	Yes	C
Caliciviridae	Single-stranded	1	+	No	Yes	No	Yes	C
Togaviridae	Single-stranded	1	+	No	Yes	Yes	Yes	C
Flaviviridae	Single-stranded	1	+	No	Yes	No	Yes	C
Coronaviridae	Single-stranded	1	+	No	Yes	Yes	No	C
Paramyxoviridae	Single-stranded	1	−	Yes	No	Yes	No	C
Rhabdoviridae	Single-stranded	1	−	Yes	No	Yes	No	C
Arenaviridae	Single-stranded	2	−	Yes	No	Yes	No	C
Bunyaviridae	Single-stranded	3	−	Yes	No	Yes	No	C
Orthomyxoviridae	Single-stranded	8	−	Yes	No	Yes	No	N
Retroviridae	Single-stranded	2 (diploid)	+	Yes	No	Yes	Yes	N
Reoviridae	Double-stranded	10–12	±	Yes	No	Yes	No	C

Key: N.A. = nucleic acid; N = nucleus; C = cytoplasm. *No* means that the characteristic does not apply to a family, whereas *yes* means that the characteristic does apply.

Table 5-4 Virion-Associated Enzymes of DNA Families

DNA virus groups	Enzyme activity
DNA viruses (ss)	
Parvovirus	Not present
DNA viruses (ds)	
Hepadnavirus	DNA- and RNA-dependent DNA polymerase (reverse transcriptase)
Papovavirus	Not present
Adenovirus	Not present
Herpesvirus	Not present
Poxvirus	DNA-dependent RNA-polymerase mRNA capping enzymes Poly (A) polymerase Nicking-joining enzyme Protein kinase Topoisomerase DNA-dependent nucleotide phosphohydrolase

Table 5-5 Virion-Associated Enzymes of RNA Families

RNA virus groups	Enzyme activity
RNA viruses (ds)	
Reovirus	RNA-dependent RNA polymerase mRNA capping enzymes Nucleotide phosphohydrolase
RNA viruses (+ss diploid)	
Retrovirus	RNA-dependent DNA polymerase (reverse transcriptase) Ribonuclease H Integrase Protease
RNA viruses (+ss)	
Picornavirus	Not present
Calicivirus	Not present
Togavirus	Not present
Flavivirus	Not present
Coronavirus	Acetyl esterase
RNA viruses (−ss)	
Orthomyxovirus	RNA-dependent RNA polymerase Neuraminidase or acetyl esterase
Paramyxovirus	RNA-dependent RNA polymerase Neuraminidase
Rhabdovirus	RNA-dependent RNA polymerase
Bunyavirus	RNA-dependent RNA polymerase
Arenavirus	RNA-dependent RNA polymerase

Viral Genetics

Earl M. Ritzi

The use of mutations in specific viral genes has permitted a more detailed understanding of viral antigenic variation, viral processes that may be amenable to antiviral therapy, mechanisms that regulate viral replication, and mechanisms of viral oncogenesis. With the exception of retroviruses, viral genetics has dealt with genomes that are haploid. The absence of duplicate alleles for vital functions leads to the conclusion that many mutations in vital functions will be lethal (nonpermissive for viral replication); therefore, conditional lethal mutants have played a central role in viral genetic studies.

The coding capacity (genetic complexity) of viral genomes has been established by assuming that 1500 nucleotides or nucleotide pairs will code for a 500-amino acid polypeptide of 50,000 mol. wt. Using this molecular weight as the average for a viral protein, estimates for coding capacity range from 3 proteins in the papovavirus family to 160 proteins in the poxvirus family. Viruses that contain RNA may code for 5 proteins in the picornavirus family to 15 proteins in the reovirus family. Such estimates of genetic complexity are minimal estimates of gene number, since some viruses utilize the same sequence to obtain more than one gene product. This may be accomplished by a displaced reading of the normal triplet reading frame (e.g., φX174 phage) or extensive messenger RNA splicing.

Viral genomes can now be physically mapped by restriction endonuclease cleavage analysis and subsequent nucleic

Table 5-6 Host Cell Surface Proteins as Animal Virus Receptors

Virus	Cell surface molecule
Poliovirus	NCAM (neuronal cellular adhesion molecule)
Rhinovirus	ICAMs (intracellular adhesion molecules)
Hepatitis A virus	Alpha-2 macroglobulin
Rabiesvirus	Neuronal acetylcholine receptor
Reovirus type 3	Beta-adrenergic receptor
Human immunodeficiency virus type 1	CD4 protein (T helper cells)
Herpes simplex virus type 1	Fibroblast growth factor receptor
Epstein-Barr virus	C3d complement receptor of B lymphocytes

acid sequencing. For RNA viruses, CDNAs (DNA molecules that are complementary base sequences of RNA genomes), have been utilized for mapping. Alternatively, viral genomes may be genetically mapped by two-factor and three-factor crosses. Such mapping relies on the basic fact that recombination frequencies are directly proportional to the distance between mutations.

A mutation is a basic requirement for viral genetic studies and may be obtained as a spontaneous mutation, one that arises by normal replication errors, or may be induced in viral genes with specific mutagens. A mutation is a change in the genotype (nucleic acid) of the virus, while its effect on a characteristic of the virus is referred to as the viral phenotype. Common viral phenotypes that have been observed include changes in drug resistance, neutralization escape, enzyme deficiency, virulence, plaque size, antigenic structure, host range, and sensitivity to inactivating substances. Point mutations resulting from single base substitutions have generated both missense mutations (insertion of the wrong amino acids) and non-sense mutations (early termination of the polypeptide chain). Deletion mutants result in defective interfering viral particles and oncogene ("onc")-containing RNA tumor viruses.

Defective Interfering (DI) Viral Particles

Often, deletion mutants with genomes shorter than wild-type (wt) virus accumulate in viral stocks. These mutants only replicate in cells that are simultaneously infected with a helper virus. While some defective particles do not interfere with wt virus replication, the majority of these deletion mutants interfere with the replication of homologous wt virus (thus, the name *DI particles*). These DI particles express normal capsid proteins, have truncated genomes, influence host-cell processes, and interfere to produce lower yields of homologous wt virus. This phenomenon was discovered by von Magnus in influenza virus studies. Influenza and vesicular stomatitis virus (VSV) are especially noted for DI-particle accumulation. Often, DI-particle interference results when shortened RNA genomes containing polymerase recognition sites replicate faster than wt genomes, thereby competing and removing RNA polymerase molecules from the pool of replicating wt genomes.

Conditional Lethal Mutations

The most useful conditional lethal mutants are temperature-sensitive mutants, or ts mutants. These mutants are usually missense mutants that can replicate at a permissive temperature but lose their ability to replicate at a higher nonpermissive temperature. With a ts mutant, the loss of a viral function at the elevated temperature normally results from an alteration in the functional confirmation of a viral protein.

A second group of conditional lethal mutants are host-dependent mutants. Generally, these mutants are non-sense mutants that can be suppressed and permitted to grow in host cells that have transfer RNA mutants. These mutants can replicate in host cells that prevent early termination of mutant gene products. The host-dependent mutants are of principal importance in genetic studies of bacteriophage in bacterial host cells.

Host-range mutants of animal viruses are also considered to be conditional lethal mutants. The mutants will replicate and form plaques in one kind of cell (permissive) and undergo abortive infection in other cell types (nonpermissive).

Genetic Interactions

Mixed infections in which more than one type of virus enters the same cell at the same time occur commonly in nature and have been routinely simulated in the research laboratory. During mixed infections, genetic (nucleic acid) interactions occur. These genetic interactions result in the production of some progeny viruses that differ from parental viruses. These altered progeny viruses have heritable changes in their viral genomes, and newly acquired characteristics are genetically stable in subsequent replication cycles. The following genetic interactions are of principal importance in viral genetic studies.

Classic Recombination

Viruses must be closely related to recombine; generally, only viruses within the same genus will undergo recombination. Two types of viral recombination are recognized. The first, intramolecular recombination, occurs by a breakage and exchange (re-union) of nucleic acid strands. This type of recombination may be intergenic (between two different genes), or it may be intragenic (within the same gene). In general, the double-stranded genomes of DNA viruses and the diploid retroviruses have the highest frequencies of intramolecular recombination. This finding can be contrasted with the single-stranded RNA virus families, which, with the exception of coronaviruses and picornaviruses, like polioviruses, experience little or no intramolecular recombination.

Genetic Reassortment

A second type of recombination (genetic reassortment) is unique for viruses with segmented genomes and occurs by a reassortment of individual viral gene segments in which progeny viruses acquire genome segments from two different parental viruses (Fig. 5-9). Higher recombination frequencies are obtained by genetic reassortment than by classic intramolecular recombination. The orthomyxo-, reo-, arena-, and bunyaviruses are subject to genetic reassortment. The pandemics and major antigenic shifts of

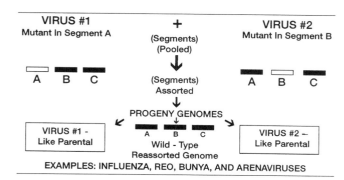

Fig. 5-9 Genetic reassortment of viruses with segmented genomes.

influenza virus are, at least in part, attributable to the process of genetic reassortment.

Marker Rescue

Marker rescue has also been termed cross reactivation because the genome of an active virion recombines with the genome of an inactive virus, resulting in viable progeny that have acquired new genetic markers from the inactivated virus. These progeny are generally stable, and rescued markers are maintained through subsequent replication cycles. This technique has been utilized with influenza viruses to rescue markers with desired antigenicity for new vaccines.

Multiplicity Reactivation

When two inactivated viral genomes recombine in the same cell to produce active, viable, and genetically stable progeny, this process is referred to as multiplicity reactivation. The probability of the occurrence of multiplicity reactivation increases with multiplicity (number of inactive particles per cell). The phenomenon has principally been noted with double-stranded DNA viruses such as vaccinia. This interaction was noted when viruses were deliberately inactivated for use as test vaccines. If greater degrees of inactivation of viral nucleic acid were utilized, then higher multiplicities of inactivated viruses were required to obtain reactivation.

Nongenetic Interactions

Nongenetic interactions do not involve an exchange of nucleic acid and do not result in heritable changes in progeny virus. Alternatively, nongenetic interactions generally refer to the sharing of viral gene products during mixed infections. The following nongenetic interactions are of principal interest.

Complementation

When two viral mutants that have mutations in different viral genes infect a cell under nonpermissive conditions, complementation is said to occur when good functional gene products are shared and progeny virus is produced. The progeny produced still have one of the original parental genomes and therefore cannot replicate without further complementation. Viral mutants can only complement each other if mutations are in different genes (intergenic complementation). Two different mutations within the same gene (intragenic) do not complement. This principle has allowed viral mutations to be subdivided into complementation groups. Mutants from each group may complement a mutant from another group, but complementation does not occur with mutants of the same complementation group. Each complementation group therefore defines a required structural or nonstructural gene of the virus. Complementation also occurs when a replication-competent helper virus, such as avian leukemia virus, supplies a functional gene product for a defective strain of avian sarcoma virus. Complementation by a replication-competent virus is responsible for the production of progeny by most of the defective sarcoma viruses; therefore, complementation may occur between an active and inactive virus or between viruses with two different defects.

Phenotypic Masking and Mixing

Phenotypic masking and mixing are special examples of complementation in structural genes. When the genome of one virus is encapsidated within the capsid of another virus, this process is referred to as transcapsidation or phenotypic masking. The progeny virus produced has the genotype of one of the parental viruses and the antigenic reactivity of the other. If the masked genome of the progeny virus is totally functional, the original parental genotype will determine and alter the antigenicity of the capsid on subsequent rounds of replication. If the genome of a viral mutant is masked, further complementation will be required for subsequent rounds of replication. Enveloped viruses also demonstrate phenotypic masking. With viruses, such as the retroviruses, mixed infections yield particles with the genome of one virus (typically a defective sarcoma virus) within the envelope of another replication-competent virus. These enveloped viral particles, referred to as pseudotypes, are also examples of structural protein complementation and phenotypic masking.

While phenotypic masking is a special form of phenotypic mixing, the term *mixing* has more accurately been used to describe a mixed infection in which progeny virus particles are produced that have a single genotype and a mosaic or mixed capsid composed of structural proteins synthesized from two different viral genomes. A diagram-

Virology

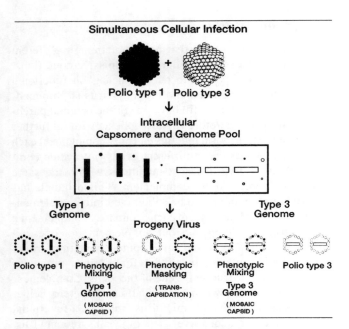

Fig. 5-10 Phenotypic mixing and masking of simultaneous cellular infection.

matic view of phenotypic masking and phenotypic mixing is depicted for the simultaneous infection of a cell by two poliovirus strains in Fig. 5-10. A phenotypically mixed capsid may have the unique property of being neutralized by sera directed against two different viruses; however, this property is lost upon further replication when capsids homologous to the genotype are produced.

Genotypic Mixing

When a single virus particle replicates to form two different parental types, this is referred to as genotypic mixing. This is a rare and unusual phenomenon that has only been noted with paramyxoviruses and may result from the encapsidation of two genomes in one particle. This property is not heritable and is lost when the progeny virus replicates.

Viruses as Foreign Gene Vectors

Detailed knowledge of viral genomes has been combined with modern molecular genetic engineering techniques to permit the following applications: (1) Foreign genes for antigens that are virulence factors, tumor antigens, or inducers of neutralizing antibodies have been inserted into viruses with powerful promoters such as vaccinia virus to create new protective vaccines; (2) foreign genes have been placed into baculovirus, a high-level expression vector, to produce large amounts of cellular or viral products that, unlike bacterial systems, are glycosylated and can be used in research; and (3) retroviruses have been engineered to carry and to insert foreign genes into the cellular genome for gene replacement therapy in individuals who suffer from disease due to specific genetic deficits.

Host Responses to Viruses

Stanley S. Lefkowitz

Most viral illnesses are self-limiting and, therefore, disease is eventually followed by recovery of the host. Host responses to viral infections consist of both specific and nonspecific responses. Immunity, as used in this section, encompasses all of the mechanisms by which a host may either specifically or nonspecifically recognize foreign viral substances and ultimately respond directly or indirectly to eliminate these foreign invaders. It should be kept in mind that the immunologic response of a host to an invading virus may be important not only for protection of that host, but also for the pathogenesis of the disease itself.

Nonspecific Defense Mechanisms Against Viruses

Anatomic Barrier

It is known that cells of the epidermis resist viral penetration. In addition, mucosal surfaces prevent invading viruses from penetrating cells. There are also internal cellular barriers, that is, the blood-brain barrier, and the layer of endothelial cells that separate blood from tissue. They normally prevent the establishment of viral infections unless a very high level of viremia occurs.

Nonspecific Inhibitors

A number of viral inhibitors are present in body fluids. This is especially true in the gastrointestinal tract, where many viruses are inactivated by acid, bile salts, and certain enzymes. In certain cases, the glycoproteins and lipoproteins, and a number of other viral inhibitors, exist that may function by preventing virus attachment to cells, directly inactivating virus, or by inhibiting virus replication. These inhibitors may be lipids, polysaccharides, proteins, lipoproteins, or glycoproteins contained in the mucus layer that are capable of combining with certain viruses and rendering them noninfectious.

Phagocytosis

It is generally considered that phagocytosis may be less effective against viral infections than against bacterial infections. Nevertheless, phagocytosis by macrophages, with or without specific antibodies, and to a lesser extent granulocytes, seem to play a role in control of viral infections. However, in other instances replication of a virus occurs within the phagocyte, allowing further systemic spread of the viral infection.

Fever and Inflammation

A modest increase in temperature can cause a very strong inhibition of virus replication. This has been observed in vitro and also occurs in vivo during infections. Therefore, the development of fever as a host response plays an important role in limiting viral infection. It has been shown retrospectively that the severity of paralysis from poliovirus infections was significantly greater in patients treated with antipyretic drugs than in untreated patients. It is also known that components of inflammation such as edema, circulatory changes, and leukocytic accumulation result in alterations that affect viral infection. Some of these changes caused by inflammation are elevated local temperature, changes in oxygen tension, altered cell metabolism, and increased acidity, which ultimately may result in a reduction of virus replication. It is clear that both febrile and inflammatory responses may be very important in virus infection by limiting spread of the virus to certain target organs.

Interferons

The interferons probably represent the most important early-protection inducible system affecting viral infections. Their role in defense is underscored by a number of observations: (1) There are correlations between interferon production and recovery from viral infections, (2) inhibition of interferon production or action results in a more severe infection, and (3) treatment with interferon seems to protect animals against a number of different viruses.

Interferons are proteins that inhibit viral replication. They have a molecular weight of approximately 17,000 in the monomeric form but may exist as larger molecules and can be synthesized in hours by virtually any nucleated cell. These substances are usually host-specific with little cross-species protection. They are induced by invading viruses, particularly double-stranded RNAs associated with certain stages of viral replication. Other inducers of diverse origin exist including both natural substances such as lipopolysaccharide (LPS) and certain synthetic molecules.

There are three major classes of interferon: (1) leukocyte or alpha interferons, (2) fibroblast or beta interferons, and (3) immune or gamma interferons. There are more than 15 different genes that code for alpha interferons and only one gene that codes for beta interferons. The former are usually produced by leukocytes and the latter by fibroblasts although this distinction is not absolute. Collectively these interferons are termed type 1. There is one gene that codes for gamma interferon, which has also been called type 2. The latter is produced by T lymphocytes in response to either lectins or antigen to which they have been previously sensitized.

Interferons do not affect viral replication directly but act by binding to specific cell surface receptors, which in turn induces antiviral proteins. A number of these new proteins function by interfering with viral protein translation. Interferon causes the induction and phosphorylation of a 67,000-kd protein kinase, which, in the presence of double-stranded RNA, phosphorylates the alpha subunit of protein initiation factor eIF-2 and inactivates it. Interferon also induces the synthesis of 2', 5'-oligo (A) synthetase, which, in the presence of ds RNA, converts adenosine triphosphate (ATP) to 2', 5'-linked oligo (A) molecules. These molecules in turn activate an endonuclease RNAase L, which cuts viral mRNAs, thereby inhibiting viral protein synthesis.

In addition to its antiviral properties, interferon has other cell regulatory functions and may turn on a cascade of reactions, including enhancement of phagocytosis, inhibition of cell division, alteration of immune responses, and increased expression of cell-membrane antigens. Gamma interferon is far more immunoregulatory than alpha or beta interferon.

Therapeutic use of interferons has already progressed beyond the experimental state. Interferons are currently approved for the treatment of hairy-cell leukemia; non-A, non-B viral hepatitis; condyloma acuminatum; Kaposi's sarcoma; and chronic glanulomatous disease. A number of other diseases have been treated with interferons; however, Food and Drug Administration (FDA) approval is currently pending. Toxic side effects have been noted when high doses of interferon have been used for antitumor therapy. These toxic effects and the association of interferons with autoimmune diseases, such as rheumatoid arthritis and systemic lupus erythematosus, demonstrate that interferons may play detrimental as well as beneficial roles in disease processes.

Specific Defenses

Specific immunologic responses to viruses can be elicited by both B lymphocytes (bursal dependent) and T lymphocytes (thymus dependent).

Humoral Immunity (B Lymphocytes)

The immunoglobin classes IgM, IgG, and IgA are associated with antiviral activity. They are produced in response to both natural infection and active immunization. Immunoglobulins of the IgG class are also involved in transplacental transfer and protection of the newborn for the first 6 to 8 months of life. Antibodies of the IgG class may persist for the life of the individual following systemic or viremic viral infections. The half-life of IgG in the bloodstream is approximately 21 days. Immunoglobulin M antibodies, which are produced first, have a shorter half-life of about 5 days. Antibodies of the IgG class are distinguished from antibodies of the IgM class by readily crossing the placental barrier, by being more avid, and by more tightly binding virus. In certain viral infections, local production of secretory IgA may be more important than high levels of circulating IgG. This is frequently true with upper respiratory infections as well as gastrointestinal infections. The presence of secretory antiviral IgA in the respiratory epithelium clearly plays an important role in host defense by both protecting against and limiting the spread of influenza virus infections.

The mechanism of protection by antibodies falls into several categories. Antibodies can neutralize a virus or render it noninfectious by (1) interfering with the penetration of the virus by coating the viral surface, thus preventing uptake by the host cell; (2) opsonizing and causing clumping of the virus, which renders it more susceptible to phagocytosis; (3) preventing uncoating of a virus after it has been phagocytized by a cell; or (4) making the virus more susceptible to lysosomal digestion. In addition to direct binding to the virus, antibodies can interact with Fc receptors on phagocytic cells or certain lymphocytes and cause target-cell destruction (antibody-dependent cell-mediated cytotoxicity).

Cell-Mediated Immunity

In addition to humoral responses, cell-mediated immunity (delayed hypersensitivity) also is involved in host defenses. Delayed hypersensitivity is of prime importance in recovery from certain viral infections. This type of hypersensitivity is mediated primarily through the T lymphocyte. The effects of delayed hypersensitivity may be direct when cytotoxic T lymphocytes recognize viral antigens present on cell surfaces or indirect when mediated through the production of specific lymphokines that function as the principal "antiviral" material (i.e., interferon, interleukins, etc.). T cells respond to viral antigen through surface receptors, resulting in a series of cellular morphologic and biochemical changes. These changes result in direct cytotoxicity to cells expressing foreign antigens, or in the elaboration of lymphokines and cytotoxins. In addition, killer cells bearing Fc receptors to which are attached specific antibodies may destroy target cells through antibody-dependent cell-mediated cytotoxicity (ADCC). Another class of leukocytes, termed natural killer cells (null cells), which also lack recognized B- and T-cell markers, may function by destroying virus-infected "target" cells without prior sensitization.

Significance of Host Responses

It is clear that people generally survive the ravages of viral infections as they do other types of infections. The host responses, both specific and nonspecific, combine to form a series of barriers that the virus must overcome in order to cause infection. It appears that substances such as the interferons play a very early role in the recovery from virus infections and antibodies and factors related to cell-mediated immunity come into play later during viral infection. Maximal cell-mediated responses may occur by day 6 whereas antibody responses may not peak for weeks. In certain viral infections, such as influenza, other upper respiratory infections, and polio, the humoral response seems to be most important, whereas in infections such as varicella, mumps, and measles, cell-mediated immunity plays the dominant role. Both "arms" of immunity are important, not only in recovery but also in prevention of repeated infections.

Poxviruses

Stanley S. Lefkowitz

General Characteristics

The poxviruses are relatively large, "brick-shaped" viral particles, which may be visible under the light microscope. They are the largest, most complex of the true viruses, being approximately 230 by 400 nm. The viral DNA is a linear, double-stranded form, which has a molecular weight of $130 \times 240 \times 10^6$ daltons. This virus contains a number of different enzymes, including a DNA-dependent RNA polymerase and as many as 100 polypeptides. Although these viruses are enveloped, they are ether resistant. At least 20 different viral antigens can be identified by immunodiffusion. All poxviruses share a common nucleoprotein (NP) antigen. In addition, a heat-labile (L) antigen and a heat-stable (S) antigen may form the LS complex. A hemagglutinin, which is not a structural component of the virion, is found in infected cell cultures. One of the more unusual aspects of the poxviruses, unlike other DNA viruses, is that they replicate in the cytoplasm, forming large intracytoplasmic inclusion bodies called Guarnieri bodies. Differentiation between viruses can be achieved by restriction enzyme cleavage of viral DNA and analysis of polypeptides in infected cells. The virus can survive in a dried condition and remain infective on clothes and other materials and in dust. The virus may persist in the environment, but there are no animal reservoirs that can lead to human infection.

The poxvirus group contains a number of different viruses that infect both humans and animals. The most important of these is the agent that causes smallpox, variola major. A milder form of the disease is caused by variola minor. Vaccinia virus is a poxvirus that has been studied in great detail and has been used as the vaccine virus for prevention of smallpox. Other closely related viruses include the cowpox virus, monkey pox, orf, milker's nodule virus, and molluscum contagiosum. The latter causes wartlike tumors on the face, arms, and body.

Pathogenesis and Disease

Exposure to variola virus is primarily by inhalation and passage through the mucous membranes of the upper respiratory tract. After utilizing a respiratory port of entry, the virus multiplies in the lymphoid tissue draining this site. The incubation period of smallpox is approximately 12 days. A transient viremia develops, and infection of the reticuloendothelial cells that move throughout the body occurs. A second phase of multiplication then occurs in these cells, leading to a secondary and more intense viremia resulting in smallpox. Skin lesions, from which the virus can be isolated, subsequently appear following the secondary viremia. The rash first appears on the face and arms as maculopapules and then on the trunk and legs. The lesions become vesicular within 24 to 48 hours and then become pustular, followed by drying and scabbing. All of the lesions present are in the same stage of development. This characteristic differs significantly from chickenpox, where lesions may be found in various stages. A modified, less severe form of the disease has been evident where there was partial immunity.

Laboratory Diagnosis

In addition to the clinical picture, which is quite characteristic, smears made from the lesions can be stained for the characteristic inclusion bodies (Guarnieri) that are found in the cytoplasm of infected cells. In addition, the virus can be readily cultured in eggs, and the characteristic lesions can be discriminated from lesions caused by vaccinia and other related viruses. Vaccinia pocks are large with necrotic centers, whereas variola pocks are smaller.

Clinically, it may be difficult to distinguish the lesions of smallpox from those of chickenpox. Differentiation may be accomplished, however, by viewing the characteristic intracytoplasmic poxvirus particles or intranuclear icosahedral herpesvirus particles of varicella-zoster virus under the light or electron microscope. Scraping of cells from lesions followed by staining reveals either the cytoplasmic inclusion bodies of poxvirus or the characteristic intranuclear inclusion bodies of herpesvirus such as varicella-zoster. Antigens from skin lesions may also be identified readily using fluorescent antibody or complement-fixing techniques.

Prevention and Treatment

It has been known since 1798 that smallpox can be prevented by vaccination with live vaccinia virus. This practice was in effect until 1979, when smallpox was declared eradicated. Eradication was possible because humans are the only natural hosts. Vaccinia is administered intradermally by puncture, scarification, or air jet. A primary response results in a papule by the third or fourth day, progressing to a pustule in 8 to 10 days. After about 3 weeks, the scab falls off leaving the characteristic pockmark. A vaccinoid or accelerated reaction is common in partially immune hosts. Risk of complications from vaccination now outweighs the possibility of contracting the disease.

A number of problems have followed vaccination. As many as 1 in 1000 primary vaccinations result in complications. Approximately 1 of each 10 million primary vaccinations result in death. Other complications include generalized vaccinia resulting in a serious systemic infection. In children who have rashes, eczema vaccinatum, a spread of lesions in the eczematous areas, may develop. Vaccinia necrosum is a progressive spread of lesions that results in a necrosis of the skin and muscle. It occurs in individuals who are immunosuppressed. Postvaccinial encephalitis is a fatal demyelinating disease of the central nervous system that occurs about 12 days after vaccination. In addition to these complications, fetal vaccinia can occur if women are exposed to the vaccine during pregnancy. Fetal infection leads to stillbirth.

In addition to prevention, the drug methisazone (Marboran) can protect an individual against infection if he or she is treated shortly after exposure to the virus. This drug seems to play a role in blocking replication at an early stage. In addition, vaccinia immune globulin (VIG) from patients hyperimmunized to the vaccinia virus can be used for the treatment of generalized vaccinia and vaccinia necrosum.

A relatively new use for vaccinia is as an effective vector for the expression of other viral genes. A number of viral genes, as well as combinations of genes, have been inserted into the vaccinia genome and appear to be effective. These include hepatitis B, herpes simplex, and rabiesvirus. Other poxviruses have also been used as vectors.

Herpesviruses

Stanley S. Lefkowitz

The herpesviruses of humans have been divided into two groups. One group consists of herpes simplex virus (HSV) type 1 and type 2 and varicella-zoster virus (VZV). The other group contains at least four distinct viruses: cytomegalovirus (CMV), Epstein-Barr virus (EBV), and two recently discovered herpesviruses that have not been completely characterized. Herpesvirus represents a very important group of human pathogens that are characterized by latency with a low percentage of apparent infections. They tend to recur and their association with the immunocompromised makes them difficult to treat and control. Their association with malignancy also underscores their importance as human pathogens. Many other types of herpesviruses infect lower animals. B-virus infection of humans is an acute, frequently fatal encephalitis. Although normally a latent virus of monkeys, it has occurred in humans following bites by infected monkeys as well as contact with contaminated cell cultures.

General Characteristics

Herpesviruses are a family of large, enveloped viruses that measure 120 to 200 nm in diameter. Nonenveloped forms are unstable with low infectivity. The double-stranded DNA has a molecular weight ranging from 85 to 150×10^6 daltons. These viruses spread from cell to cell, replicating in the cell nucleus, where they form characteristic inclusion bodies. They are characterized by both latent and recurrent infections, with an affinity for skin and nerve cells or for lymphocytes. There is no common family antigen, but all are morphologically identical.

Herpes Simplex Virus Type 1 and Type 2

Herpes simplex viruses type 1 and type 2 replicate in the nucleus, forming intranuclear inclusions (Cowdry type A). They will readily cross the species barrier and replicate in other animals and on the chorioallantoic membrane of hen eggs (CAM). There is approximately 50 percent homology between the nucleic acids of type 1 and type 2, which accounts for some serologic cross-reactivity. These viruses can be distinguished by antigenicity, temperature sensitivity, and cellular restrictions in host range.

Pathogenesis and Disease

Seroprevalence rates to type 1 range to 90 percent or more in certain populations. The majority of infections caused by HSV type 1 and type 2 are subclinical. The virus replicates at the site of entry and may pass through the regional lymph nodes, enter the bloodstream, and proliferate in the skin or mucous membranes, or it may travel up the sensory nerves to the corresponding sensory ganglia. The virus is readily transmitted by touching, kissing, intercourse, fomites, and so forth. Generally, direct contact with infected secretions is required. The virus may remain in the latent stage at the site of the primary exposure and be activated by factors such as sunlight, menstruation, fever, or stress. The almost universal presence of antibodies to HSV seems to have little effect on recurrent herpes.

Specific lesions of the skin and mucous membrane include herpetic stomatitis (gingivostomatitis) and herpes labialis. The former is primarily a disease of children aged 1 to 5 years and is characterized by a painful vesicular ulceration of the buccal mucosa and tongue, as well as mucocutaneous borders of the mouth, coupled with fever. Herpes labialis represents the classic fever blisters (cold sores), which tend to recur at the same site. The permanent site of latent infection is the trigeminal ganglion. In addition, herpes cornealis, or keratoconjunctivitis (eye), appears as dendritic keratitis or corneal ulcers that may lead to blindness. Herpetic whitlow (finger) and herpes genitalis (vulvovaginitis or progenitalis) are also associated with herpetic infection. Herpes genitalis is primarily associated with HSV type 2, which frequently presents as infections "below the waist." The presence of type 2 is correlated with sexual activity. Its incubation period is 2 to 7 days, and recurrence is common. Lesions may be most severe during the primary episode.

In addition to these types of disease, other clinical syndromes include eczema herpeticum, otherwise known as Kaposi's varicelliform eruption. This disease occurs primarily in children with eczema and represents a cutaneous form of the disease. Finally, a disseminated herpes or neonatal herpes can occur when the newborn is exposed to the virus during passage through the birth canal. Open lesions in the mother may necessitate delivery by cesarean section, as mortality in the newborn can range from 50 to 80 percent. Lesions of the central nervous system include aseptic meningitis, encephalitis, or both.

Laboratory Diagnosis

Examination of infected cells in tissues or smears reveals giant cells with characteristic intranuclear conclusions (Cowdry type A). In addition, the virus may be directly isolated from lesions, vesicle fluid, the throat, saliva, or corneal scrapings using cell culture and may be identified using colorimetric, fluorescent, or radioactive indicators.

Treatment

The purine analogue vidarabine inhibits viral DNA polymerase. It was the first antiviral agent for herpes encephalitis and neonatal herpes. Acyclovir targets HSV-infected cells and is phosphorylated by HSV-encoded thymidine kinase. Acyclovir is subsequently converted to the triphosphate form and becomes incorporated into viral DNA chains by the viral DNA polymerase resulting in chain termination. Fortunately, this compound inhibits the viral DNA polymerase more than host DNA polymerases.

Acyclovir is available for intravenous, oral, or topical administration. For serious infections, parenteral administration is favored particularly for immunocompromised patients and those with severe primary genital herpes. For treatment of herpes encephalitis or neonatal herpes, acyclovir is favored over vidarabine. Oral acyclovir is effective against primary and recurrent genital herpes. It reduces viral shedding, promotes healing, and reduces pain. Use of acyclovir for treatment of herpes labialis is not as well defined.

Herpes keratitis can be treated topically with idoxuridine, trifluridine, or deoxythymidine analogues. Idoxuridine and trifluridine are both incorporated into viral DNA; however, the former also inhibits thymidine kinase. A number of other compounds are currently being tested for effectiveness against herpes infections including isoprinosine and foscarnet.

Varicella-Zoster Virus

General Characteristics

Varicella-zoster virus is strongly cell-associated and is not released during replication. The virus does not infect laboratory animals, and is not infectious for embryonated eggs.

Pathogenesis and Clinical Features

Varicella-zoster is the cause of chickenpox in the nonimmune child and recurs as shingles in the previously infected adult. Primary exposure to this highly contagious virus is usually through the respiratory tract. The incubation period is approximately 2 weeks. The virus replicates initially in the mucosa, after which viremia develops and the virus localizes in the skin. A person is infectious 1 day before the appearance of the rash and during the week after rash onset. The rash appears on the trunk first, then the scalp, and then spreads to the extremities. The rash is followed by the development of macules that develop into papules and eventually into vesicles. This process parallels a fever of 38 to 39°C. It is important to understand that there are different stages of lesions present at any one time, which distinguishes chickenpox clinically from smallpox. The development of chickenpox in the immunosuppressed individual is severe and frequently fatal.

The other disease associated with VZV is zoster, or shingles. The disease manifestations, primarily seen in elderly and immunosuppressed patients, represent an activation of latent virus that has remained dormant in the sensory cells of the dorsal root ganglion. Activation can be triggered by alterations in immunity, aging, or concurrent infections. The exact mechanism is not known. Active zoster lesions in patients are infectious and may cause chickenpox in nonimmune children who are in close contact. Typical zoster lesions appear primarily on the trunk and chest and occasionally on the forehead, face, and neck. The eruption is characteristically unilateral, associated with a specific spinal nerve dermatome, and is quite painful.

Laboratory Diagnosis

In most cases, the disease picture is quite characteristic, and diagnosis can be made clinically. However, it may be necessary to distinguish the disease from herpes simplex, vaccinia, and smallpox infections. Since herpesviruses replicate in the nucleus, scrapings from lesions show characteristic intranuclear inclusions. The detection of antigen or virus particles in vesicle fluid and lesions may be determined by immunofluorescence.

Prevention and Treatment

Varicella is usually treated with supportive measures. Both vidarabine and acyclovir are licensed for treatment of zoster in immunocompromised patients. A live attenuated vaccine, which was developed in Japan, is currently being tested. Results indicate that it is effective in protecting against development of chickenpox. However, questions remain as to both the extent and longevity of protection. It is anticiapted that it will be available soon.

In children who are receiving immunosuppressive therapy, a lethal infection can develop following exposure to this virus. Zoster immune globulin (ZIG) obtained from convalescing zoster patients is very effective in limiting the spread and severity of the disease in immunocompromised patients. High-dose interferon treatment has also proved efficacious in reducing viral replication and disease severity.

Cytomegalovirus

General Properties

Cytomegalovirus causes severe congenital anomalies in about 10,000 infants in the United States each year; however, it is also found in normal, healthy individuals. This virus replicates in human cells only and does not infect laboratory animals. A number of other CMVs infect different species of animals but are not pathogenic for humans.

Pathogenesis and Disease

Latent infection is common, as 80 percent of adults have antibody to this virus. The virus is localized in the salivary gland and has been termed "salivary gland virus." In addition to saliva, virus may be found in other body fluids including urine, semen, breast milk, vaginal secretions, and is associated with sexual transmission in adults. It is a highly necrotizing virus that ultimately kills the cells that it

Virology

infects. Cytomegalic inclusion disease (CMID) is caused by congenitally acquired virus that passes through the placenta. Manifestations of CMID include premature birth, jaundice, hepatosplenomegaly, hepatitis, and mental retardation in survivors. Infection of adults is usually inapparent except in immunocompromised or transplant patients. Cytomegalovirus mononucleosis (heterophile-negative) may occur after open heart surgery or following frequent blood transfusions. Cytomegalovirus infections are also associated with late stages of acquired immunodeficiency syndrome (AIDS) and may result in life-threatening complications.

Laboratory Diagnosis

Generally the virus is recovered by inoculation of material from the nasopharynx or urine into tissue culture. Fluorescent antibody techniques can be used to localize antigen in infected cells and tissues. Staining of urine sediments may indicate the presence of the large "owl eye" intranuclear inclusions that are characteristic of this virus. The measurement of complement-fixing antibodies is also of diagnostic value.

Treatment and Prevention

The antiviral agents ganciclovir and foscarnet are the most useful for treating CMV disease. The use of high-titered anti-CMV immunoglobulin in combination with ganciclovir has also proved efficacious. Two live attenuated CMV vaccines have been developed and may offer some protection.

Epstein-Barr Virus

General Properties

Epstein-Barr virus does not grow readily in tissue culture. It is not as highly cytopathic as other herpesviruses and replicates in B lymphoid cells. Most infections are inapparent or subclinical, particularly in infants and children, and antibodies can be found in more than 90 percent of the adult population.

Transmission and Clinical Features

The virus is readily transmitted from person to person by the oropharyngeal route, probably through saliva. The virus appears to replicate in the parotid gland and is disseminated by viremia. The incubation period of EBV is approximately 4 to 7 weeks, and the principal disease manifestation is infectious mononucleosis. The clinical features include headaches, fever, chills, sore throat, and swollen cervical lymph nodes. Tonsillopharyngitis is common and is accompanied by a thick exudate. Splenomegaly occurs in about 50 percent of patients. A skin rash may also be associated with the disease. A majority of patients

recover completely in 1 to 4 weeks. Blood-cell analysis indicates a leukocytosis of up to 40,000 per cubic millimeter, of which 50 to 90 percent are mononuclear cells. Half of the leukocytes (most of which are T cells) are present as atypical forms.

Complications in the normal host are rare; however, neurologic complications that result in death include the Guillain-Barré syndrome, meningitis, and encephalitis. Other complications of infections include spleen rupture, anemia, agranulocytosis, and thrombocytopenia. This virus has also been associated with a poorly defined chronic syndrome that has been termed "chronic fatigue syndrome."

With severe immunocompromised patients, EBV may reactivate, resulting in a severe "mononucleosis state." This virus is associated with several B-cell lymphoproliferative diseases, including Burkitt's lymphoma, Hodgkin's lymphoma, and B-cell lymphoma in immunocompromised hosts. In addition, nasopharyngeal carcinoma (NPC), which is a malignant tumor found in the orient and other parts of the world, also correlates with EBV infection. Specific EBV DNAs as well as antigens and antibodies serve as markers for these malignant diseases.

Treatment

Treatment for EBV infection is usually supportive since infections are generally self-limited.

Laboratory Diagnosis

Diagnosis consists of a positive heterophil agglutination test. In approximately 80 percent of infected patients, antibodies to sheep erythrocytes develop. A number of slide agglutination kits are available that also detect heterophil antibodies. Other indications of infectious mononucleosis are a leukocytosis of 10,000–20,000 per cu. ml. with 10 to 40 percent atypical lymphocytes, as well as the elevation of a number of liver function tests. One of the first antigens to appear is the viral capsid or structural antigen (VCA). Early antigens (EA) produced by the virus are nonstructural antigens formed early in viral replication but do not persist. Another group of antigens are the membrane antigens (MA), which appear in the cell membranes of infected lymphocytes during acute infections. Antibodies to Epstein-Barr nuclear antigen (EBNA) appear during the convalescent phase and are not usually found until 1 or 2 months after acute infection. These antigens may be detected by immunofluorescence.

Human Herpesvirus 6 (HHV-6)

This herpesvirus was isolated from patients with lymphoproliferative disorders in 1986. Infection appears to be widespread, with at least 75 percent of the population having antibodies to this virus. At present, this herpesvirus is associated with the development of roseola exanthem subitum, a disease of infants and children. This disease is characterized by the development of a maculopapular rash on the trunk and neck following several days of fever and upper respiratory symptoms. Primary infection of adults is associated with a mononucleosis-like syndrome.

Human Herpesvirus 7 (HHV-7)

This virus was isolated from human T lymphocytes in 1990. Its association with disease remains obscure to date.

Adenoviruses

Stanley S. Lefkowitz

General Characteristics

Adenoviruses were first isolated from human adenoid tissues. They have a strong affinity for lymph nodes and a predilection for latency. Adenoviruses have a double-stranded, linear DNA with a molecular weight of 20 to 25 $\times 10^6$ daltons. Viral capsids are 70 to 90 nm in diameter, icosahedral, and nonenveloped. There are more than 46 subtypes of human adenoviruses, which are divided into 7 groups. The distinction between the various adenovirus types involves very minor antigenic differences. The surface structure of the virus is composed of 252 capsomers that consist of three different types of subunits: the fiber, penton, and hexon. Both the fiber and the hexon units have type-specific antigenic determinants and can be neutralized with serotype-specific antisera. All adenoviruses share a common antigen that is present on the hexon unit. Therefore, detection of this antigen by complement fixation is indicative of an adenovirus infection. The subunits are made in excess during viral replication. Many of the adenovirus types have hemagglutinins as part of the virion or as separate structures. In addition to being associated with latent infections, adenovirus types 12, 18, and 31 have been shown to cause tumors after injection into newborn hamsters. Both tumor cells and cells transformed by adenoviruses in vitro contain "T" antigens, which play a role in cell transformation. Although "early" T antigens are expressed in transforming infections, progeny virus is not produced. A small, defective parvovirus that has been called adenoassociated virus (AAV) has frequently been found in adenovirus-infected cells. Adenoviruses are helper viruses for AAV.

Pathogenesis and Disease

Adenovirus infections are predominantly upper respiratory infections that affect cells of mucous membranes, the cornea, and other organ systems. They are also associated with gastrointestinal symptoms and infection of the genitourinary tract. Transmission primarily involves person-to-person spread by respiratory and pharyngeal droplets or by direct contact with contaminated objects. The fecal-oral route has also been shown to be important in the transmission of certain serotypes particularly in children. The predominant feature of adenovirus infections is their unapparent or subclinical nature. Few individuals develop clinical symptoms. Symptoms range from very minor respiratory illness, similar to the common cold, to much more complex clinical syndromes. Adenovirus type 8 is associated with epidemic keratoconjunctivitis, which has been called "shipyard eye" because of its occurrence in shipyards during World War II. Other types may also cause ocular infections. Pharyngitis is a common symptom associated with infection. More complex clinical syndromes include pharyngoconjunctival fever. This syndrome is characterized by a high fever with both pharyngitis and conjunctivitis. A clinical syndrome called acute respiratory disease (ARD) is a flulike illness that occurs primarily in military recruits during the first few days or weeks of basic training. It is caused by types 3, 4, 7, 14, and 21 and is of major concern to the military. In several studies, it was noted that 10 percent of recruits in basic training were hospitalized for adenovirus infection. Up to 72 percent of all respiratory illness in the winter is caused by this group of viruses. Adenoviruses have also been associated with severe pneumonia and systemic disease, particularly in newborns and infants, and can result in a lethal infection during this stage of development. Gastrointestinal infections including infant diarrhea are caused by the fastidious enteric adenoviruses types 40 and 41. Acute hemorrhagic cystitis has been associated with types 11 and 21.

Laboratory Diagnosis

Virus infection can be readily diagnosed serologically by a fourfold rise in antibody titer between acute and convalescent sera using complement-fixation or neutralization methods. Direct viral isolation from infected tissue scrapings or stool specimens is done by inoculation of cell cultures. Characteristic intranuclear inclusions can be seen in infected cells stained with hematoxylin and eosin. Fluorescent antibody techniques are also frequently used to detect viral-specific antigens in infected cells. Indirect immunofluorescence using a monoclonal antibody to the cross-reacting hexon antigen can be used for rapid viral diagnosis by demonstrating common antigens in infected cells. Enzyme immunoassays are also used to detect soluble viral antigens in feces or nasopharyngeal secretions. The noncultivatable enteric adenoviruses can be identified from fecal specimens by immune electron microscopy.

Virology

Prevention and Control

A single attack usually results in long-term immunity to a given virus type. Adenovirus infections do not constitute a sufficiently important health problem in the general population to warrant the use of a vaccine; however, this is not true in the military. The military has tested several experimental vaccines. Problems in vaccine safety developed when adenoviruses hybridized with simian virus 40 (SV40), an oncogenic virus contaminant of monkey kidney cell cultures, were used to support growth of vaccine virus. These hybrids contained both adenovirus and all or part of an SV40 genome within an adenovirus capsid. A vaccine has been prepared for the military against types 4 and 7 using live virus grown in human diploid cells. It is administered orally in a capsule to liberate the virus in the intestine. There is also a subunit vaccine that is available to the military. This vaccine consists of adenovirus protein subunits and has been found to be relatively safe.

Papovaviruses

Stanley S. Lefkowitz

General Characteristics

Papovaviruses are icosahedral nonenveloped viruses from 45 to 55 nm that have a ds circular DNA genome with 5000 to 8000 base pairs. They are classified into two subfamilies. Polyoma viruses are in one subfamily and papilloma viruses are in the other. A number of animal viruses are in each group.

Polyoma Viruses

The polyoma virus SV40, which was discovered in normal rhesus monkey cells during the early studies with poliovirus, is the best characterized. At the present time, two human polyoma viruses have been designated, the JC and BK viruses after the initials of the patients from whom they were originally isolated. It is likely that primary infection occurs by the respiratory route. The JC virus was isolated from brain tissue from a patient with progressive multifocal leukoencephalopathy (PML). The BK virus has been isolated from the urine of immunosuppressed patients following kidney transplantation and has subsequently been isolated from a number of immunocompromised patients. Latent infection appears to be common with both agents (approximately 80%), with reactivation and disease occurring following immunosuppression. Both viruses are oncogenic in newborn hamsters, hemagglutinate human O cells, and react serologically with SV40.

Treatment

There is no treatment for PML; however, leukocyte interferon has been used to treat BK and JC virus infections in patients who have undergone transplantation.

Papilloma Viruses

Papilloma viruses are the etiologic agents of warts in humans and other animals. Inability to propagate these viruses in vitro has interfered with rapid progress toward our understanding of their characteristics. In addition to strict species specificity these viruses have a specific tropism for squamous epithelial cells and maturation of virus occurs in the terminally differentiated layers. To date more than 70 virus types infecting humans have been classified on the basis of DNA duplex formation with all known types in a liquid reassociation kinetics reaction under stringent conditions.

Wart viruses are usually acquired through mechanical injury such as minor abrasions and many have a long incubation period of several months. A number of types are associated with common, plantar, or flat warts. Epidermodysplasia verruciformis, a familial disease that is associated with depression of cell-mediated immunity, may result in malignant conversion of warty lesions. Virus types 6 and 11 are associated with condylomata acuminata, or genital warts, which are transmitted sexually. These same virus types also cause juvenile laryngeal papillomatosis. Virus types 16 and 18 and to a lesser extent types 31, 33, 35, and 39 are usually found in association with cervical neoplasia and are considered as cofactors in the etiology of cervical cancer.

Treatment

Removal of warts is the most frequently used modality of treatment. This can be implemented by the application of caustic agents, such as podophyllin; surgery; cryosurgery; and laser therapy. Alpha interferon, administered both intralesionally and systemically, has also been used with some success.

Parvoviruses

Stanley S. Lefkowitz

General Characteristics

Parvoviruses are small, linear ssDNA viruses 18 to 26 mm in diameter that are nonenveloped with icosahedral symmetry. Both plus and minus DNA strands may be encapsidated. There are two genera associated with human infections. One genus, the Dependovirus, consists of defective agents that replicate in the presence of adenoviruses and are also known as adenoassociated viruses. They are not presently known to cause disease. The other genus, Erythrovirus, is associated with diseases in both humans and animals. The virus, designated B19, is the cause of erythema infectiosum, or fifth disease.

Pathogenesis and Disease

The respiratory tract is the usual port of entry of B19; however, the virus can also be transmitted by blood or blood products. In volunteers exposed to this virus, a viremia developed that was associated with fever, malaise, myalgia, and a headache. This was followed by a rash with or without subsequent arthritis and arthralgia. A temporary fall in hemoglobin also developed in these volunteers. The virus appears to replicate in rapidly dividing erythroid precursor cells. Patients with hemolytic anemia are at risk for an aplastic crisis. On the basis of these observations it is logical to assume that these agents are the cause of erythema infections.

Natural infections may result in a rash on the face described as "a slapped-cheek" appearance. The rash may involve the upper and lower extremities and may persist for several days. The arthritis and arthralgia, which are usually transient, may occur more commonly with adults. The most serious consequences of parvovirus infection include aplastic crisis in patients with anemia and hydrops fetalis in pregnant women when the virus has crossed the placenta. Previous infection protects against subsequent infections.

Diagnosis

Parvovirus has been detected in sera by immune electron microscopy and radioimmunoassays. Currently the use of dot-blot hybridization involving cloned viral DNA is the most sensitive test. Serologic diagnosis is accomplished by measuring IgM-specific antibodies and is the test available through the Centers for Disease Control.

Treatment and Prevention

No specific treatments or preventive measures are available for this disease.

Orthomyxoviruses (Influenza)

Stanley S. Lefkowitz

General Characteristics

Orthomyxoviruses are single-stranded RNA viruses approximately 100 nm in diameter. Influenza viruses are spherical or pleomorphic, surrounded by a lipoprotein envelope. Two types of glycoprotein projections protrude from the envelope, which function as hemagglutinins or have neuraminidase activity. The former is associated with attachment to specific receptors on cells and agglutination of erythrocytes; the latter is an enzyme associated with the digestion of neuraminic acid residues (receptors) on host-cell surfaces and is involved in viral release. This interaction is important in viral pathogenesis as well as replication. The genome, although single-stranded, is made up of eight pieces of RNA with a molecular weight of 3.9×10^6 daltons. Each piece codes for a distinct protein. In addition, a specific RNA polymerase is present in association with the genome. The production of large numbers of defective viral particles that interfere with infectivity is known as the von Magnus phenomenon. This occurs under certain conditions of viral replication.

An internal antigen (nucleocapsid), also known as "soluble" antigen, identifies the group antigen, designated A, B, or C. Type C differs from types A and B and is not an important human pathogen. Externally, the hemagglutinin (HA) and neuraminidase (NA) spikes have been termed the viral or V antigen. Changes in the V antigens (primarily HA) are responsible for changes associated with influenza antigenicity that eventually lead to epidemics and pandemics. There are some 12 distinct HA subtypes and 9 NA subtypes, most of which are not associated with human infections.

Pathogenesis and Disease

The virus is transmitted readily by droplet secretions through the upper respiratory tract. Viral replication occurs in the epithelial cells of the upper respiratory tract. Viremia is not associated with influenza. Systemic symptoms of influenza are due to the presence of viral antigens, which are toxic, to the liberation of endogenous pyrogens, and to the products of host cells including interferon. The incubation period is very short, usually 1 to 2 days. Characteristic symptoms are chills, rhinitis, and body aches and pains, particularly headaches with characteristic retroorbital pain. High fever is frequently associated with influenza, ultimately followed by weakness and a lengthy convalescence. The disease is more severe in the elderly and those who have other underlying medical problems. Complications such as bronchial pneumonia may occur and may be associated with secondary bacterial infections.

A number of disease syndromes may follow influenza infection or vaccination. These include Guillain-Barré syndrome, which is an ascending paralysis that results in a demyelination of the peripheral nervous system. This disease has been statistically associated with mass vaccination programs, such as the "swine flu" vaccination of 1976. Another disease that may follow influenza or chickenpox, and certain other viral infections, is Reye's syndrome, which occurs in infants and adolescents. This is a serious disease, characterized by vomiting, lethargy, and progressive mental deterioration. Reye's syndrome can ultimately lead to death in 50 percent of affected individuals.

Laboratory Diagnosis

Precise diagnosis of influenza is impossible without laboratory tests. Diagnosis may be accomplished through isolation of the virus. Isolation involves the inoculation of throat washings or nasal swabs into cell culture or hen eggs. After appropriate incubation, testing for the hemagglutinins, which identify the viral antigens, is diagnostic of influenza infection. Specific identity of the virus can be accomplished by using hemagglutination inhibition (HI) assays with known antisera. In addition, serologic means can be used to confirm the diagnosis of influenza. Either complement-fixation or HI techniques are used. In general, a fourfold rise in antibody titer in the convalescent serum, as compared with acute serum, is considered positive. Finally, confirmation can be made by immunofluorescence of infected cells from the nasopharynx. A fluorescein-conjugated antisera directed against influenza virus is used.

Epidemiology

Historically, epidemics have occurred, resulting in natural disasters. During the pandemic of 1918 to 1919, more than 20,000,000 people died. Outbreaks of influenza result from changes in antigenicity of the influenza virus. A major change in antigenicity of either the hemagglutinin or neuraminidase, or both, is called *antigenic shift*. This shift can occur by the dual infection of two different strains of virus in a single host. This results in a "genetic reassortment" of the various subunits of RNA, resulting in a high recombination frequency. Genetic reassortment of the various subunits can result in the formation of a new virus. Many of these changes occur in the Orient and arise in ducks or other birds that live "close" to humans. Antigenic shifts with type A influenza may occur approximately every 10 to 11 years. Major changes in type B occur less frequently.

Minor antigenic changes, which occur frequently in influenza viruses, may result from only one or two amino acid substitutions. These point mutations in the genome occur sporadically. Minor changes of this type have been termed *antigenic drift*. They occur frequently in the hemagglutinin. Antigenic drift occurs in response to changes in immunity of the population (herd immunity). As the number of susceptible individuals decreases, new antigenic variants become the dominant viruses in the population, and the population again becomes susceptible to infection.

There appear to be a finite number of antigenic variant possibilities, since variants tend to recur periodically. There is evidence, for example, that the H_2N_2 Asian strain of 1957 shared antigens with viruses prevalent during 1889. The "doctrine of original antigenic sin" is associated with the immune reaction of individuals to influenza virus infection. This doctrine refers to the restimulation of antibodies to the original or first influenza virus infection following secondary exposures to different strains of the virus.

Viruses are designated by the major group, location of first isolation, and year of isolation, followed by a characterization of the hemagglutinin and neuraminidase, for example, A/Philippines 82 (H_3N_2).

Treatment and Prevention

Amantadine hydrochloride, if administered orally shortly after exposure to the virus, will prevent penetration of influenza A into cells and limit virus replication, resulting in milder infections and reduced dissemination of the virus. Treatment within 48 hours of onset is recommended.

Standard vaccines consist of inactivated virus and are formulated each spring depending on the anticipated viral strains in the population. They are presently trivalent antigens from A/H_1N_1, A/H_3N_2, and B strains. The vaccine is injected subcutaneously and is effective for about 60 to 80 percent of the population for up to 6 months. A library of recombinant strains has been prepared should the viruses be needed for preparation of new vaccines. Allergy to egg proteins is a contraindication to use of the vaccine. In addition, fever, local inflammation, and systemic toxicity can occur following vaccination. In general, the vaccine is recommended for the elderly, those with high-risk medical problems, and those individuals, such as health care providers, who are in frequent contact with influenza patients.

In addition to the standard whole-virus vaccine, other preparations are being employed for immunization. For example, viral subunit vaccines (split virus) containing purified neuraminidase and hemagglutinin are used particularly in children under 13 years of age. Antibody to hemagglutinin subunits can neutralize virus, completely inhibiting infection. Antibody to neuraminidase results in reduction of virus replication, a decrease in transmission, and a reduction of symptoms. In addition to viral subunits, a number of experimental attenuated, live-virus vaccines can be administered by aerosol. These are frequently temperature-sensitive mutants that do not replicate beyond the superficial epithelial cells in the nasopharynx. Because of the high recombination frequency of influenza virus and the potential danger of an attenuated virus reverting to virulence, live-virus vaccines have not been adopted for general use. There is, however, a major effort to develop recombinant vaccines and genetically engineered strains of virus that will protect against the disease.

Paramyxoviruses

Earl M. Ritzi

General Characteristics

The paramyxoviruses are larger than the orthomyxoviruses and are characterized by a nucleocapsid diameter of 18 nm and a virion diameter of 120 to 150 nm. The RNA genome of paramyxoviruses is a single molecule of negative polarity. This genome is not infective alone and must be associated with the virion RNA-dependent RNA polymerase for infectivity. The genome, which does not function as a message, is transcribed by the virion-associated polymerase into shorter-than-genome-length messages upon entering the host cell. The paramyxoviruses are enveloped, helical viruses. A matrix protein lies under the lipid bilayer of the envelope, and two functional glycoproteins, HN and F, are inserted into the lipid bilayer as spike proteins. The HN glycoprotein has both hemagglutinin and neuraminidase activities, whereas the F glycoprotein is a hemolysin and promotes fusion of cell membranes. The F protein has been useful in promoting cellular fusions and has aided in the study of somatic cell genetics. With respect to glycoprotein function, measles and respiratory syncytial virus (RSV) have sometimes been referred to as pseudomyxoviruses because measles lacks neuraminidase activity, while RSV lacks hemagglutinin and neuraminidase activities. In general, the paramyxovirus group can establish persistent noncytocidal infections of cell cultures and provide interesting models for studying diseases such as subacute sclerosing panencephalitis (SSPE).

The parainfluenza viruses (PIVs types 1–4), mumps, measles (rubeola), and RSV are the paramyxoviruses most commonly associated with human disease. Further division indicates that the PIVs 1 to 4 and mumps are in the *Paramyxovirus* genus; RSV is the only human pathogen in the *Pneumovirus* genus and measles virus is in the *Morbillivirus* genus.

Parainfluenza Viruses

PIVs 1 to 3 most commonly cause croup. Four vital serotypes of parainfluenza were isolated between 1955 and 1958. Parainfluenza viruses produce minimal cytopathic effect in cell cultures and produce localized respiratory infections of humans in which viremia is rarely detected. Parainfluenza virus type 1 is most commonly associated with croup (laryngotracheobronchitis) in children 6 months to 3 years of age. Infected adults generally have only a febrile illness similar to the common cold. Viral-induced croup in children may be life threatening due to edema and blockage of the windpipe. The cough often sounds like a barking seal. While croup is the principal manifestation of type 1 viruses, the full range of symptoms (pharyngitis, bronchitis, bronchiolitis, or pneumonia) may be noted. Sendai virus and hemadsorption virus type 2 (HA-2) are PIV 1 representatives. The HA-2 virus is more commonly isolated from patients with croup. Parainfluenza virus type 2 is also associated with croup (in fact, a type 2 representative is named *croup-associated virus*). Second only to RSV, PIV type 3 is most commonly associated with bronchiolitis and pneumonia in infants less than 1 year old. Children 1 to 3 years of age infected by type 3 may experience croup. Parainfluenza virus type 4 is less frequently isolated, has only been associated with minor common cold symptoms, and is not a serious disease threat. The HN protein mediates PIV attachment to cell membranes whereas the F protein mediates fusion of the viral envelope and the plasma membrane. Host-cell proteases cleave the F glycoprotein, determining susceptibility and tissue tropism.

Mumps

Infection by the mumps virus produces systemic disease with enlargement of one or both parotid glands (epidemic parotitis). Mumps virus infections are also characterized by glandular or nervous tissue involvement. Two theories exist for the development of viremia during mumps virus infections. One suggests that the virus travels from the mouth through Stensen's duct to the parotid gland, where it undergoes primary multiplication in the parotid gland. Secondarily, the virus infects other organs as a result of a generalized viremia. The second theory places more emphasis on respiratory droplet infection and places primary multiplication in the respiratory epithelium. This course of viral infection argues for a simultaneous infection of salivary glands and other organs as a result of generalized viremia. After an incubation period of 16 to 18 days and early symptoms of fever, anorexia, and unilateral or bilateral parotitis, generalized viremia may secondarily lead to infection of the testes, ovaries, pancreas, and brain. A viruria frequently develops during mumps virus infections. The following are possible mumps virus complications:

1. Orchitis (atrophy of the testis) is the most common secondary effect of mumps virus infection. Orchitis occurs in 20 to 35 percent of men past the age of puberty but is usually unilateral and therefore does not gener-

ally result in sterility. Infections of the ovary never lead to secondary sterility in women.

2. Aseptic meningitis results from infection of the meninges of the brain. About 10 to 15 percent of aseptic meningitis cases are attributed to mumps virus infection.

3. Meningoencephalitis is a more severe infection of the central nervous system but permanent damage is rare. Only 2 to 5 cases per 1000 mumps virus infections lead to aseptic meningitis or meningoencephalitis.

4. Other less common manifestations are unilateral nerve deafness, thyroiditis, and nephritis.

Although inflammation of the testes, brain, or other organs leads to secondary complications in mumps infection, uncomplicated mumps with associated parotitis produces little tissue damage and few permanent effects.

Measles (Rubeola)

Disease following measles infection is characterized as an acute, highly infectious, exanthematous disease with fever and respiratory symptoms. Although the measles virus might appear to be a dermatropic virus localized to the skin, measles virus is a systemic infection characterized by viremia. The virus enters the body and first replicates in cells of the upper respiratory tract or the conjunctival sac of the eye. A generalized viremia follows, and vesicles form in the buccal mucosa (Koplik's spots) before appearance of a rash. The virus localizes and causes characteristic measles multinucleate giant cells in the skin, lymph nodes, spleen, tonsils, lungs, and kidneys. In approximately 1 case per 1000, measles will localize in the central nervous system causing encephalitis.

The prodromal period of a measles virus infection is characterized by fever, coughing, coryza, conjunctivitis, Koplik's spots, and lymphopenia. The rash of measles is distinguishable from that of rubella virus by being a darker red in color, less discrete, and more coalescing. The maculopapular rash of measles begins as a discrete pink rash that rapidly becomes red and coalescing, spreading over the entire body in 2 to 4 days. The rash finally becomes brownish and desquamative.

The following secondary complications of measles virus infection are of principal concern:

1. Encephalomyelitis (1 : 1000 cases) may occur during or immediately following the rash. A 10 to 30 percent mortality is noted, and 40 percent of survivors have sequelae such as seizure disorders or psychoses.

2. Subacute sclerosing panencephalitis is only detected in individuals previously infected by measles virus.

Disease is most common in children 5 to 10 years of age. It is believed to be the result of a persistent measles infection. This progressive, demyelinating disease which results in mental deterioration and death, is usually detected 5 or more years after a measles virus infection. Measles virus nucleoprotein antigen is found in nerve cell inclusion bodies, and measles virus has been grown by cocultivation of HeLa cells with SSPE brain biopsy material. SSPE is confirmed by finding measles virus antibodies in cerebrospinal fluid, while elevated levels are detected in serum.

3. Secondary infection of the respiratory tract, principally by hemolytic streptococci, occurs in 15 percent of cases. These infections lead to pneumonia, bronchitis, and otitis media.

Respiratory Syncytial Virus

RSV is the single most common infectious cause of death in the first year of life and the single most serious cause of bronchiolitis and pneumonia in infants less than 6 months of age. About 40 percent of infants less than 6 months of age with bronchiolitis and 20 percent with pneumonitis yield RSV when cultured; however, RSV is rarely isolated from healthy infants. Respiratory syncytial virus is extremely fragile and difficult to isolate in cell culture, but it produces a characteristic syncytium with cytoplasmic inclusion bodies. Cultures infected with RSV characteristically lack hemadsorption properties. The transmembrane virion surface F glycoprotein promotes cell-to-cell fusion, whereas both F and G glycoprotein carbohydrate side chains are required for RSV infectivity. The infection of RSV is characterized by a short incubation period (1–4 days), a very localized infection of the ciliated epithelium of the airways, and an absence of viremia. Symptoms of fever, lethargy, and apnea result as sloughing of epithelium and exudate occlude the lumen of airways. Croup is less common with RSV infections but is seen in children 1 to 3 years of age. Repeat RSV infections are the rule but are typically less severe and accompanied by an anamnestic immune response. Primary host immune responses are not completely protective. Historically, maternal RSV antibody and immune responses to inactivated vaccines did not protect infants and actually may have exacerbated the disease. The immune complexes formed by anti-RSV and infecting virus may induce inflammatory responses that lead to clinical disease in young infants. While high levels of RSV-IgE and histamine signal more severe disease, some studies suggest that neutralizing antibodies are beneficial and high-titer immune globulin may be useful; however, further study is required. In hospitalized infants, a mortality of about 2 to 5 percent is noted. Otitis media is also a possible complication of RSV infection.

Epidemiology

The parainfluenza viruses are transmitted by aerosols of respiratory droplets. Type 1 virus infections occur in fall epidemics, whereas type 2 infections are more sporadic. While children and adults may be reinfected, producing colds, most children have antibody to all three serotypes by age 10.

Humans are the only reservoir of mumps virus, and mumps infections occur predominantly in individuals between the ages of 5 and 15 years. Mumps virus is not as contagious as varicella or measles and is transmitted by direct contact, respiratory droplets, saliva, and possibly urine. Mumps virus is transmitted from about 4 days before to 1 week after symptoms occur. Inapparent infections occur in 30 to 40 percent of cases.

Measles virus is highly contagious and causes epidemics when sufficient numbers of susceptible individuals accumulate. Measles is endemic worldwide and occurs chiefly in nonimmune children in late winter and spring; however, susceptible persons of any age may be infected. While measles vaccine caused a decrease in indigenous measles in the United States, present-day measles outbreaks of unimmunized young in inner cities, older students in high schools and college campuses, and cases imported from foreign countries have been typical. Measles is spread by nasal or pharyngeal droplets, produced by sneezing or coughing, and spreading may occur during the interval from 1 to 2 days before the rash to a few days after the rash fades. Measles can also be transmitted through the placenta.

Respiratory syncytial virus spreads in infants and young children during the winter months. Nurseries and hospitals are sites of nosocomial infections. Attack rates for RSV are high in families.

Laboratory Diagnosis

The parainfluenza viruses can be isolated in primate or human cell cultures and detected by the hemadsorption method. Immunofluorescence or enzyme-linked immunosorbent assay (ELISA) can be used to detect PIV antigen, whereas complement fixation (CF), hemagglutination inhibition, neutralization, and ELISA tests can be used for antibody titers.

Mumps virus can be isolated from saliva, cerebrospinal fluid, or urine when inoculated into monkey kidney cells. The virus produces multinucleated giant cells in culture and can be identified by hemadsorption inhibition with mumps-specific antisera. In addition, complement fixation can be utilized to detect a fourfold rise in antibody titer to mumps virus. A delayed hypersensitivity test is available for mumps virus; however, it is less reliable than other serologic tests for determining immune status.

Measles infections are generally clinically diagnosed by the presence of Koplik's spots and the distinctive measles maculopapular rash. A variety of serologic techniques such as ELISA and immunofluorescence assays can be utilized to diagnose the 5 percent of infections that lack Koplik's spots. The virus may be isolated from the blood or nasopharynx from 1 day before symptoms to 1 day after the rash occurs.

The respiratory syncytial virus can be isolated in human or primate cell cultures, where it produces a characteristic syncytial effect, and can be differentiated from parainfluenza viruses by the absence of hemadsorption. An indirect immunofluorescent test or ELISA is used to detect RSV antigen in exfoliated cells of nasal washes. Fourfold rises in RSV antibodies can also diagnose RSV infection in CF tests, neutralization assays, plaque reduction assays, and ELISA.

Prevention and Treatment

Infection by PIV does not confer immunity to reinfection. While seroconversion has been achieved with formalin-inactivated parainfluenza virus vaccines, no vaccine is presently recommended or protects against parainfluenza virus infections. Neutralizing secretory IgA plays a critical role in protection against parainfluenza virus infections as well as RSV infections. The treatment of viral-associated disease is supportive and may involve decongestants or mechanical means of opening a child's airway, such as steam, vaporizers, or, less commonly, a tracheostomy. Oxygen can also be used for dyspneic infants.

Unlike parainfluenza virus cases, the number of mumps virus and measles virus cases has been greatly reduced by the use of two live, attenuated virus vaccines. In the United States, the measles vaccine has additionally reduced SSPE from 20 to 40 cases per year to a rarely detectable case. A second dose of measles vaccine has been recommended to reduce the primary vaccination failures, thereby reducing outbreaks in college-aged individuals. Mumps, measles, and rubella may be present in a combined vaccine, or measles can be used as a monovalent vaccine. In either case, measles immunization should not occur before 15 months of age to prevent maternal antibodies from interfering with the induction of immunity by the live-virus vaccine. Measles virus infections in nonimmune individuals can be treated with immune human gamma globulin early in the incubation period. A small dose of immunoglobulin reduces the severity of disease and permits immunity to develop, whereas a large dose protects against disease but leaves the individual without lasting immunity.

Immune human gamma globulin is not effective in the treatment of mumps-associated orchitis.

The severity of RSV infections has created an urgent need for an effective vaccine; however, killed RSV vaccines have been more detrimental than beneficial and live-virus RSV vaccines have failed to protect against RSV, although a subunit vaccine against the F glycoprotein is being tested. The F glycoprotein elicits neutralizing antibodies. The antiviral agent ribavirin is utilized in an aerosol form to treat infants hospitalized with RSV-induced bronchiolitis or pneumonitis, but its efficacy for PIV infections is not documented. Antivirals are not recommended for mumps or measles viruses.

Coronaviruses

Stanley S. Lefkowitz

General Characteristics

Coronaviruses are single-stranded, pleomorphic RNA viruses with helical nucleocapsids. They range from 80 to 130 nm in diameter and possess an unsegmented genome with a molecular weight of 7×10^6 daltons. The virus is enveloped with characteristic 20-nm petal- or club-shaped projections on its surface (solar corona). This virus is fastidious as well as labile. Routine isolation is difficult except in certain types of organ cultures. Optimal temperature for cultivation is between 33 and 35°C. A hemagglutinin is associated with the surface of the virus. A number of viral subtypes exist, but their exact number is unknown.

Pathogenesis and Disease

Coronaviruses are transmitted by aerosol and respiratory droplets and cause common colds in adults as well as febrile upper respiratory tract illness. As many as 20 percent of cases of the "common cold" have been attributed to coronaviruses, particularly in winter. Acquired immunity develops poorly, and reinfection with the same subtype is common. The virus is also associated with lower respiratory tract disease in hospitalized children. The presence of large numbers of coronavirus particles in fecal specimens as well as their frequent association with gastroenteritis and diarrhea suggests their potential importance in other diseases.

Laboratory Diagnosis

Diagnosis is made primarily by serology using complement-fixation or viral neutralization tests with paired sera. As noted, virus isolation is difficult and is not routinely done.

Picornaviruses and Caliciviruses

Earl M. Ritzi

Picornaviruses

General Characteristics

The picornaviruses are small, naked capsid viruses with cubic symmetry. The single-stranded RNA genome of these viruses consists of a single molecule with positive (messenger RNA) polarity. This positive-stranded viral RNA genome is infective when extracted from the virion and acts as messenger RNA upon entering the host cell. A single giant polyprotein of 200,000 daltons is synthesized and subsequently cleaved by proteases to generate four structural proteins, Vp 1 to 4 and a replicase. Virion-associated polymerases are not found in picornaviruses. The picornaviridae family is composed of two major genera of importance to humans: the enterovirus group, which grows in the intestine, and the rhinovirus group, which grows in the upper respiratory tract. Other genera of interest include the aphthovirus (foot-and-mouth disease virus of cattle) and the cardiovirus (encephalomyocarditis virus [EMC]), a rodent virus occasionally associated with aseptic meningitis in humans. In addition, the virus of infectious hepatitis (hepatitis A virus) is a picornavirus. The enterovirus group that typically infects humans includes the viruses described in Table 5-7. The enteroviruses are stable in acid (pH 3.0–5.0) for 1 to 3 hours and are distinguished from the rhinoviruses, which are acid labile and differ in buoyant density. The human rhinoviruses consist of 113 different serotypes. The following enteroviruses are involved in human disease.

Poliovirus

A typical course of poliovirus infection begins with ingestion of serotype 1 or 3 and is followed by initial replication of the virus in the oropharyngeal mucosa and intestinal mucosa. The virus is then found in the throat and shed in feces. The virus spreads through the lymph system (tonsils

Table 5-7 Medically Important Human Enteroviruses of the Picornaviridae Family

Enteroviruses	No. of serotypes	Serotypes
Polioviruses	3	1, 2, and 3
Coxsackievirus A	23	1–22, 24
Coxsackievirus B	6	1–6
Echoviruses	32	1–9, 11–27, 29–34
Human enteroviruses	4	68–71
Human hepatitis A virus	1	72

and Peyer's patches) to the bloodstream, forming a transient viremia. Other susceptible extraneural tissues become infected, and sufficient virus may be produced to establish a persistent viremia. This persistent viremia is responsible for hematogenous spread to the central nervous system (CNS). While the principal route of CNS infection appears to be through the bloodstream, poliovirus may also spread through peripheral nerves to the CNS. The majority of poliovirus infections (90–95%) as well as other enterovirus infections are subclinical and are demonstrated only by seroconversion. A small percentage of cases (4–8%) are abortive infections without CNS involvement, and only 1 to 2 percent of infections may be clinically recognized as a CNS illness. Clinical disease may be manifest as aseptic meningitis (nuchal rigidity and back pain) or more serious disease forms, including spinal poliomyelitis leading to paralysis (due to infection of the anterior horn cells of the spinal cord), bulbar poliomyelitis leading to fatal cardiac or pulmonary failure (due to lesions in the medulla and brain stem), and encephalitic poliomyelitis (due to lesions in the motor cortex). The paralytic form of disease, as opposed to a mild or subclinical infection, is favored during infection by surgical trauma (e.g., tonsillectomy), injection, fatigue, pregnancy, or increased age of the patient. The immune response against virus-infected neurons in the CNS is responsible for neuronophagocytosis, which contributes, in large part, to neuron destruction, brain lesions, and the development of asymmetric paralysis, which affects lower extremities more than upper.

Coxsackieviruses

The single most common coxsackievirus disease syndrome (type A or B) is aseptic meningitis. Often meningitis is accompanied by a mild paresis that, unlike polio, produces no permanent paralysis. Groups A and B also produce febrile summer or fall illnesses. Table 5-8 describes coxsackievirus manifestations of disease.

Some diseases are chiefly associated with only one of the coxsackievirus groups. The principal manifestation of group A coxsackieviruses is herpangina (vesicular pharyngitis). The characteristic symptom of herpangina is the formation of 10 to 20 gray-white vesicles with a red areola surrounding them. Vesicles appear in the posterior part of the oral cavity on the tonsillar pillars and proceed to form punched-out ulcers with an intense erythema. Group A coxsackieviruses (particularly A16) have also been associated with hand-foot-and-mouth disease. This disease manifestation is characterized by oral and pharyngeal ulcers as well as a vesicular rash on the palms and soles that spreads to the arms and legs. Uniquely, vesicles heal without crusting. This disease results from a human coxsackievirus infection and is distinguished from the foot-and-mouth disease of cattle, which is occasionally transmitted to humans by an

Table 5-8   Coxsackievirus Manifestations of Disease

Differences		Similarities between Type A and B
Type A	Type B	
Herpangina	Pleurodynia (Bornholm disease, epidemic myalgia)	Aseptic meningitis (most common)
Hand-foot-and-mouth disease	Myocarditis	Mild paresis Transient paralysis
Acute hemorrhagic conjunctivitis	Pericarditis Diabetes (mice) (humans?) Severe systemic illness of newborns	Upper respiratory tract infections (colds) Summer or fall febrile illness Rash

aphthovirus. A number of the group A coxsackieviruses have also been associated with an acute upper respiratory infection similar to the common cold.

Disease-specific relationships have also been documented for different serotypes of the group B coxsackieviruses. Pleurodynia, also referred to as epidemic myalgia or Bornholm disease, is an acute disease caused by group B coxsackieviruses. The characteristic symptom of this uncommon infection is a severe paroxysmal chest pain that is felt over the ribs or sternum, or substernally, and is accentuated by deep breathing or movement. Infections of group B coxsackieviruses are also manifest as a general disease of the newborn. During the first week of life, an infant may experience loss of appetite, cough, vomiting, and myocarditis or pericarditis. Cardiac and respiratory problems may rapidly lead to death, or the infant may recover completely. The group B coxsackieviruses have most recently been implicated in primary myocardial disease of adults. These viruses may affect the endocardium, pericardium, myocardium, or all three. Approximately 5 percent of symptomatic group B infections produce heart disease. A weaker association with heart disease has been noted for group A coxsackieviruses and echoviruses. Studies have also suggested that coxsackievirus B4 infection may predispose individuals to the abrupt onset of diabetes mellitus. In addition, a variant of coxsackievirus A24 (enterovirus 70) has been implicated as one of the etiologic agents of acute hemorrhagic conjunctivitis.

Echoviruses (Enteric Cytopathogenic Human Orphan Viruses)

Initially, echoviruses were distinguished from coxsackieviruses by their *failure* to produce a coxsackievirus-like paralysis in newborn mice; however, this principle does not hold true for all echoviruses and coxsackieviruses. Due to

Virology

this confusion, new virus isolates are classified as numbered enteroviruses rather than echoviruses or coxsackieviruses. The echoviruses have commonly been associated with exanthematous febrile illnesses and aseptic meningitis with or without rash. In fact, echoviruses are a leading cause of asceptic (viral) meningitis. The common rashes of type 9 and 16 have been referred to as Boston exanthema. In addition to aseptic meningitis and rashes, which are most common in children, echoviruses (particularly 18) are associated with infantile diarrhea.

Hepatitis A Virus (HAV; Enterovirus 72)

This virus is a major cause of viral hepatitis and jaundice. It is transmitted like polioviruses by the fecal-oral route (contaminated food). It causes acute disease and not chronic liver disease as noted with hepatitis B virus. This picornavirus is discussed further in the hepatitis virus section.

Rhinoviruses

The pathogenesis of the rhinoviruses differs markedly from that of the enterovirus group. Rhinoviruses produce very localized infections of the upper respiratory tract without any detectable viremia. The virus is commonly found in the throat and nose but is not isolated from feces. The lower temperature and pH of the upper respiratory tract favor rhinovirus replication. These viruses are acid labile and grow best at 33°C in cell culture rather than 37°C. The rhinoviruses have a short incubation period (2–4 days), typical of a localized infection, and histopathologic changes are only noted in the surface epithelium and submucosa of the upper respiratory tract. The rhinoviruses, as well as other viruses such as the coronaviruses and parainfluenza viruses, cause colds; however, the rhinoviruses, including 113 serotypes, are generally considered the major cause of the "common cold." Individuals are not made more susceptible to infection by being chilled or wearing wet clothing; however, chills are a symptom of rhinovirus infection. Natural immunity developed during rhinovirus infection is dependent on secretory IgA and is only fleeting. This may explain why individuals with serum antibody directed against a rhinovirus may be reinfected. Rhinovirus infections are generally apparent (3 : 2 ratio) as compared to most enterovirus infections, which are inapparent and subclinical.

Epidemiology

The enteroviruses such as polio are transmitted by the fecal-oral route, and a sufficient number of susceptibles are required for epidemics. While vaccines have greatly reduced the incidence of poliovirus cases in the United States, poliovirus may still produce epidemics in under-developed countries where a sufficient number of susceptibles exist. As hygiene and sanitation methods improve in developing countries where widespread vaccination is not practiced, older individuals rather than young children are infected, and a greater number of more serious poliovirus cases will be detected. The coxsackie-, echo-, and polioviruses are more frequently detected in the summer and autumn months. Enterovirus infections are more typical in the young than in the old, and familial exposure is considered important in the spread of echo- and coxsackieviruses.

The rhinoviruses differ from enteroviruses by causing late-autumn, winter, and early-spring outbreaks of colds. Rhinoviruses are spread more easily by children than by adults, and transmission can occur by two modes. Respiratory droplets *were* formerly considered most important but now hand contamination from virus on objects or other hands followed by self-inoculation is the most likely natural route of transmission.

Laboratory Diagnosis

Enteroviruses replicate well in cell culture and may be recovered from throat swabs, rectal swabs, or cerebrospinal fluid. Polioviruses, unlike coxsackie- and echoviruses, are difficult to recover from cerebrospinal fluid. Rises in titer of neutralizing and complement-fixing antibodies are useful in poliovirus infections; however, serology is generally impractical in coxsackievirus and echovirus infections unless antigen has been isolated from a particular epidemic serotype. The coxsackieviruses are classified as group A or B depending on the induction of flaccid or spastic paralysis in suckling mice.

Prevention and Treatment

Passive immunization of susceptibles with immunoglobulin is effective in the prevention of poliovirus paralytic disease; however, both a killed poliovirus vaccine (Salk) and a live-virus vaccine (Sabin) are available for induction of lasting immunity. The killed-virus vaccine is protective against disease and induces serum immunoglobulin production; however, it does not induce secretory nasal or duodenal IgA, and it does not prevent viral multiplication in the gut on exposure to the virus. The live oral polio vaccine, which is a trivalent vaccine that contains all three serotypes, replicates in the recipient, is disseminated among individuals in the community, and induces a complete spectrum of antiviral immunity including secretory IgA that will prevent reinfection of the gut. The attenuated polioviruses used for vaccine may in extremely rare cases (1 per 3 million) mutate upon replication and revert to virulence. Table 5-9 summarizes key differences between killed and live polio vaccines.

Table 5-9 Summary of Key Differences in Polio Vaccines

	Salk (killed)	Sabin (live)
Induces secretory IgA	No	Yes
Prevents viral replication in the gut	No	Yes
Interrupts transmission in community	No	Yes
Vaccine spreads to immunize others	No	Yes
Useful for immune compromised (or unimmunized adults)	Yes	No
Refrigeration in tropics	No	Yes
Enterovirus infection can induce interference (multiple doses given)	No	Yes
Route of administration	Injection	Oral
Lengths of immunity	Shorter	Longer
Prevents paralysis	Yes	Yes
Induces humoral IgG	Yes	Yes

Note: Vaccines are not available for coxsackieviruses, echoviruses, or rhinoviruses because the large number of serotypes makes vaccine development impractical. Echovirus infections are best prevented by avoiding contact with febrile patients, particularly those with a rash.

Caliciviridae

General Characteristics

These are naked capsid icosahedral viruses slightly larger than picornaviruses (35–40 nm diameter). They are positive-polarity single-stranded RNA viruses that are transmitted by the fecal-oral route. The strategy of genome expression, however, differs from that of picornaviruses. Two viruses that infect humans are probable caliciviruses. One is the Norwalk agent and the other is the hepatitis E virus (HEV).

Norwalk Agent

This is a group of morphologically similar but antigenically different viruses that cause epidemic gastroenteritis, consisting of vomiting, abdominal cramps, and diarrhea in school-aged children, family contacts, and adults. Adult manifestation of diarrhea clearly differs from rotavirus, the cause of infantile diarrhea. The inability to grow these viruses in tissue culture has prevented extensive study.

Hepatitis E Virus

HEV is a virus found outside the United States in developing countries. It is enterically transmitted non-A, non-B (NANB) hepatitis that is responsible for epidemic outbreaks, often due to contaminated water; therefore, it is also called *water-borne hepatitis*. This virus is discussed further in the section on hepatitis viruses.

Laboratory Diagnosis

Immune electron microscopy (IEM) of stool samples has been utilized to detect both of the caliciviruses.

Togaviruses, Flaviviruses, Bunyaviruses, and Arenaviruses

Earl M. Ritzi

General Characteristics

The togaviruses and flaviviruses are single-stranded RNA viruses with genomes of positive (messenger RNA) polarity. Both virus families have an enveloped icosahedral structure, replicate in reticuloendothelial cells, and produce viremia in hosts. The togavirus family consists of two important genera, the alphaviruses and rubivirus (rubella). The flaviviruses are a separate family. Some differences between togaviruses and flaviviruses are presented in Table 5-10. Formerly, the alphaviruses and flaviviruses were respectively termed the group A and group B arboviruses.

The bunyaviruses are also arboviruses, and all replicate in arthropods; however, the virion structure and replication strategy of bunyaviruses differ markedly from those of togaviruses. Bunyaviruses have a single-stranded RNA genome composed of three segments. This genome is of negative polarity and requires a virion-associated transcriptase for replication. Bunyaviruses possess helical symmetry, bud into cytoplasmic vacuoles, and hemagglutinate goose cells with spike projections composed of two distinct viral glycoproteins.

The arenaviruses also possess a unique virion structure. These single-stranded RNA viruses have a segmented genome of negative polarity with two circular nucleocapsids. The most unique characteristic of arenaviruses is the presence of electron-dense granules (host-cell ribosomes) within the pleomorphic enveloped particles. Arenaviruses form persistent infections of a single rodent host that differs from virus to virus, and only occasional spread to other mammals or humans is noted. Table 5-11 lists the important diseases caused by these four virus families.

Table 5-10 Comparison of Togavirus and Flavivirus Characteristics

Togavirus	Flavivirus
Larger in size, 60–70 nm	Smaller in size, 45–55 nm
Budding from plasma membrane	Budding involves cytoplasmic membranes
Expression involves subgenomic mRNA species	Subgenomic mRNA is not detected

Table 5-11 Summary of Important Human Viruses by Family

Togaviridae	Flaviviridae	Bunyaviridae	Arenaviridae
Eastern equine encephalitis	St. Louis encephalitis	California encephalitis complex (LaCrosse virus)	Lymphocytic chorio-meningitis (LCM)
Western equine encephalitis	Powassan agent	Bunyamwera	Lassa fever
Venezuelan equine encephalitis	Yellow fever		Hemorrhagic fever viruses (junin, Machupo)
Rubella	Dengue fever Hepatitis C		

Togaviruses

The alphavirus genus of the togaviridae includes the important mosquito-borne agents of eastern equine encephalitis (EEE), western equine encephalitis (WEE), and Venezuelan equine encephalitis (VEE). Disease is most severe following EEE infection and may be characterized by generalized illness, fever, headache, diffuse encephalitis, coma, convulsions, and residual CNS damage. Mortality is high (50–70 percent) and mental retardation, epilepsy, or paralysis is common in survivors. A higher disease incidence is noted in children, and few infections are inapparent in nature. Eastern equine encephalitis is transmitted along the eastern Atlantic Coast and Gulf Coast by the *Aedes* mosquito.

Western equine encephalitis may also produce encephalitis; however, the disease is generally less severe, with mortality of 2 to 3 percent. Disease following WEE infection is predominantly found in the western portion of the United States and is more severe in children. Fewer infections of children are inapparent in nature as compared to infections of adults.

The characteristics of the Venezuelan equine encephalitis infection differ markedly from those of EEE or WEE. The disease is generally mild or influenza-like, encephalitis is rare, and sequelae are unknown. Encephalitis is generally only seen in horses.

The genus *Rubivirus* represents rubella virus. This is the only togavirus that does not have an animal reservoir and does not utilize mosquito or tick vectors in transmission. Rubella virus is the agent of German measles and the congenital rubella syndrome. Rubella is discussed further in the following section.

Flaviviruses

The Flaviviridae are mosquito-borne or tick-borne viruses and include the following three groups of diseases: (1) encephalitis, (2) systemic diseases of the viscera (hemorrhagic fevers), and (3) mild systemic diseases with rash and arthralgia. The St. Louis encephalitis virus (SLE) is a mosquito-borne flavivirus and one of the most common etiologic agents of encephalitis in the United States. St. Louis encephalitis produces a higher incidence of disease in the elderly than in young children. Mortality of 5 to 10 percent has been noted, as well as mental and emotional sequelae. The Powassan agent, a tick-borne encephalitis agent, is the only flavivirus related to Russian spring-summer encephalitis virus that has been isolated in the United States.

A second group of flaviviruses, the hemorrhagic fever viruses, is represented by a historically important prototype, the yellow fever virus. Yellow fever is a systemic disease of the viscera in which hemorrhagic fever, hepatitis, and nephritis develop. Symptoms include liver-cell inclusion bodies (Councilman bodies), gastrointestinal black vomit, extensive hemorrhages, jaundice, and proteinuria.

A third group of flaviviruses causes undifferentiated fever, arthralgia, and rash. The prototype for this group is the dengue fever virus. There are four clinically important serotypes of dengue virus. This disease syndrome, typically referred to as breakbone fever, is characterized by headache, lymphadenitis, and pains in the back, muscles, and joints. Covalescence is prolonged following infection, and a secondary exposure may lead to dengue shock syndrome, which is characterized by gastrointestinal hemorrhages that are often fatal. Dengue shock syndrome is hypothesized to result from an immune hypersensitivity reaction.

The agent of posttransfusion hepatitis (PTH), hepatitis C virus (HCV), has been described as a flavilike virus. This virus is further discussed in the hepatitis virus section.

Bunyaviruses

These were formerly the group C arboviruses. Their medically important virus is often called the California encephalitis virus; however, 14 different antigenically related mosquito-borne viruses, including a more virulent strain termed the *LaCrosse virus*, compose the California encephalitis complex. Presently, California encephalitis is one of the most common US encephalitis agents; however, disease distribution has shifted, and illness now occurs more frequently in the Great Lakes region and eastern United States than in California. California encephalitis is characterized by a severe frontal headache, fever, lethargy, disorientation, and convulsions. Although convalescence is generally prolonged, fatalities and neurologic sequelae are rare.

Arenaviruses

While the arenaviridae family includes the hemorrhagic fever viruses (Argentinian hemorrhagic fever [junin] and Bolivian hemorrhagic fever [Machupo]), the lassa fever virus and the lymphocytic choriomeningitis virus (LCM) are of greater interest in the United States. The lassa fever virus is highly contagious and human contact is the mode of transmission in the hospital setting. The lassa fever virus produces very high fever, skin rash, severe hemorrhages, encephalitis, and damage to several organ systems. Mortality from lassa fever ranges from 36 to 67 percent. The second arenavirus of importance is LCM. This virus normally exists as a lifelong, persistent infection of mice; however, under crowded conditions, the urine and other excretions of dense mouse populations will transmit LCM to humans. Lymphocytic choriomeningitis infections of humans are associated with aseptic meningitis and influenza-like symptoms.

Epidemiology

Arboviruses obtained by ingestion of blood from a viremic vertebrate replicate in mosquito or tick vectors and are transmitted to other vertebrates, which act as animal reservoirs. Generally, humans are an accidental or dead-end host in the natural transmission cycle. Yellow fever and dengue fever are exceptions, having urban transmission cycles that involve humans. With EEE, WEE, and SLE, wild birds serve as reservoirs, and mosquitoes are vectors. Human epidemics generally parallel horse epizootics, and the horse can be considered a sentinel for infection. Horses are not involved in normal viral transmission cycles with the exception of Venezuelan equine encephalitis, for which horses become an important reservoir during epidemic outbreaks. The California encephalitis virus is also a mosquito-borne virus; however, it differs from togaviruses by using rabbits and small mammals rather than birds as an animal reservoir. Arbovirus infections generally occur in the summer months.

Laboratory Diagnosis

Viral isolation is difficult in togavirus or flavivirus infections, since viremia only occurs early in the infection, before the appearance of symptoms. In fatal cases, the virus may be isolated from brain tissue by inoculation of suckling mice or of vero cells. Neutralizing (N) and HI antibodies persist for many years after infection, while CF antibodies may begin to decrease in 6 months. All three serologic tests (N, HI, and CF) can be utilized with paired blood samples. Lassa virus has been isolated in vero cell cultures from patients' blood.

Prevention and Treatment

An attenuated vaccine for yellow fever virus (17D strain) has been used for many years, but human vaccines for the encephalitis viruses are not available. An attenuated VEE vaccine has been successfully utilized on equines to limit the spread of disease. Vector control, spraying mosquitoes with malathion, has also been effective in controlling arbovirus disease. No specific treatments are available for toga-, flavi-, bunya-, or arenavirus infections.

Rubella (German Measles)

Stanley S. Lefkowitz

General Characteristics

The rubella virus is a single-stranded RNA, enveloped particle approximately 60 nm in diameter with a 30-nm dense core. It is the only member of the *Rubivirus* genus in the family *Togaviridae*. A hemagglutinin for some avian erythrocytes is present as projections on the surface of the virion. The virus is ether sensitive, unstable at room temperature, and susceptible to inactivation by a number of chemical and physical agents. Its recognition as a cause of congenital defects was credited to an ophthalmologist, Sir Norman Gregg, in 1941.

Pathogenesis and Disease

Transmission of this virus is primarily by droplet infection through the upper respiratory tract. The incubation period is approximately 2 weeks. Rubella replication in the cervical lymph node leads to a viremia. This occurs approximately 7 to 14 days after exposure and is subsequently followed by a rash that lasts 2 to 3 days. Rubella can also occur without a rash. The virus may be found in the urine and feces during the viremia and can be isolated from the nasopharynx after development of the rash. The disease is characterized as a 3-day rash with a generalized lymph node involvement. Following the rash, transient episodes of arthritis and joint pain are frequently experienced.

The effects of viral replication, although relatively benign in adults, are very serious in the fetus. Transplacental infection can cause a number of problems, including abortion, miscarriage, stillbirth, and fetal anomalies associated with rubella syndrome. The most frequent anomalies associated with congenital rubella syndrome are ophthalmologic (cataracts, glaucoma, chorioretinitis), cardiac (patent ductus arteriosus, pulmonary artery stenosis, and various septal defects), auditory (sensorineural deafness), and neurologic (mental retardation, meningoencephalitis, microcephaly). Other problems include growth retardation, hepatosplenomegaly, and thrombocytopenia purpura. Danger to the fetus occurs primarily during the first trimester. If infection of the fetus occurs during the first month, approximately 80 percent of the children will have abnormalities. By the third month of the first trimester, abnormalities may develop in approximately 15 percent of those exposed.

The virus circulates in the blood, crosses the placenta, and localizes in the embryonic cells. Multiplication of the virus causes abnormal development of fetal cells through alteration of the growth rate. The virus persists in the fetus and is found in the newborn, from whom it may be excreted in the feces and urine for 12 to 18 months.

Laboratory Diagnosis

Clinical diagnosis of rubella is unreliable and should be followed by a definitive laboratory diagnosis. The principal laboratory method measures an increase in antibody titer to rubella virus using hemagglutination inhibition, or ELISA. Inhibition of hemagglutination at an antibody dilution of 1:8 indicates immunity. Other laboratory methods used include latex agglutination, fluorescence immunoassay, passive hemagglutination, hemolysis in gel, complement fixation, and neutralization. Before the development of these methods, an interference test for rubella virus was used. In this test, monkey kidney cells infected with a possible rubella isolate were subsequently infected with a cytopathic virus such as echovirus 11. Interference of cytopathology by echovirus 11 indicates prior infection with rubella. While this assay is based on rubella's noncytopathic interaction with monkey kidney cells, there are some cell cultures that develop cytopathology after direct infection with rubella virus.

Interpretation of serologic events may be required to make a definitive diagnosis. Nonpaired sera may be tested to determine the susceptibility of a patient. In some cases, it is necessary to determine the class of antibody present to determine if there is a current infection. In congenital rubella, the fetus produces IgM. Therefore, the presence of IgM, specific for rubella, is indicative of rubella infection in the newborn. The absence of specific IgM in cord blood argues against diagnosis of congenital rubella infection. Presence of rubella-specific IgG at birth followed by its decline in about 6 months indicates antibodies of maternal origin. Persistence of antibody throughout the first year of life, including frequent shedding of virus in the urine and feces, is indicative of congenital rubella infection.

Prevention and Treatment

A live vaccine grown in human diploid cells is administered as a single subcutaneous injection. The current vaccine of choice, RA 27/3 was licensed in 1979. It can also be used in combination with measles and mumps vaccine. Multiplication of the vaccine virus may be symptomless or may cause transient arthritis, lymphadenopathy, headache, and fever. A small amount of virus may be shed, but the virus does not readily spread to contacts. A number of congenital infections have occurred in pregnant women inadvertently immunized with vaccine strains. The virus appears to spread to the fetus, but no malformations have resulted. In spite of its apparent safety, rubella vaccine should not be administered to pregnant females. Antibody develops in 95 percent of vaccinated individuals, but the antibody titers are lower than those produced in a natural infection. Protection is solid for a number of years but eventually declines.

In the United States, it is recommended that all preschool children be immunized in order to reduce or eradicate rubella. Infants less than 1 year old should not be immunized. However, in other parts of the world only the prepubertal and postpartum females are immunized. The advantages of the latter policy are that naturally acquired immunity is greater and longer lasting. Immunizing all children deprives women of the natural boosters of the wild-type virus, which are more effective. A routine two-dose vaccination schedule may be implemented.

The administration of immune serum globulin to rubella contacts to achieve prophylaxis has been disappointing. In some cases, disease is prevented, but rubella infection is not. This treatment is considered unreliable and unpredictable.

Reoviruses, Rotaviruses, and Orbiviruses

Earl M. Ritzi

General Characteristics

Each of the three genera of the Reoviridae family (orthoreo-, rota-, and orbiviruses) have double-stranded RNA genomes composed of 10 to 12 segments. The name *reo* is an acronym of respiratory enteric orphan, since reoviruses were not associated with any disease. These viruses contain a virion-associated transcriptase but lack a true envelope. The capsid structure is instead a double protein shell of which the inner shell has icosahedral symmetry and the outer shell is indistinct. The capsid of rotaviruses, as viewed in electron micrographs, has a wheel-like appearance with spokes radiating inward to a hublike core, whereas the orbiviruses have larger circular capsomers that have a ringlike appearance. Viruses of the Reoviridae family replicate in the cytoplasm, strongly induce the formation of interferon, and synthesize a single polypeptide from each genome segment. The reoviruses and rotaviruses are acid stable (pH 3.0) and are transmitted by the fecal-oral route, whereas the orbiviruses are acid-labile arboviruses.

Pathogenesis and Disease

The three serotypes of human reoviruses have been easily detected in the bowel and are found in sewage. Reoviruses are recovered in the respiratory and enteric tracts of healthy children as well as children with mild respiratory and gastrointestinal problems. To date, an etiologic relationship between reoviruses and human illness has not been demonstrated.

Since the discovery of rotavirus in 1973 in duodenal biopsies of pediatric patients, it has been associated with a large share of cases involving severe, nonbacterial infantile diarrhea. In fact, rotaviruses are considered to be the single most common agent of epidemic diarrhea in infants 6 to 24 months of age. In developing countries, the rotavirus syndrome of vomiting, significant dehydration, electrolyte imbalance, and diarrhea is life threatening and is a major cause of infant death. The human rotaviruses have been difficult to grow in tissue culture; however, genetic reassortment of the 11 segments of human and animal rotaviruses has allowed new reassortant viruses to be formed. Animal rotaviruses and reassortant rotaviruses (containing human and animal RNA genome segments) can be grown easily in tissue culture and are potentially useful for vaccines.

The orbiviruses cause a number of animal infections, such as bluetongue virus infection of sheep, but the disease of principal interest to humans is Colorado tick fever. Disease is transmitted by the wood tick (*Dermacentor andersoni*), while the ground squirrel serves as a vertebrate reservoir for the Colorado tick fever virus. Infection of humans tends to occur during months of tick infestation (April to June) in Colorado and the northwestern United States. Colorado tick fever is characterized by a diphasic fever, headache, muscle and joint pains, anorexia, nausea, vomiting, and leukopenia. Disease is usually self-limiting, and recovery is complete. In a small percentage of cases, this mild febrile illness may lead to encephalitis.

Epidemiology

The reoviruses are ubiquitous but show little association with disease. They may be involved in very mild respiratory or gastrointestinal disease. Rotavirus diarrhea is limited to infants. Adults have an anamnestic immune re-

sponse but do not have diarrhea. Rotavirus antibody is present in 90 percent of infants by 24 months of age. Breast feeding and breast milk offer greater protection during epidemics than does formula feeding. In temperate climates such as the United States, rotavirus infections in nurseries and pediatric wards peak during cold months (December to March) whereas infections occur year-round in the tropics.

Laboratory Diagnosis

Rotavirus infections have been diagnosed by the use of electron microscopy and IEM to detect the virus in stool specimens. Fastidious human rotaviruses can be isolated in culture from clinical specimens using embryonic rhesus monkey kidney cells (MA104 cells). An ELISA and a latex agglutination test have been developed and are commercially available for viral antigen detection and quantitation in stool specimens. Reovirus infections can be detected by ELISA for IgG, IgA, and IgM.

Colorado tick fever is diagnosed by a history of tick exposure, a fourfold antibody rise, isolation of the virus from a patient's blood sample, or detection of viral antigen in red blood cells.

Prevention and Treatment

Rotavirus vaccines are being developed and subjected to clinical trials. Oral vaccines of bovine and monkey origin, as well as reassortant viruses containing the human VP7 gene and 10 animal virus genes, are being tested. The VP7 human gene is believed to be responsible for protective immunity. A bovine rotavirus vaccine has been shown to be immunogenic in humans; however, rotavirus vaccines are not yet licensed or in general use in the United States. Rotavirus infections may be controlled by improving sanitation methods and limiting exposure and possible nosocomial infections in pediatric hospital settings. Antiviral treatments for rotavirus are not available. Treatment of rotavirus infections generally involves fluid replacement and maintenance of proper electrolyte balance. No specific treatment is available for Colorado tick fever virus; however, infection is prevented by avoiding areas infested with wood ticks.

Rhabdoviruses (Rabies)

Stanley S. Lefkowitz

General Characteristics

Rabiesvirus is bullet-shaped and 130 to 240 nm by 65 to 80 nm in size. It is surrounded by an envelope with 6- to 7-nm

Virology

projections. The genome is a negative sense ssRNA with a molecular weight of 4.6×10^6 daltons. Virions contain an RNA-dependent RNA polymerase and are extremely stable. Only one serotype is known.

Pathogenesis and Disease

The rabiesvirus is transmitted either by a bite of a warm-blooded animal or by inhalation. Transmission has occurred by inhalation of aerosolized bat feces in caves and through transplantation of corneal grafts. All warm-blooded animals are susceptible to infection with this virus. Bats are symptomless reservoirs. The virus multiplies slowly in muscle or connective tissue and spreads through peripheral nerves to the CNS. Following further replication of the virus in the CNS, centrifugal spread along nerves leads to infection of the salivary gland. Viremia is rare in rabies infections.

In dogs, the incubation period lasts from 10 days to 2 months. During the prodrome, the animal frequently develops changes in temperament. This is followed by an excitable phase during which the animal may be irritable, restless, or very active. Subsequently, a paralytic phase ensues, and the animal becomes immobile. In humans, the incubation period can be as short as 2 weeks or as long as 1 year. The early prodromal phase includes symptoms of malaise, headache, and fever and is followed by a sensory phase during which the individual becomes quite nervous with specific sensations at the site of exposure. This is followed by an excitement phase, with sympathetic overactivity and excessive salivary secretions. Finally, the paralytic phase develops and is characterized by hallucinations and seizures.

Laboratory Diagnosis

Diagnosis is made by finding specific Negri bodies in the cytoplasm of cells from the anterior horn of the suspect animal's brain. A smear is made from the Ammon's horn and stained with Seller's stain. In rabies infections, characteristic Negri bodies approximately 2 to 10 μ in diameter occur that are red with blue granules. Fluorescent antibody techniques are frequently used and are far more sensitive. Fluorescein-conjugated specific antibody to rabies antigen is incubated with an impression smear from the animal's brain, and, in animals positive for rabies, specific fluorescence can be observed using a fluorescent microscope. Another method that can be used is direct isolation of virus from the brain or saliva of the suspected animal. The virus is detected after intracerebral inoculation in mice. These animals are then observed for several days for the development of paralysis.

Epidemiology

Because of the severity of this disease, it is extremely important to understand its epidemiology. The risk of death following the development of symptoms due to rabies is virtually 100 percent. In the United States, only a few cases occur annually. Worldwide there may be as many as 1000 cases. Every year in the United States, approximately 25,000 persons receive prophylactic treatment for rabies. Only about 150 cases of rabies in dogs occurred in 1982; however, the disease in wildlife, especially skunks, foxes, raccoons, and bats, accounted for more than 85 percent of animal rabies. Bites by wild animals should be treated as if the animals were rabid until they are proved negative by laboratory tests. Dogs and cats that have been previously immunized and have minimal chance to contract rabies should be observed for at least 10 days before administration of postexposure prophylaxis to the bite victim.

Prevention and Treatment

Historically, a number of vaccines have been used. The Pasteur vaccine was a nerve-tissue vaccine that consisted of dried spinal cords from infected rabbits. Later, the Semple or phenol inactivated virus was used as a vaccine. There was always the danger of allergic encephalitis resulting from its use. The duck embryo vaccine (DEV) has been used until recently. This was an inactivated virus grown in duck embryo cells. The currently used vaccine is an inactivated virus preparation grown in human diploid cells. It is much safer, and antibody titers following its use are higher than those produced with other vaccines. Terms found in the literature referring to rabies include street virus and fixed virus. Street virus is used to identify any recent clinical isolate, whereas fixed virus refers to an attenuated virus of low virulence obtained by passage in animals. The Flury rabies virus is a live, attenuated virus used in many veterinary vaccines.

Today two types of products are used for immunization: vaccines that induce an active immune response and globulins that provide rapid but passive protection. In the United States, human diploid-cell rabies vaccine (HDCV) is an inactivated virus vaccine prepared from rabies virus grown in WI-38 or MRC-5 human diploid cells. Globulins include rabies immune globulin (RIG) from hyperimmunized human donors.

For preexposure prophylaxis, three intramuscular injections of HDCV are administered. This treatment is indicated for persons at high risk of contact with rabid animals. For postexposure prophylaxis, immediate and thorough washing of all bite wounds with soap and water is essential. Both antibody (RIG) and vaccine should be administered. One half of the RIG is administered into the wound area and the balance is given intramuscularly. This should be followed by five 1-ml intramuscular doses of HDCV. The first dose should be administered immediately and the balance on days 3, 7, 14, and 28.

Other rhabdoviruses may also be associated with human disease. Vesicular stomatitis virus, usually associated with cattle, pigs, and horses, can also infect humans. In laboratory employees who work with the agent, an acute febrile illness associated with fever, myalgia, and malaise may develop.

A family of agents known as Filoviridae has been separated from the rhabdoviruses. They are associated with severe hemorrhagic shock and bleeding. The Marburg agent (African hemorrhagic fever) has been found in green monkeys. Cell cultures prepared from these animals have been a source of virus, causing serious diseases in animal handlers and laboratory workers. Ebola is another virus in this group that has caused considerable mortality during several major outbreaks in Africa. The viruses of rabies, Marburg, and Ebola have a high case-fatality ratio, which may approach 100 percent.

Slow Virus Infections

Stanley S. Lefkowitz

A number of viruses or "viral-like" agents have been linked to chronic degenerative diseases of the CNS. These diseases are characterized by (1) long incubation periods, (2) a regular protracted course that usually results in death, (3) involvement of a single host species, and (4) pathologic lesions limited to a single organ or tissue system.

It has been suggested that certain diseases of humans may be associated with chronic virus infections with or without an autoimmune component. These include Parkinson's disease, amyotrophic lateral sclerosis, multiple sclerosis, and systemic lupus erythematosus. Two retroviruses that produce slow-virus diseases of sheep are visna and progressive pneumonia (maedi).

Spongiform Encephalopathies

The spongiform encephalopathies are slow infections of the central nervous system that have a number of features in common. These include incubation periods ranging from months to years and the transmission of the agent by injection of infected tissue into animals. Pathology is restricted to the brain, which develops characteristic, intracytoplasmic vacuoles in the axonal and dendritic processes of neurons, resulting in coalescence of vacuoles and destruction of cells. The diseases ultimately progress to

death of the host. They are caused by a new type of infectious agent, which has been termed *prion* or *protein infectious agent*. No recognizable viral particles are associated with the infectious agent. Infection is caused by a unique 27 to 30 kD protein that has been termed *PrP 27–30*. Interestingly, the gene coding for this protein has been found in both normal and infected animals. It is speculated that a posttranslational error may convert the normal protein to the infectious PrP 27–30. This protein is associated with host cell membrane structures but not with specific nucleic acids. It is extraordinarily resistant to heat, 10% formaldehyde, nucleases, and ultraviolet light. Infectivity is destroyed by phenol, ether, sodium hypochlorite, and other protein-disrupting agents. There is no measurable host cellular or humoral immunity to this agent. A number of naturally occurring diseases are caused by the agent, including in humans, kuru, Creutzfeldt-Jakob disease, and Gerstmann-Sträussler-Scheinker syndrome, a familiar variety of Creutzfeldt-Jakob disease. In animals, a number of diseases have been described, including scrapie in sheep, transmissible mink encephalopathy, bovine spongiform encephalopathy, and chronic wasting disease in captive mule deer and elk.

Kuru

Kuru is a fatal disease that occurs only in the Fore tribe in New Guinea. It is a degenerative disease of the CNS that is similar to scrapie, and consists of progressive cerebellar ataxia, tremors, and ultimately death. It has occurred more frequently in women and is associated with ritual cannibalism. It is believed to have been transmitted from contaminated brain tissue through cuts or sores during "preparation." The incubation period ranges from 4.5 to over 30 years. Since cannibalism is not currently practiced by this group, the disease has all but disappeared. Kuru can be readily transmitted to experimental animals, and titers of greater than 10^9 infectious doses per gram of brain tissue have been reported.

Creutzfeldt-Jakob Disease

Creutzfeldt-Jakob disease (CJD) is a subacute presenile dementia that was first reported in 1920. Its pathology is similar to that of kuru. Onset is gradual with progressive dementia, ataxia, and somnolence that leads to death. This disease is readily transmitted to chimpanzees and has been transmitted accidentally from person to person through corneal transplantations and contaminated electrodes following brain surgery. It has also been transmitted through the use of contaminated human growth hormone. The disease may occur sporadically or tend to recur in certain families, which carry specific genetic alterations of these proteins.

Table 5-12 Recognized Hepatitis Viruses

Virus	Family	Nucleic acid	Routinely cultivated successfully in vitro	Identified principally through viral gene cloning	Genomes cloned or sequenced	Identified by electron microscopy	Tests for antigen or antibody
HAV	Picornaviridae (enterovirus 72)	+ ssRNA	Yes	No	Yes	Yes	Yes
HBV	Hepadnaviridae (hepadnavirus type 1)	ds circular DNA with a ssDNA gap	No	No	Yes	Yes	Yes
HCV	Flaviviridae	+ ssRNA	No	Yes	Yes	No	Yes
HDV	Defective RNA virus	− ssRNA	No	No	Yes	Yes	Yes
HEV	Caliciviridae	+ ssRNA	No	Yes	Yes	Yes	Yes

Scrapie

Scrapie is a disease of sheep that has been known for hundreds of years. In sheep, the incubation period is from 1 to 3 years. Susceptibility is dependent on the breed, which can be completely resistant or more than 80 percent susceptible. The disease can be readily transmitted to mice, with an incubation period of several months. A number of different strains have been recognized. Early symptoms include tremors and lack of coordination. The disease progresses to spasticity, paralysis, and ultimately death.

A disease in cattle called bovine spongiform encephalopathy was first recognized in the United Kingdom in the middle 1980s. The pathology and clinical manifestations are similar to those observed in scrapie, including ataxia, excitability, and aggressiveness, followed by progressive wasting and ultimately death. The source of infection is believed to be scrapie-infected sheep carcasses used in cattle feed. Isolation of PrP 27–30 protein from infected cattle reveals an amino acid sequence that differs in only one amino acid between the mouse and CJD proteins. This protein is not found in healthy cattle.

Hepatitis Viruses

Earl M. Ritzi

General Characteristics

Five types of viral hepatitis have now been recognized; however, additional viruses may still be characterized from the old non-A, non-B classification. One classic type of disease, infectious hepatitis, or short-incubation hepatitis, has been attributed to HAV infection. The second classic disease, serum hepatitis, or long-incubation hepatitis, is associated with hepatitis B virus infection (HBV). The recognition that hepatic disease could be transmitted by blood products, containing neither type A nor type B virus,

led to the designation of NANB hepatitis. One of the major viruses responsible for this NANB parenteral transmission is HCV. This flavilike virus was detected through cloning of a viral gene for its principal immunoreactive viral peptide. This use of cloning to detect an uncharacterized pathogen is unique and can be considered a first in pathogen identification. Hepatitis C virus is the major cause of PTH. In addition to these three viral forms, a fourth defective RNA virus, referred to as the delta agent or hepatitis D virus (HDV), was discovered in hepatitis B surface antigen (HB$_s$AG)-positive individuals. This virus replicates in the presence of HBV and therefore has similar transmission routes. A fifth virus to be defined from the non-A, non-B grouping is hepatitis E virus (HEV). This calicilike virus is considered to be responsible for enterically transmitted NANB hepatitis and this agent has also been referred to as water-borne hepatitis. The hepatitis viruses and their principal characteristics are found in Table 5-12.

Hepatitis A Virus

Hepatitis A virus is responsible for about 67 percent of acute hepatitis cases. The physicochemical characteristics of HAV are identical to those of picornaviruses such as polio- and coxsackieviruses. For this reason, HAV has been classified in the picornaviridae family as enterovirus 72. The entire HAV has also been referred to as the HA antigen. This antigen is present in liver and stool preparations.

Hepatitis B Virus

Hepatitis B virus is more structurally complex than HAV and has been placed in the hepadnavirus family. Similar viruses of the woodchuck, squirrel, and duck belong to this family. Three different morphologic forms of HBV have been identified in patient sera. The complete 42-nm infectious particle containing a DNA genome is least abundant and is referred to as the Dane particle. The other two morphologic forms, a 22-nm sphere and a 22-nm filament (100–700 nm long), are very abundant, lack a DNA genome, and are composed of HB_sAG. The envelope of the Dane particle is also composed of HB_sAg (previously referred to as Australia antigen), whereas the core antigen is termed HB_cAg. HB_sAG has one group-specific determinant (a) and two sets of mutually exclusive subtype determinants (d and y, r and w). This leads to four serotypes—adw, adr, ayw, and ayr—which can be utilized in epidemiologic studies. A hidden antigenic determinant of the HBV core is referred to as HB_eAg. The e antigen is exposed in serum, and HB_eAg persistence becomes a useful diagnostic marker commonly associated with chronic or persistent infections. The Dane particle possesses a unique circular, double-stranded DNA genome with a single-stranded gap. A DNA polymerase associated with the Dane particle is capable of both RNA and DNA-directed DNA polymerase activity. HBV is unique in being able to reverse transcribe its (+) strand DNA from an RNA template suggesting a similarity to the retroviruses. Antibody directed against HB_sAG will agglutinate all three HBV morphologic forms that circulate in blood. Anti-HB_s is involved in viral neutralization and the development of immune protection; however, antibodies to core protein (anti-HB_c) or e antigen (anti-HB_e) have not been associated with immune protection.

Hepatitis C Virus; Parenterally Transmitted Non-A, Non-B Hepatitis

The presence of different viral structures in electron micrographs of NANB agents, variance in the length of viral incubation periods, multiple recurrences in humans, and a failure in animal challenge experiments for one NANB agent to cross-protect immunologically against another have led to the conclusion that a number of NANB hepatitis agents exist. Hepatitis C virus (a flavilike virus) has been cloned and identified by an antibody test for anti-HCV. HCV is the leading cause of PTH.

Hepatitis D Virus, Delta-Associated Agent

This is a defective ssRNA virus defined by the delta antigen and delta antibody system. It has an RNA core with delta antigen that is found enveloped in blood by the HB_sAG of HBV.

Hepatitis E Virus; Enterically Transmitted Non-A, Non-B Hepatitis

Hepatitis E virus is not found in the United States, but this calicilike virus may be the major worldwide cause of

Table 5-13 Missing Features of Viral Hepatitis in Hepatitis A Virus Infections

1. Extrahepatic manifestations
   a. Arthralgias, arthritis
   b. Polyarteritis nodosa
   c. Nephritis
   d. Immune-complex diseases (serum sickness–like)
2. Chronic hepatitis infections
3. Long-term viral carrier state
4. Cirrhosis
5. Primary hepatocellular carcinoma

hepatitis. It is an important cause of waterborne epidemics in the Far East. It is detected by IEM of stool specimens.

Pathogenesis and Disease

The hepatitis viruses produce an acute inflammation and necrosis of liver cells. The symptoms (fever, chills, nausea, vomiting, anorexia, abdominal discomfort, and jaundice) as well as the histopathologic lesions of acute infections cannot be distinguished from one another with respect to virus type. It should also be noted that 30 to 80 percent of acute HAV, HBV, and HCV infections are asymptomatic. In addition to an acute, self-limiting viral infection, HBV, HCV, and HDV viruses may also cause chronic hepatitis.

Hepatitis A Virus

Although hepatitis A is the most common cause of an acute clinical disease syndrome, HAV is distinguished from other hepatitis viruses because it lacks certain features of other hepatitis virus infections. The important missing features are presented in Table 5-13.

Unlike HBV, HAV has an abrupt clinical onset, a short incubation period (average 4 weeks), a short elevation of liver transaminases (1–3 weeks), and a complete recovery in nearly all cases with the lowest mortality case rate ($<0.5\%$) for the hepatitis virus group. The virus is present for a short period in the blood, but this does not develop into a persistent viremia as noted in HBV infections; therefore, blood is not a major route of transmission. The virus is most easily transmitted just before symptoms of jaundice, when the virus is detected at its highest concentration in feces. Anti-HAV antigen appears first in the IgM fraction during acute infection and later during convalescence in the IgG fraction. The IgG anti-HAV that results from natural infection is protective against reinfection and persists for many years.

Virology

Table 5-14   Features Typically
Associated with Hepatitis B Virus Infections

1. Extrahepatic manifestations
   a. Arthralgias, arthritis
   b. Polyarteritis nodosa
   c. Glomerulonephritis
   d. Serum sickness–like disease (skin rash and urticaria)
2. Chronic carrier state [asymptomatic, HB_sAg (+)] (infected newborns, immunosuppressed, and non whites > likelihood)
3. Chronic disease (liver injury, HB_sAg and HB_eAg persist > 6 months)
4. Chronic aggressive disease (same as 3, very high anti-HB_cAg titer, lymphocyte infiltration, and bridging necrosis)
5. Cirrhosis
6. Primary hepatocellular carcinoma (HBV DNA is integrated into tumor-cell DNA)
7. High incidence of perinatal infections when mothers are HB_eAg (+)
   (95% at time of birth, 5% transplacental)
   (90% of infected become chronic infections)

Hepatitis B Virus

Hepatitis B virus is responsible for only 25 percent of acute infections but plays a major role in chronic liver disease and its associated immunologic complications. The incubation period is extended for HBV, averaging 10 weeks, and the clinical onset of disease symptoms is very gradual. Infection with HBV may be acute and self-limiting, or in a small percentage of cases, infections may lead to persistent viremia, producing cases of chronic liver disease or chronic carrier states. Table 5-14 lists important features of hepatitis infections often associated with HBV or accompanying HDV infection.

Hepatitis C Virus

HCV may produce both acute and chronic hepatitis; however, HCV infection causing PTH becomes chronic in 54 percent of cases. Therefore, this leading cause of PTH also causes the highest frequency of chronic disease. HCV is also associated with cirrhosis but an association with liver cancer is still questionable. Manifestations of the HBV- and HCV-mediated disease may be accentuated when the immune status of suppressed patients improves, thus indicating that the immune system plays a role in the pathology of these infections.

Hepatitis D Virus

HDV infection has most of the features of HBV infection since it only exists as a coinfection or superinfection of HB_sAg (+) individuals. Hepatitis D virus infection is found with more severe HBV infections and more often leads to chronicity.

Hepatitis E Virus

HEV is a major food- or water-borne epidemic virus of underdeveloped poorer countries. Little is known about this virus; however, to date, it has not been found to be associated with extrahepatic manifestations, chronic infections, cirrhosis, or cancer.

Epidemiology

The routes of transmission and persons at risk differ markedly with regard to virus type. Hepatitis A virus infections are transmitted by the fecal-oral route (blood product transmission is rare). The majority of HAV infections are subclinical, and peak incidences are noted in autumn, particularly in crowded households or institutions. The contamination of clams by sewage has also implicated shellfish in type A infections. A higher incidence of infection in homosexuals has suggested that HAV may be sexually transmitted; however, this transmission is more likely fecal-oral due to oral-anal interactions.

The mode of transmission for HBV is predominantly parenteral (involving blood products or injections); however, secondary routes of transmission also exist. Sexual contact is an important secondary route of infection. Person-to-person transmission can occur through contact with bodily products such as saliva, tears, semen, vaginal secretions, cord blood, or breast milk. Transplacental infection by HBV is rare, but neonatal infection from HBV-infected mothers does occur with high frequency. Mother-to-child transmission plays a much greater role in the spread of disease in areas of the world outside the United States. The individuals at highest risk by HBV infection are percutaneous drug users, hemodialysis patients, blood bank laboratory personnel, and homosexuals. Screening blood has nearly eliminated the risk of HBV infection in blood transfusion recipients.

Since the delta agent only replicates in HB_sAg (+) individuals, HDV coinfection or superinfection involves the same routes of transmission as HBV.

Hepatitis C virus is parenterally transmitted by transfusion and intravenous drug use. The availability of a serologic screening test should greatly reduce HCV-mediated PTH in the near future.

Hepatitis E virus is enterically transmitted NANB hepatitis. Contaminated water in countries outside the United States often is responsible for the fecal-oral spread of this virus in epidemics. Table 5-15 summarizes principal routes of transmission for the five known hepatitis viruses.

Table 5-15 Routes of Hepatitis Virus Transmission

HAV	HBV	HCV	HDV	HEV

Fecal-oral
Sexual
  Homosexuals' oral-
    anal interactions
	Parenteral
	  Blood
	  Blood by-products
	  IV drug use
	  Occupational (working
	    with blood or
	    infected patients)
	Sexual
	Vertical infection of
	  newborn
	Saliva
		Parenteral
		  Transfusion
		  IV drug use
		  Occupational
			Parenteral
			  Blood
			  Blood by-products
			  IV drug use
			  Occupational (working
			    with blood or
			    infected patients)
			Sexual
			Vertical infection of
			  newborn
			Saliva
				Fecal-oral
				  (no other known route)

Laboratory Diagnosis

Tests for abnormal liver function such as serum transaminase levels and bilirubin levels are used extensively for diagnosis of hepatitis. A sharp rise in serum alanine aminotransferase (ALT) at the time of fever onset distinguishes HAV infection from HBV and NANB virus infections. The latter viral infections are characterized by a gradual, prolonged elevation in ALT. A second transaminase that may be elevated during acute disease is serum aspartate transaminase (AST; formerly serum glutamic oxaloacetic transaminase [SGOT]). Levels of AST are generally lower than ALT during acute viral hepatitis.

Specific viral markers detected by radioimmunoassay (RIA) or ELISA have been useful in the diagnosis of both type A and type B hepatitis. Type A infection produces an elevation in IgM (greater than HBV or NANB infections) and is best diagnosed early during disease onset by an RIA specific for IgM anti-HAV antigen. This specific IgM is short-lived and disappears in 2 months. Shortly after the first appearance of IgM, IgG anti-HAV antigen becomes a diagnostic marker that persists for many years. The detection of specific IgM is indicative of current HAV infection whereas specific IgG is a marker of prior infection but not necessarily a current infection.

The use of viral diagnostic markers is more complex for HBV, since the number of markers is greater and the utility of a diagnostic marker is dependent on the stage of infection and the nature of the infection (acute versus chronic). During acute self-limiting infection, viral antigens can be detected early in the blood. During the incubation periods before disease onset, HB_sAg, HB_eAg, Dane particles, and DNA polymerase are present in the blood; however, HB_sAg (detected by RIA) is generally most abundant and utilized in diagnosis. At the time of clinical onset, anti-HB_c appears and is used as a marker, in addition to HB_sAg. The detection of IgM anti-HB_c of high titer argues for acute infection. At this time, HB_sAg and HB_eAg may still be detected but antigen concentrations in the acute self-limiting infections have begun to decline in the bloodstream. The period of convalescence in self-limiting infections is marked by the appearance of anti-HB_e and anti-HB_s, disappearance of HB_sAg, and continued high levels of anti-HB_c. In early convalescence, IgM anti-HB_c is a useful marker, whereas in later convalescence both IgG anti-HB_c and anti-HB_s act as diagnostic markers. The behavior of viral markers and the time course of appropriate tests are presented for a self-limiting HBV infection in Fig. 5-11.

In chronic infections (chronic active liver disease or a chronic carrier state), HB_eAg and HB_sAg persist in the blood for prolonged periods, and anti-HB_s is not detected in the chronic carrier state. Since HB_eAg is the first antigen to disappear in self-limiting infections, the continued or prolonged presence of HB_eAg has been used as an indication of increased infectivity and the establishment of a chronic infection. In chronic carriers, HB_eAg may be replaced over a period of years by anti-HB_e.

Diagnosis and prevention of NANB disease were severely limited by the complete lack of a reliable viral diagnostic test that could be used on blood or blood by-products; however, HCV, one of the principal NANB viruses and main cause of PTH, can now be detected by a serologic test for anti-HCV antibodies. This test for HCV can be used to screen blood along with other NANB surrogate markers (such as ALT > 75 IU/ml, history of high-risk activities, HIV antibodies, or history of hepatitis). Anti-HCV may indicate a prior HCV infection rather than a current infection and may be difficult to detect in HIV-1–infected immunosuppressed patients.

The presence of hepatitis delta antigen (HDAg) in woodchuck livers has permitted development of solid-phase RIA and ELISA assays for detection of antihepatitis delta antigen (anti-HDAg) in serum. An antibody class capture RIA has been developed to specifically detect IgM anti-HDAg. An early sharp rise in titer of IgM anti-HDAg is

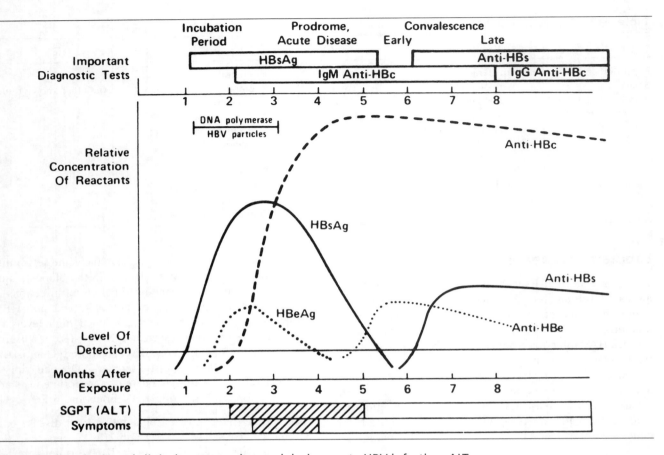

Fig. 5-11 Serologic and clinical patterns observed during acute HBV infection. ALT, alanine aminotransferase; SGPT, serum glutamic pyruvic transaminase. (From F. B. Hollinger and J. L. Dienstag. Hepatitis Viruses. In E. H. Lennette, A. Balows, W. J. Hausler, Jr., et al., *Manual of Clinical Microbiology* (4th ed.). Washington, DC: American Society for Microbiology, 1985. Pp. 813–835. Reprinted with permission.)

diagnostic of acute HDV infection in both HBV acutely infected individuals and in HBV carriers.

A serologic test for anti-HEV has also been developed to detect HEV in stool specimens. This enterically transmitted NANB virus has been detected by IEM. Table 5-16 summarizes key results of hepatitis serology and their diagnostic implications.

Diagnosis of undefined NANB viruses is established by eliminating other agents such as HAV, HBV, HCV, HDV, HEV, Epstein-Barr virus, and cytomegalovirus.

Prevention and Treatment

The prevention of HAV infections involves a careful control program to prevent fecal contamination of food or water supplies. In addition, the spread of HAV to susceptibles can be blocked in both pre- and postex-

posure settings by the administration of normal immune serum globulin (ISG). Before exposure, ISG should be given when traveling to an endemic area. In postexposure settings, ISG should be administered to susceptibles in day-care centers, institutions, and hospitals, and to household contacts, sexual contacts, exposed primate handlers, and those kitchen personnel associated with a common-source outbreak such as contaminated food. In common-source food-related outbreaks, ISG must be administered before the onset of clinical symptoms to achieve prophylaxis.

Inactivated hepatitis A vaccines are currently being developed. One vaccine for hepatitis A virus is a formalin inactivated alum-adjuvanted preparation of the HM175 hepatitis A strain. These inactivated viral vaccines, while promising, are not yet licensed and available for routine use.

While standard ISG is effective in HAV prophylaxis, ISG is only recommended for nonparenteral exposure and

Table 5-16   Interpretations of Serodiagnostic Tests for Hepatitis

Interpretation			Marker(s)		
Acute hepatitis A infection			Anti-HAV IgM (+)		
Hepatitis C virus infection			Anti-HCV (+) [other viruses (−)]		
Hepatitis E virus infection			IEM (+) for anti-HEV [other viruses (−)]		

	HB$_s$Ag	HB$_e$Ag	Anti-HB$_c$	Anti-HB$_e$	Anti-HB$_s$
HBV vaccine response or passive hepatitis B hyperimmune globulin treatment	(−)	(−)	(−)	(−)	(+)
Early in acute HBV infection	(+)	(−)	(−)	(−)	(−)
HBV chronic carrier [e (+) > infectivity]	(+)	(+) or (−)	(+)	(−)	(−)
Acute HBV infection *or* chronic HBV infection with high infectivity (e +)	(+)	(+)	(+)	(−)	(−)
Acute HBV infection (HB$_e$Ag cleared) *or* chronic HBV with low infectivity (e −)	(+)	(−)	(+)	(+)	(−)
Convalescence after HBV infection	(−)	(−)	(+)	(±)	(+)

Interpretation	Marker(s)
More likely acute HBV than chronic HBV infection	High-titer anti-HB$_c$ IgM detected and RIA of paired samples over time shows HB$_s$Ag *decline*
More likely to become chronic HBV than acute HBV infection	High-titer anti-HB$_c$ IgM detected and HB$_s$Ag does *not* decline over 2–3 mo
Strongest indication of chronic HBV infection	HB$_s$Ag (+) that persists for more than 4 to 6 months after clinical onset of illness, HB$_e$Ag may be (+) or (−)
Hepatitis D virus (delta agent) infection	HB$_s$Ag (+) individual tests (+) for IgM anti-HDAg

does not play a major role in the prevention of HBV infections. However, hepatitis B hyperimmune globulin (HBIG), which has a high anti-HB$_s$ titer, is indicated for prophylaxis after exposure to blood or saliva of an HB$_s$Ag-positive patient, after transfusion of HB$_s$Ag (+) blood, after intimate sexual contact with an HB$_s$Ag (+) individual, or immediately after birth of a neonate from an HB$_s$Ag-positive mother. The incidence of posttransfusion HBV infections has been markedly decreased by screening blood for HB$_s$Ag. The great abundance of the HB$_s$Ag in the plasma of carriers provided a source of viral antigen for vaccine development. The use of inactivated human plasma (containing HB$_s$Ag) was unique to the manufacture of HBV vaccine and prompted extensive safety testing. The original HBV vaccine, known as Heptavax-B, has been both efficacious and lacking in undesirable side effects.

This vaccine has been superseded by two vaccines created by recombinant DNA technology. These vaccines, Recombivax HB and Engerix-B, both consist of purified HB$_s$Ag. Preexposure recommendations for vaccine use include health care workers, medical students, staff of mental institutions, hemodialysis patients, active homosexual males, active IV drug users, individuals with multiple sexual contacts, recipients of certain blood products,

household and sexual contacts of HBV carriers, and individuals in contact with endemic HBV populations. These vaccines are also being considered as a general vaccination for all newborn infants. In a postexposure setting, HBV vaccine is recommended for newborns of HB$_s$Ag (+) mothers, for sexual exposure with an HB$_s$Ag (+) partner, or for percutaneous exposure to blood of an HB$_s$Ag (+) patient. Booster immunizations for HBV are not recommended in normal hosts for at least 7 years. Protective immunity induced by natural infection or vaccines resides solely in the anti-HB$_s$Ag response. Vaccination against HBV should also aid in reducing the incidence of HBV-associated hepatocellular carcinoma. In addition, the use of HBV vaccines eliminates the possibility of defective HDV infection.

Vaccines do not exist for HCV and HEV. No specific antiviral therapy is recommended for acute hepatitis. Corticosteroids such as prednisone have been used with human interferon to improve treatment of chronic hepatitis. In chronic hepatitis due to HBV, positive responses have been reported with vidarabine, azidothymidine (AZT), dideoxycytidine (ddc), and acyclovir with or without interferon; however, these treatments are still experimental and further proof of efficacy is needed.

Virology

Tumor Viruses and Oncogenes

Earl M. Ritzi

The oncogenic viruses can be divided into two groups, the DNA tumor viruses and the RNA tumor viruses. Members of papova-, adeno-, herpes-, hepadna-, and poxviruses compose the DNA tumor virus group, whereas only members of the Retroviridae family are authentic RNA tumor viruses.

DNA Virus Associations with Animal and Human Cancers

The polyoma virus genus of the Papovaviridae family includes agents such as SV40 and polyoma virus. These agents produce tumors when injected into newborn mice or hamsters and have been extensively studied as animal models for viral-induced cellular transformation and tumor induction. The human polyoma viruses, JC and BK viruses, can transform human fibroblast cultures, but have not been associated with human cancers. Both BK and JC viruses are neurotropic and cause tumors in animals; however, only JC virus is associated with progressive multifocal leukoencephalopathy (PML). In contrast to the polyoma virus genus, the members of the papilloma virus genus are strongly associated with human tumors. Shope papilloma virus produces papillomas and carcinomas in rabbits, whereas human papilloma viruses (HPVs), existing in more than 50 types, may produce genital warts (condyloma acuminata) that lead to squamous cell carcinoma of the penis or cervical carcinoma. Human papilloma virus genomes have six open reading frames (ORFs) for encoding regulatory proteins. The ORFs, E6 and E7, together comprise the papilloma virus "oncogene," these two proteins together can transform cells in culture. While these oncogene products transform cells in culture, cofactors (such as herpes simplex virus type 2 [HSV-2]) may still be involved in natural tumor causation. HPVs of differing serotype are associated with corresponding disease manifestations in Table 5-17.

The adenoviruses have not been associated with human cancers but produce tumors in newborn hamsters. Adenovirus serotypes have been subgrouped as highly oncogenic (types 12, 18, and 31), weakly oncogenic (types 3, 7, 14, 16, and 21), and nononcogenic (types 2 and 5). Adenoviruses have also been utilized in model systems for studying viral transformation of cells.

The neoplastic diseases of animal herpesviruses include chicken lymphomatosis (Marek's disease virus), frog renal adenocarcinoma (Lucké virus), and monkey lymphoma (herpesvirus *Saimiri*). Human neoplastic diseases are asso-

Table 5-17   Benign and Malignant Human Papilloma Virus Manifestations

HPV Types*	Manifestations
16, 18	Strongly associated: Cervical intraepithelial neoplasia (CIN) and cervical cancer (condylomata)
31, 33, 35, 45, 51, 52, 56	Moderately associated: CIN and cervical cancer
6, 11	Genital warts (condylomata acuminata), laryngeal papillomas in children
7	Meat-handlers' warts
5, 8, 9, 12	Epidermodysplasia verruciformis (skin cancer with ultraviolet exposure)
1, 2, 3, 4	Benign warts (common, plantar, flat, and butcher's)

*Only a partial list of the most typical HPV types is presented.

ciated with EBV, HSV-2, and human cytomegalovirus (HCMV). EBV is associated with African Burkitt's lymphoma and nasopharyngeal carcinoma. This virus also transforms human B lymphocytes and has been used to create immortalized lymphocyte cell lines. Epstein-Barr virus is the only truly oncogenic human herpesvirus since it possesses a viral oncogene, LMP1. EBV causes rapid fatal lymphoproliferative disease in immunosuppressed patients, and EBV-induced papillomatous proliferation of epithelial cells in patients with AIDS is referred to as oral hairy leukoplakia. EBV-induced tumors, such as Burkitt's lymphoma, are associated with the presence of EBNA, the presence of episomal closed circles of EBV DNA, and elevated expression of the c-myc protooncogene.

Unlike EBV, the herpes simplex virus type 2 and human cytomegalovirus apparently lack viral oncogenes. HSV-2 and HCMV are associated with human cervical carcinoma; however, the evidence is primarily epidemiologic in nature. These viruses, when inactivated with ultraviolet (uv) radiation, transform cells in culture. HSV-2 and HCMV may induce or predispose cells to malignancy by acting as insertional mutagens or by acting as abnormal activators of transcription for normal cellular genes.

The proxviruses, not generally thought of as tumor viruses, can induce hyperplastic growth of cells and tissues, producing fibromas or myxomatosis in rabbits. The Yaba virus produces benign skin tumors in rhesus monkeys; however, poxviruses have not been associated with human cancers.

The hepadnavirus, HBV, is strongly associated with increased incidence of primary liver cancer (hepatoma) in chronically infected patients. In 75 to 85 percent of hepatoma cells, HBV DNA is found integrated in host-cell DNA.

Hepatitis B virus does not contain a known oncogene or cause oncogene activation and chromosomal translocation as does EBV. HBV mechanisms of tumor induction are still under study; however, HBV may act as a direct insertional mutagen or as an indirect mutagen that generates oxidants as by-products of chronic inflammatory infection.

Transformation by DNA Tumor Viruses

The process by which a DNA tumor virus induces a heritable change in the cellular properties of an infected cell without bringing about cell death is referred to as transformation. Simian virus 40 has been utilized as a DNA tumor virus prototype for detailing the transformation process. DNA tumor viruses will generally replicate well in permissive cells of the natural host and fail to replicate in nonpermissive cells of other species that they transform. Simian virus 40 replicates in monkey cells, leading to cell death, but it transforms mouse cells, leading to the expression of altered cell properties, which are referred to as the transformed phenotype. Permissive cells can only be transformed if a polyoma virus deletion mutant (defective particle) or UV-inactivated virus is utilized for infection. Therefore, viral multiplication must be stopped in a cell to allow for polyoma virus transformation. The "early" events of a nonproductive transforming infection are similar to those of a lytic infection in permissive cells. Viral temperature-sensitive mutants exist that cannot transform cells; therefore, a single viral gene and its gene product can control transformation. In general, only one or two viral genes are involved in cellular transformation, even when larger DNA viruses such as adenoviruses are involved. A central feature of viral transformation (either DNA or RNA) is the integration of a short segment of DNA or a genome-length segment of DNA into the host-cell genome. In DNA virus infections, the integrated portion of the viral genome contains a viral oncogene that is necessary for the initiation and/or maintenance of cellular transformation. The polyoma viruses, papilloma viruses, and adenoviruses have early viral gene products that function to immortalize and/or transform cells. One of the most important mechanisms employed by these viruses involves the binding of a viral oncogene product to a tumor suppressor gene product (formerly referred to as an antioncogene product). Tumor suppressor gene products such as p53 and pRB (retinoblastoma gene product) function to maintain normal cellular growth. When bound to a viral oncogene product, the function of p53 or pRB, or both, namely to maintain homeostasis, is lost and cell transformation ensues. Polyoma virus and EBV are exceptions to these mechanisms. Table 5-18 details some of these important viral oncogene products, their functions, and important protein-protein interactions.

In transforming cells, these early viral protein interactions are of primary importance since nonproductive transforming infections of most DNA viruses are also characterized by a failure to express "late" (capsid) proteins or to produce progeny virus. Instead of progeny production and cell death, DNA synthesizing and proliferating cells with altered cellular properties emerge from infection. These stable transformants have many altered properties, which are known as the transformed phenotype. Table 5-19, details well-studied characteristic alterations of viral transformed cells.

What Are Tumor Suppressor Genes?

A group of genes, called *tumor suppressor genes (TSGs)*, have been discovered that express proteins that exert a negative control on cell growth and proliferation. These genes have the opposite effect of oncogenes, which, when activated, positively influence cell growth and promote tumor formation. For this reason, these genes were first called antioncogenes. The TSG products function to maintain normal cell growth; however, when these genes are mutated or deleted, or when the function of their gene products is abrogated by protein binding or complex formation, the *loss* of these TSG functions may result in cell transformation or tumor induction. The following are some of the important tumor suppressor genes: retinoblastoma (RB), p53, Wilms' tumor (WT-1), neurofibromatosis (NF-1), DCC (deleted in colorectal carcinoma), and APC (familial adenomatous polyposis coli). As indicated in the preceding section, the viral oncogenes of many DNA tumor viruses bind RB, p53, or both TSG products resulting in a loss of TSG product function and the induction of cellular transformation. The discovery and understanding of TSGs have not only provided insight into the mechanism of transformation for most DNA tumor viruses, but also have provided a group of "antioncogenes" that help to explain the roles of cellular oncogenes (c-oncs) that have been transduced by the RNA tumor viruses. Therefore, TSGs and their protein products are central in the understanding of mechanisms of transformation by DNA and RNA tumor viruses. In addition, knowledge of TSGs helps to explain the failures in opposing oncogene and tumor suppressor gene controls that result in human cancers.

General Characteristics of RNA Tumor Viruses

The retroviruses have a 70S RNA genome that is diploid, being composed of two identical 35S RNA subunits (3500–9000 nucleotides). The genome is a single-stranded RNA of positive polarity, but extracted virion RNA is not infective. The retrovirus particle is unique among RNA viruses

Virology

Table 5-18   DNA Viral Oncogenes and Cell Transformation

Virus	Gene product	Function(s)	Protein bound or associated
SV40	Large T antigen	1. Stimulates host-cell DNA synthesis 2. Initiates viral DNA replication 3. Transcriptional transactivator 4. Immortalizes primary cells 5. Transforms cells	pRB p53 (tumor suppressor gene products [TSGP])
	Small T antigen	1. Causes loss of contact inhibition 2. Causes increased plasminogen activator production 3. Complements large T antigen in transformation	
Polyoma virus	Middle T antigen	1. Alone it transforms cell completely (acute transforming protein) 2. Stimulates the activity of membrane kinases (phosphorylates cellular proteins)	pp60 c-SRC p62 c-yes (protooncogene products)
Human papilloma virus type 16 (HPV-16)	E7 protein	1. Jointly transforms cells with E6 2. Transcriptional transactivator	pRB
	E6 protein	1. Jointly tranforms cells with E7	p53 (TSGP)
Adenovirus	E1A proteins	1. Immortalize cells but do not completely transform 2. Transcriptional transactivators	pRB
	E1B proteins	1. Transform cells	p53
Epstein-Barr virus (EBV)	EBNA-2	1. Transcriptional transactivator [inducer of latent membrane protein (LMP)]	
	LMP (LMP1)	1. Transforms B lymphocytes 2. Plasma membrane association with cytoskeleton 3. Acts with LMP2A and LMP2B to effect protein phosphorylation	Vimentin (cytoskeleton)

Table 5-19   Properties of the Transformed Phenotype

1. Possession of at least part of the viral genome (either integrated or as nuclear episomes)
2. Increased tumorigenicity in susceptible hosts
3. More rounded and refractile morphology
4. Growth in a less oriented manner
5. Loss of anchorage dependence for cell growth (colony formation in soft agar)
6. Disaggregation of actin filaments
7. Loss of contact inhibition of cell growth
8. Decreased density-dependent regulation of growth (increased saturation densities)
9. Continued cell growth (immortalization)
10. Reduced requirement for serum growth factors
11. Appearance of new antigens (both viral and cellular)
12. Increased agglutinability of cells by plant lectins due to receptor clustering
13. Increased membrane transport of sugars
14. Increased anaerobic glycolysis
15. Changes in glycolipid and glycoprotein chemical composition of plasma membranes
16. Loss of fibronectin (LETs protein)
17. Increased secretion of plasminogen activator (a protease)
18. Decreased cyclic adenosine monophosphate levels
19. Induction of cellular DNA synthesis often coincides with induction of the transformed phenotype
20. Chromosomal changes, including duplications, amplifications, deletions, and translocations of portions of or entire chromosomes (altered karyotype)
21. The ability to rescue integrated cryptic viral genomes by fusion of viral transformants with permissive cells (does not apply to transformants that possess only a portion of the viral genome)

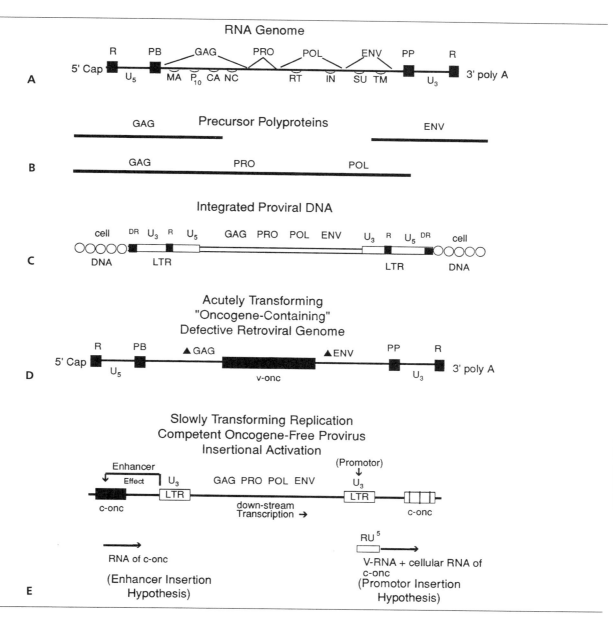

Fig. 5-12 Basic retroviral structures.

and contains an RNA-directed DNA polymerase (reverse transcriptase) that is capable of synthesizing DNA from RNA. The 35S RNA subunits are held together by hydrogen bonds of a palindromic sequence that is located approximately 80 nucleotides from the 5' ends of each subunit. Host-cell transfer RNAs are associated with the viral genome and act as primers to initiate transcription of RNA into negative-strand DNA. A single subunit of a nondefective genome is depicted in Fig. 5-12A. Four genes are typically found, namely the *gag, pro, pol,* and *env* genes. The *gag* gene encodes either three or four proteins. The following three *gag* proteins are always present: (1) the

matrix protein (MA), a myristylated N-terminal domain that associates with the plasma membrane for budding; (2) the capsid protein (CA), which is the main structural protein of the core/shell; and (3) the nucleic acid binding protein (NC), a basic protein that associates with the RNA genome. The *pro* gene encodes a protease for cleavage of polyprotein precursors. The *pol* gene encodes a reverse transcriptase (RT) and an integrase (IN). The *env* gene encodes a surface protein (SU), which is highly glycosylated, binds to receptors, and contains viral neutralization epitopes. In addition, *env* encodes a transmembrane protein (TM), which anchors the exterior glycoprotein spike

Table 5-20 Functions of Representative Oncogenes

Functional Grouping	Oncogene	Viral Origin	Function
Analogues of growth factors	v-sis	SiSV	B chain of platelet-derived growth factor (PDGF) analogue
	int-2	None	Fibroblast growth factor-like
		"Mouse mammary tumor activated" in cell DNA	
Growth factor receptors with tyrosine protein kinase activity	erb B	AEV	Truncated epidermal growth factor (EGF) receptor
	erb B$_2$ a. HER$_2$ (human) b. neu (mouse)	None	Related to EGF receptor
	fms	FeSV	M-CSF or CSF-1 receptor
Hormone receptors	erb A	AEV	Thyroid hormone receptor antagonist
Membrane-associated tyrosine kinase	src	RSV	src family of tyrosine kinase (TK +)
	abl	Abelson-MULV	TK +
	fes	FeLV	TK +
	yes	ASV-Y73	TK +
Cytoplasmic serine and threonine kinases	mos	Moloney MuSV	Kinase, cytostatic factor (CSF)
Membrane-associated guanine nucleotide-binding proteins (G proteins)	ras a. Ha-ras b. Ki-ras	 Harvey MuSV Kirsten MuSv	GDP/GTP binding: GTPase (signal transduction)
Nuclear factors (transcription factors and DNA-binding proteins)	jun	ASV17	Combines with fos to form AP-1, a transcription factor
	fos	FBJ-MuSV	Forms AP-1
	myb	AMV	Specific DNA-binding protein
	myc	MC29	Specific DNA-binding protein

and possesses a less glycosylated hydrophobic domain. Flanking these four genes are regulatory regions with a repeat sequence (R) and unique sequences termed *U5* and *U3*. A tRNA primer binding site (PB), near the 5′ end of the genome, serves to prime reverse transcription of negative-strand DNA while a purine-rich sequence (PP), near the 3′ end of the genome, primes positive-strand DNA synthesis.

Replication

While retroviruses enter cells by receptor-mediated endocytosis, the following steps differ from those of all other RNA viruses. Replication involves a DNA intermediate that may form a circular DNA duplex, as well as a double-stranded linear molecule. The double-stranded linear DNA that is synthesized in nucleocapsids in the cytoplasm moves to the nucleus for integration into host-cell DNA. The integrase is responsible for removing two base pairs from each end of the linear proviral DNA during the integration process. Integration produces a 4–6 base-pair duplication of cellular DNA, which flanks the integrated genome. These cellular repeat sequences are referred to as

direct repeats (DR). The integrated form of the genome is referred to as a DNA provirus and is depicted in Fig. 5-12C. The integrated DNA provirus differs from the viral RNA genome by possessing long, terminally redundant repeats of 5′ and 3′ noncoding sequences on each side of the provirus. These long terminal repeats (LTRs) contain a viral promoter for transcription of the integrated provirus, as well as many sequences for regulation of genome functions (capping, polyadenylation, etc.). Transcription of the integrated provirus produces both genome RNAs for progeny virus particles and messenger RNAs for viral protein synthesis. Viral proteins are formed as polyproteins and subjected to posttranslational cleavage to produce individual gag proteins, protease, envelope proteins, and RNA-dependent DNA polymerase. The typical polyprotein precursors are depicted in Fig. 5-12B.

Morphology

The RNA tumor viruses (subfamily Oncovirinae) can be divided into four morphologic groups (types A, B, C, and D). The type A particles have electron-lucent centers and are found only within cells either as intracytoplasmic A particles or intracisternal A particles. Some type A particles are immature type B particles. The remaining three morphologic groups are extracellular retrovirus particles. The type B particle buds as a preformed nucleoid that becomes eccentric upon maturation (e.g., mouse mammary tumor virus). The type C viruses have centrally located nucleoids that undergo maturation during and after budding. Most animal sarcoma and leukemia viruses are of type C morphology. The type D viruses bud like type B viruses but have centrally located nucleoids (e.g., Mason-Pfizer monkey virus). Retroviruses of the subfamily Lentivirinae (such as HIV-1) have cylindrical nucleoids.

Endogenous Retroviruses

The endogenous retroviruses are transmitted within a host species from generation to generation as DNA proviruses. These proviruses behave as normal cellular genes, are present in 1 to 10 copies per cell genome, and are inducible by different types of mutagens or carcinogens. Endogenous retroviruses are found in nearly all species (RAV-O in chickens, RD114 in cats, and baboon endogenous virus in baboons). Endogenous viruses are replication-competent viruses but are generally not directly associated with cancers. These viruses may, through recombination mechanisms, generate the more highly oncogenic exogenous retroviruses.

Mechanisms of Retroviral Carcinogenesis

Acute Transformation by Highly Oncogenic Viruses

The leukemia and sarcoma viruses that produce acute disease, such as avian myeloblastosis virus, murine sarcoma viruses, feline sarcoma virus, and simian sarcoma virus, express a gene that is not required for viral replication. This gene has been termed a *transforming* or *oncogene (onc)*. Retrovirus oncogenes were principally derived from normal host-cell growth controlling genes. By recombination, retroviruses were able to acquire cellular onc sequences from cellular protoncogenes as integral parts of their viral genomes. The activation of these nucleic acid sequences by point mutation, deletion, or rearrangement led to the increased oncogenicity of these sequences, which can be referred to as *retroviral oncogenes (v-oncs)*. These v-oncs, which are under viral promoter control, are highly transcribed and often expressed at elevated levels. High-level oncogene expression leads to acute retroviral transformation of the host cell and enhanced tumorigenicity. Most viruses that contain oncogenes, particularly sarcoma viruses, are defective for replication and require a helper virus (Rous sarcoma virus [RSV] is a notable exception to this rule). An example of a typical defective "oncogene-containing" retrovirus genome is presented in

Fig. 5-12D. The v-onc that expresses the transforming protein may replace varying portions of the *gag, pro, pol,* and *env* genes in different acutely transforming viruses. The protein products of these viral oncogenes differ from virus to virus, but a limited number of oncogenes appear to exist. The retroviral oncogenes (v-oncs) fall into different classes of altered cellular growth control genes. Table 5-20 presents a few well-studied representatives of each functionally different oncogene group.

Tumor Induction by Retroviruses that Lack a Viral Oncogene

The following mechanisms often apply to retroviruses with slow or delayed onset of tumor.

Insertional Mutagenesis or Activation

Viruses such as avian leukosis virus (ALV) and mouse mammary tumor virus (MMTV) lack viral oncogenes but induce tumors by integrating their genomes into the host cell at positions that allow for activation and expression of host-cell oncogenes. The diagram in Fig. 5-12E demonstrates two hypothesized mechanisms. The first is known as the promoter insertion hypothesis and is depicted on the right whereas the second can be considered an enhancer insertion hypothesis and is depicted on the left. The promoter insertion hypothesis argues that the viral promoter in the right-hand LTR can transcribe viral sequences, as well as downstream cellular onc sequences, thus leading to the enhanced expression of a cellular oncogene. The second theory argues that an enhancer element, such as the MMTV hormone response element, is capable of activating the expression of cellular oncs (such as INT1 and INT2) at greater distances and in upstream, as well as downstream, positions. In either case, activation and expression of cellular oncogenes lead to tumor. In addition, retroviruses can mutagenize by integrating in a c-onc sequence (such as c-erb B) to alter the gene product and thereby "activate" the c-onc. Integration by retroviruses can also induce tumors by inactivating tumor suppressor genes.

Recombination with Endogenous Viruses to Generate Mink Cell Focus-Forming (MCF) Viruses

Viruses that lack oncogenes can develop increased oncogenicity by recombining with endogenous retroviruses to alter their envelope gene. Such MCF viruses have altered cellular host range and induce leukemia in mice.

Induction of Human Adult T-Cell Leukemia by Human T-Cell Leukemia Virus Type 1 (HTLV-1)

While HTLV-1 is unquestionably an oncogenic retrovirus, it does *not* possess a viral oncogene and does *not* employ insertional activation to produce disease. Instead, it is likely that transacting transcriptional activation of T-cell proliferation genes by the *tax* gene protein of HTLV-1 leads to cell proliferation and disease.

Cellular Protooncogenes and Human Tumor-Cell Oncogenes

The viral oncogenes in genomes of transforming retroviruses appear to be closely related to cellular oncogenes that have been cloned from human tumor-cell lines. The V-Ha-ras oncogene of Harvey sarcoma virus is a homologue of an oncogene isolated from a human bladder carcioma cell line; V-Ki-ras of Kirsten sarcoma virus is a homologue of oncogenes isolated from human lung and colon carcinomas. In theory, normal cellular protooncogenes could be activated by nonviral causes (carcinogens or mutagens) as well as by viruses that alter normal gene expression. When normal cellular protooncogene sequences are compared to oncogene homologues in transforming RNA tumor viruses or human tumors, results indicate that these protooncogene sequences have most often been "activated to oncogenicity" by point mutations. Oncogene overexpression in human tumors is caused by the following two mechanisms: chromosomal translocation and DNA amplification of regions that contain c-oncs.

C-Type Retroviruses Associated with Human Cancers

Human T-cell leukemia virus type 1 is an exogenous C-type retrovirus that transforms T cells in culture, allowing them to grow in the absence of IL-2. HTLV-1 is the cause of adult T-cell leukemia (ATL) and tropical spastic paraparesis (HTLV-1–associated myelopathy). This virus is endemic in southern Japan, central Africa, and the Caribbean basin including southern Florida. A second rarer isolate is HTLV-2. While this virus was isolated from a patient with hairy-cell leukemia, its role in human disease is not well documented. These two human-type C retroviruses are related to bovine leukemia virus (BLV) and simian T-cell leukemia virus (STLV). They have two regulatory genes that are rather unique for C-type retroviruses. The *tax* gene product is a transactive transcriptional activator and the *rex* gene product controls splicing of the viral mRNA.

Human Immunodeficiency Virus, Lentiviruses, and Acquired Immunodeficiency Syndrome

Earl M. Ritzi

General Characteristics

In 1983, the etiologic agent of epidemic AIDS was identified as human immunodeficiency virus (HIV-1). While this was one of the first human retroviruses discovered, it differed significantly from other C-type human T-lymphotrophic viruses (HTLV-1 and HTLV-2). HIV-1 is not a C-type virus, and does not transform cells or act as an RNA tumor virus. Instead, it is a cytocidal virus with T-cell tropism that destroys cells of the immune system. HIV-1 buds as a long stalk and has a morphology that is similar to that of lentiviruses, a subfamily of the Retroviridae composed of viruses such as visna and maedi viruses of sheep. HIV-1 has a cylindrical nucleoid resembling visna virus. HIV-1 demonstrates the following similarities to lentiviruses: (1) It shows extensive sequence homology with lentiviruses, (2) it produces a persistent and chronic course of infection after a long latent period that results in a progressively deteriorating disease with CNS involvement, and (3) it shows envelope gene drift or great heterogenicity in the *env* gene product. These characteristics place HIV-1 with the following related lentiviruses: visna-maedi virus, caprine arthritis encephalitis virus, equine infectious anemia virus, simian immunodeficiency virus mac (SIV$_{mac}$), and feline immunodeficiency virus. A second form of HIV, termed *HIV-2*, has been identified. HIV-2 is only 50 to 60 percent related to HIV-1, is endemic in West Africa and does not have a worldwide distribution like HIV-1, is closely related to SIV$_{sm}$ and SIV$_{mac}$, and is somewhat less virulent than HIV-1. It is not known whether HIV evolved from related simian viruses or whether they evolved in parallel; however, SIVs exist that produce a similar immunodeficiency syndrome in rhesus macaques. *Neither* human *nor* simian immunodeficiency viruses can be considered endogenous viruses of their species. HIV-1 persists in an integrated state and its many regulatory genes provide for controlled expression, latency, and persistence of infection.

HIV-1 Replication, Genome Structure, and Regulation

Infection of cells by HIV-1 depends on both the presence of cell-surface CD4 (the HIV receptor) and the tropism conferred by the HIV *env* protein (gp 120), which binds to CD4. The gp120 molecule also possesses the epitope responsible for neutralization in its V3 loop; however, neutralizing antibodies, which are low titer (1 : 20 to 1 : 200), have not been sufficient to protect against disease. Early in infection, HIV isolates tend to show greater tropism for monocytes and macrophages, whereas later in infection, HIV shows a tropism for helper/inducer T cells. The early infection of macrophages and peripheral blood monocytes has been referred to as the *Trojan horse mechanism* of viral dissemination. Monocytes and macrophages, lacking sufficient CD4 on their cell surfaces, do not typically form syncytia or die as a result of infection; there

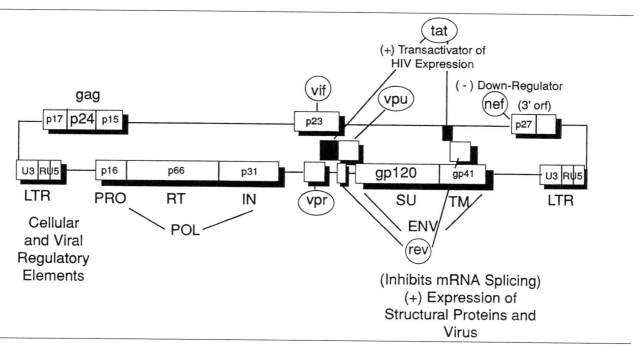

Fig. 5-13 HIV-1 DNA provirus.

fore, virus can replicate, remain hidden, and be disseminated by these cells throughout the body. Subsequent to macrophage infection, CD4-expressing T₄ cells are infected. Since cell killing is related to CD4 density on a cell's surface, T_4 cells tend to form syncytia and die. Viral replication can continue in localized sites such as lymph nodes during the incubation period or so-called latent period of AIDS when virus is not detected in blood. In addition to macrophages and helper T cells, microglia and astrocytes located in the brain are infected. In general, CD4-positive cells are the predominant cells infected and destroyed, in particular, helper T_4 lymphocytes. HIV's entry into cells occurs by a process of membrane fusion involving the gp41 transmembrane protein. This process is unique as compared to other retroviruses and produces giant cells or syncytia. The HIV reverse transcriptase is highly error prone and produces viral isolates that, over time, differ by as much as 10 percent in the same patient. The linear double-stranded DNA formed by reverse transcription integrates randomly into the host-cell DNA to yield a DNA provirus as depicted in Fig. 5-13. The proviral HIV genome is clearly unique for it possesses six regulatory genes not typically present in RNA tumor viruses. Some of these genes are also unique bipartite genes (*tat* and *rev*), which are expressed as a doubly spliced mRNA. The following functions have been associated with these important regulatory gene products: (1) *P14 tat* is an essential

powerful (+) transactivator of HIV transcription; (2) *P19 rev* is an essential enhancer of viral structural protein expression by controlling transport of large unspliced or singly spliced transcripts to the cytoplasm (controller of posttranscriptional viral mRNA splicing), *rev* protein acts through an antirepression mechanism by binding a sequence called the *rev* response element (RRE) or CAR (cis-antirepressor) in the *env* gene RNA; (3) *P27 nef* is a GTP-binding protein with GTPase activity; it appears to act through signal transduction to downregulate [(-) controller] of HIV transcription; (4) *P18 VPR* is a weak transactivator of transcription; (5) *P23 Vif* is required for viral infectivity; and (6) *P15 Vpu* is still under study to define its function.

HIV-1 Transcriptional Control and Coinfection

HIV transcriptional control is extremely complex. The u3 region of its LTR contains binding sites for at least six cellular transcription factors including the important lymphocyte activation factor, NF-κB. In addition, the viral transactivator *tat* can bind an RNA stem loop called TAR and act to enhance transcription 100-fold or more. The viral response element TAR is actually downstream [position (+) 19 − (+) 42] of the transcription start site. The cis-acting regulatory elements in the HIV LTR are extremely important since activation of T cells by foreign antigens inducing NF-κB, or cytokines such as IL-2, TNF-α, or IFN-γ will bring about a transcriptional activation of the latent HIV provirus. Coinfection by other sexually transmitted agents such as *Haemophilus ducreyi* may immediately supply such T-cell activation. Two special cases of coinfection should be noted. First, HTLV-1 coinfection results in a powerful transactivation of the HIV-1 genome. The *tax* gene of HTLV-1 induces a cellular factor that can transactivate HIV-1 through the NF-κB binding site. A second unique coinfection is human herpesvirus type 6 (HHV-6). This virus uses the same CD4 receptor on T cells and, like HTLV-1, has a transactivator to specifically enhance HIV expression.

Clinical Manifestations of AIDS

While seroconversion to HIV AB positive at 3 to 12 weeks postinfection signals the infection of individuals, a period of 7 to 10 years, which is asymptomatic or characterized by lymph adenopathy syndrome (LAS) or AIDS-related complex (ARC), or both, may occur before the onset of more serious conditions. It is now believed that virus replication occurs in lymph nodes during the period that was previously thought to be a latent period for virus replication. Often, a *decline* in antibody to the p24 core antigen, *anti-p24*, and a *rise* in blood *p24 antigen* provide a prognostic signal for the onset of a broad spectrum of more serious clinical conditions. An inversion of the T_4/T_8 cell ratio ($T_4/T_8 < 1$) and a decline in T-cell counts (<200) is indicative of the primary T-cell deficiency. The following clinical spectrum is seen in HIV infections: (1) a lymphadenopathy or wasting syndrome (LAS and ARC) characterized by fever, lymphadenopathy, diarrhea, weight loss, and appetite loss; (2) Kaposi's sarcoma, non-Hodgkins lymphoma, and/or squamous cell carcinoma of the anus or mouth; (3) a large number of opportunistic infections of which *Pneumocystis carinii* (pneumonia) is the most common; and (4) neurologic involvement, including AIDS dementia, encephalopathy, vacuolar myelopathy, and aseptic meningitis.

Opportunistic Infections that Serve as Indicator Diseases of AIDS

Most of the AIDS-associated agents are ubiquitous and relatively harmless in healthy individuals; however, in the immunosuppressed they can cause life-threatening diseases. These agents are protozoa, fungi, viruses, and bacteria. The protozoal group includes the following: (1) *Pneumocystis carinii*, which causes pneumonia (the most

frequent manifestation of AIDS), (2) toxoplasmosis of the brain; (3) cryptosporidiosis with diarrhea; and (4) isosporiasis with diarrhea. The fungal infections include the following: (1) candidiasis of the esophagus, (2) cryptococcosis that is extrapulmonary, (3) disseminated histoplasmosis, and (4) disseminated coccidioidomycosis. The viral infections most noted are as follows: (1) cytomegalovirus infection, (2) persisting or disseminated herpes simplex virus infection, and (3) progressive multifocal leukoencephalopathy. The bacterial infections include (1) disseminated *Mycobacterium avium* complex, (2) "atypical" mycobacterial disease, (3) extrapulmonary tuberculosis, (4) recurrent *Salmonella* septicemia, and (5) recurrent pyogenic bacterial infections. Many pathogens have disease manifestations that are unique to HIV-infected individuals. These manifestations and the unique aspects of treatment are detailed in other sections of this book.

Immunologic Features of AIDS

The primary deficit of AIDS is due to a destruction of T_4 cells. The T_4 cells decrease and the T_4/T_8 cell ratio becomes less than 1. All tests for T-cell activity, such as the delayed-type hypersensitivity (DTH) skin test, cell proliferation in response to mitogens, and cell production of cytokines (IL-2 and IFN-γ), are diminished or negative. A defect in natural killer cell (NK cell) activity is noted as well. A secondary effect of T-cell loss is a polyclonal B-cell activation. This polyclonal humoral response results in hypergammaglobulinemia (elevated levels of total serum immunoglobulins). The increase in antibody is nonspecific and humoral B-cell responses to specific antigens are defective. Increased levels of beta-microglobulin and IFN-α have been noted.

Transmission of HIV and Populations at Risk

The following modes of HIV transmission are well established: (1) sexual contact; (2) parenteral transmission by blood, blood products, or syringes; and (3) transmission from mother to newborn infant. The largest risk group to date has been homosexual or bisexual males. Anal intercourse and high numbers of sexual partners increase risk. Heterosexual transmission has predominated in developing countries, but it is usually associated with the transmission of other venereally transmitted diseases, especially those that produce genital ulcers. Heterosexual transmission is increasing in the United States. Intravenous drug users and women are showing the greatest rates of increase in HIV infection. The increase in infected women is paralleled by an increase in HIV-infected newborns. Screening tests for HIV antibodies have greatly reduced the risk of blood transfusion–related AIDS. The transmission rate of infection from HIV-positive mothers to offspring is approximately 30 percent. Congenital HIV infections of infants born to seropositive mothers can occur in the following ways: (1) transplacental infection, 2) exposure to infectious blood and fluids at the time of birth, and (3) exposure to mother's breast milk. Nosocomial HIV infections may occur as a result of needle stick or blood exposure; however, the number of medical personnel infected has been relatively small and medical personnel are not considered a high-risk group. While rates of increase have been controlled for the largest risk group, homosexual and bisexual men, the group of IV drug users is increasing worldwide and their HIV infection rate is increasing in a concurrent fashion.

Diagnosis of HIV Infection

The most frequently used method for screening blood and serum samples is an ELISA test using whole disrupted virus as bound antigen to detect antibodies to HIV. To exclude false positives, western blotting, which detects serologic reactivity with individual HIV proteins, is used as a confirmation test. Western blotting is the standard for confirmation of a positive diagnosis. Virus isolation by cocultivation with healthy donor T lymphocytes or T-cell lines is possible, but takes weeks to complete and is only done in patients such as seropositive infants when the diagnosis is in question. An antigen test for the core antigen p24 in blood can be used to detect rare antibody-negative HIV infections; however, it has limited use since p24 antigen blood screening is less sensitive and in most cases is not more effective than the routine ELISA for HIV antibodies. Before seroconversion at 3 to 12 weeks, or when diagnosis is in question, sensitive polymerase chain reaction (PCR) techniques can be used to amplify and detect proviral DNA. The diagnosis of infection in infants of infected mothers has been complicated by the presence of maternal antibody. For this reason, the following tests have been developed: a western blotting technique that is specific for infant IgM antibodies to HIV proteins and a PCR technique to amplify and detect the HIV proviral DNA in infected infant cells.

Treatment and Experimental Approaches

The principal treatments recommended are nucleoside analogues that inhibit reverse transcription of viral RNA. The best-known and most widely used drug is AZT (Retrovir, Zidovudine). It was initially given to patients with *Pneumocystis carinii* pneumonia and individuals with T_4 counts less than 500/mm², however, now AZT is being utilized earlier in asymptomatic seropositive individuals. Earlier use of AZT may increase the risk of developing AZT-resistant HIV. AZT may cause anemia with continued use. The analogues ddc and dideoxinosine (ddi) have also been approved for use and produce side effects of peripheral neuropathy and pancreatitis, respectively.

Treatments of HIV-infected patients are often directed at, or used for, prevention of specific AIDS-associated opportunistic infections. *Pneumocystis carinii* is treated with aerosolized pentamidine or trimethoprim-sulfamethoxazole combined with dapsone. Candidiasis of the esophagus is treated with ketoconazole or fluconazole. Cytomegalovirus is treated with ganciclovir. Herpes simplex or zoster is treated with acyclovir, and acyclovir-resistant strains are treated with vidarabine or foscarnet.

Experimental Approaches to HIV Treatment

The following experimental approaches to HIV therapy are being investigated: (1) development of reverse transcriptase inhibitors, (2) prevention of HIV adsorption to T lymphocytes by blocking with soluble CD4 or a CD4 recombinant protein modified to prevent rapid clearance, (3) blocking HIV adsorption with anti-idiotype IgG mimicking CD4 or gp120, (4) inhibiting viral expression with antisense RNA directed against the *rev* gene, (5) inhibiting viral expression by transdominant variants of *tat* and *rev* that produce proteins that bind to response elements without producing the normal *tat* and *rev* responses, (6) blocking HIV expression by blocking the unique HIV protease that cleaves precursor proteins, and (7) using ricin or *Pseudomonas* exotoxin bound to monoclonal antibodies to CD4 or envelope gene products, thereby absorbing toxic complexes on HIV-infected cell surfaces for subsequent internalization.

Development of Vaccines

High genetic variability of the *env* gene product gp120, which contains the 4 amino acid neutralization epitope, and the documented progression of disease in individuals with neutralizing antibodies argue that vaccine development may be difficult and that a humoral response alone may not be sufficient for protection. Vaccines are primarily being designed to produce antibodies against epitopes in gp160, gp120, and gp41. The membrane-associated core protein p17 is an alternate possibility. The following experimental approaches are being pursued: (1) live attenuated HIV (unlikely due to high mutation rate of HIV), (2) whole inactivated HIV, (3) live vaccinia or adenovirus recombinants expressing selected *env* epitopes, (4) synthetic peptides of *env* or p17 epitopes combined with adjuvant, (5) recombinant DNA products of gp160 or gp120 with adjuvant, (6) native purified envelope or core proteins (subunit vaccines), (7) anti-idiotypes that mimic *env* epitopes, and (8) passive immunization.

Laboratory Diagnosis of Viral Infections

Stanley S. Lefkowitz

Diagnostic virology has become relevant to patient therapy because of the development of new antiviral chemotherapies. Newer methods, employing monoclonal antibodies and immunofluorescence, enzyme immunoassays (EIA), DNA hybridization, and PCR technology, have made rapid diagnosis possible. Laboratory diagnosis of viral diseases involves detection of at least one of the following: virus, viral components, or an immune response to the virus, usually antibodies.

Specimens for viral isolation should be obtained as early as possible after the onset of symptoms. Typical sources of viral cultures include nasopharyngeal secretions, urine, stool, blood, cerebrospinal fluid, and tissue samples and scrapings. Specimens should be kept on ice for brief periods or frozen at −70°C if storage is required before processing.

Viral isolation is probably one of the most sensitive assays available since theoretically a single virus particle can infect a culture. However, isolation and growth of virus is slow and time consuming, and requires considerable expertise. Direct examination and antigen detection represent somewhat less sensitive but more rapid methods of identifying viral proteins or antigens. Direct histopathology that recognizes "specific" giant cells or inclusion bodies, or both, is useful, particularly in identifying members of the herpesvirus group. Electron microscopy, although relatively insensitive, is useful for identifying certain types of viruses (particularly those found in stools that cause diarrhea and gastroenteritis), which are difficult to isolate and grow. By using centrifugation and specific antisera, these viruses have been visualized and identified in clinical specimens. Included in this group are the Norwalk agent, caliciviruses, rotaviruses, and the enteric adenoviruses.

Direct antigen detection in clinical specimens, using immunofluorescence, represents one of the most rapid and widely used techniques utilized in the diagnostic laboratory. Tissue specimens, scrapings, infected cells, and so forth are exposed to specific antibody conjugated with fluorescein isothiocyanate (FITC) and the preparation is viewed under a fluorescent microscope. A positive specimen is identified by a yellow-green fluorescence after extensive washing. An indirect procedure can also be used by exposing the specimen to unconjugated antibody followed by a second anti-immunoglobulin antibody that is conjugated with FITC. Immunoperoxidase staining is similar in principle to immunofluorescence, but utilizes the light microscope instead.

Solid-phase immunoassays rely on the immobilization of either antibody or antigen on a surface of a bead or micro-titer plate well followed by a series of steps using the reciprocal to bind to and subsequently identify the specific agent. The agglutination of antigen-coated latex particles in the presence of specific patients' antisera can be used to measure immunity to rubella virus. Radioimmunoassays are very rapid and sensitive methods for the detection and measurement of either antibodies or viral antigens, but they have been largely supplanted by EIA, which has a longer shelf life and lower cost, and does not use radioisotopes. Enzyme immunoassays are able to detect 10^3 to 10^4 virus particles. EIAs for antigen detection utilize an antibody bound to either a bead or microtiter plate. The viral antigen in the clinical specimens is "captured" by the specific antibody. A second antibody conjugated with a specific enzyme is added to the system. This is followed by the addition of an appropriate substrate that will be degraded by the bound enzyme, resulting in a color change that can be measured spectrophotometrically. The procedure can be reversed to detect antibodies by using viral antigen–coated "supports," which bind patient antibodies. A second antihuman IgG, coupled to the enzyme, is then added.

Another procedure for the identification of viruses is nucleic acid hybridization. This procedure utilizes a probe, representing viral nucleic acid. The probe is labeled with an isotope or other marker that anneals with specific viral DNA found in infected cells. The PCR is another technique, which is so sensitive that a single DNA molecule can be amplified, and viral DNA is detected by hybridization. However, this test is not routinely available in most viral diagnostic laboratories.

An increase in antibodies normally occurs following viral infections. A diagnosis of infection is usually considered positive if a fourfold increase in serum antibody titer occurs between the acute and convalescent stages of the disease. Conventional serologic tests include the complement-fixation tests, hemagglutination tests, and neutralization tests (NT). Although the latter may be one of the most sensitive assays, it is complex because it relies on the use of cell culture and the ability of antibodies to render the virus particles noninfectious.

Assays Used in Viral Serology

Neutralization

Neutralization is loss of viral infectivity by binding of antibodies directly to viruses. This is an extremely sensitive procedure for measuring an increase in antibodies, or it can be used to identify an "unknown" virus.

Complement Fixation

The ability of complement to bind to a specific antigen-antibody complex can be used to diagnose the increase in antibodies that occurs during infection. The test is commonly done by assessing the amount of complement that does not bind. Free complement is measured in a second antigen-antibody reaction using sheep erythrocytes (SRBC) and homologous antibody (anti-SRBC). This test is not as sensitive as neutralization.

Hemagglutination Inhibition

Certain viruses are capable of agglutinating erythrocytes. Specific antibodies to these viruses block agglutination of the erythrocytes. Patients with infections caused by the viruses produce the antibodies that block hemagglutination.

Immunofluorescence

Immunofluorescence is a very sensitive and rapid method to identify viral antigens. It consists of coupling a fluorescent dye, such as FITC, to specific antibodies. The presence of viral antigens in smears of cells can be detected by visualizing the antibodies bound to specific antigens. The antibodies will fluoresce when viewed microscopically with an ultraviolet light source.

ELISA

This assay is performed by first conjugating an enzyme to either an antibody or an antigen. The bound enzyme is then attached to a solid phase. Immune complexes and free antibody or antigen are measured, indirectly, by determining the amount of substrate converted to product by the bound enzyme. Chromogenic substrates are used to assay enzyme activity. The color change is a direct function of bound enzyme activity, which in turn relates to the amount of antigen or antibody present.

Radioimmunoassays

One of the most sensitive assays for quantitation of protein antigens that may be present in biologic materials. Binding of a radioactively labeled antigen to its antibody is inhibited by known amounts of unlabeled antigen or labeled anti-Ig binds to antibody which is complexed with antigen. Standard curve is generated to which unknown samples are compared.

Western Blot

Viral proteins, which are separated by gel electrophoresis, are transfered (blotted) onto a nylon membrane. Specific antibodies to that virus bind to proteins and may be detected by a labeled anti-Ig.

Rapid Diagnosis

In recent years, emphasis has been placed on rapid diagnosis of viral infections in a matter of hours rather than the use of assays that require days to complete. Immunofluorescent technqiues, as well as solid-phase EIA, provide rapid identification of either antigens or antibodies. The latter is particularly suited to screening large numbers of specimens. Antibody detection of viral antigens, especialy where acute and convalescent specimens are involved, is of little help in the early stages of infection; however, assays for viral-specific IgM are becoming increasingly useful to indicate current or recent infections since this immunoglobulin species does not persist beyond several months after infection.

Questions

1. All of the following are distinctive characteristics of viruses **except**:
   A. Viruses lack the machinery for protein synthesis
   B. Viruses require living cells for replication
   C. Viruses were called filterable agents
   D. Viruses replicate by a process of binary fission
   E. Viral genomes are either DNA or RNA but not both
2. All of the following statements about icosahedral viruses are true **except**:
   A. As triangulation number increases, the number of capsomers in a capsid increases
   B. Their capsid encloses a maximum volume with a minimum surface area
   C. The presence of hexons at vertices relieves stress on the capsid
   D. Repeating subunits are utilized in their construction
   E. They have fivefold, threefold, and twofold rotational symmetry

For each numbered phrase, select the *one* lettered choice (A–I) that is most closely associated with it. *Each lettered choice may be used once, more than once, or not at all.*
   A. Poliovirus
   B. Adenovirus
   C. Cytomegalovirus
   D. Retrovirus
   E. Rotavirus
   F. Poxvirus
   G. Influenza virus
   H. Togavirus
   I. Hepatitis B virus

3. A (-) single-stranded segmented RNA virus
4. An enveloped icosahedral virus with tegument
5. A naked capsid icosahedral virus with both hexons and pentons
6. A DNA virus of complex symmetry
7. An enveloped icosahedral RNA virus
8. A double-stranded segmented RNA virus
9. A naked capsid icosahedral RNA virus composed entirely of identical capsomers
10. An RNA virus with a DNA-replication intermediate
11. Dane particles with both DNA- and RNA-directed DNA polymerase activity
12. Which of the following proteins is most likely to contain an epitope for neutralization of viral infectivity?
    A. Reverse transcriptase
    B. Hepatitis B core antigen (HBcAg)
    C. DNA-directed DNA polymerase
    D. Retroviral SU (gp120-like surface glycoprotein)
    E. Retroviral NC (nucleic acid binding protein)
13. All of the following viral families have icosahedral symmetry **except**:
    A. Reoviridae
    B. Rhaboviridae
    C. Picornaviridae
    D. Papovaviridae
    E. Adenoviridae
14. All of the following unique aspects of genome structure are correctly matched **except**:
    A. Adenovirus genome—5′ covalent linkage to 55kd protein
    B. Herpesvirus genome—inverted terminal repeat sequences (ITRS)
    C. Adenovirus genome—inverted terminal repeat sequence (ITRS)
    D. Poxviruses—covalent cross-linking of double-stranded genome ends
    E. Retrovirus genome—terminal redundancy (repeat sequences near genome ends)
15. Which of the following virus pairings is composed of a DNA virus that replicates in the cytoplasm and an RNA virus with a nuclear replicative phase?
    A. Polyoma viruses and picornaviruses
    B. Herpesviruses and paramyxoviruses
    C. Adenoviruses and reoviruses
    D. Poxviruses and orthomyxoviruses
    E. Papilloma viruses and flaviviruses
16. All of the following statements about viral replication are true **except**:
    A. mRNA splicing controls late adenovirus protein expression
    B. RNA extracted from virions of (+) stranded RNA viruses is infectious in nucleic acid infections
    C. A DNA-dependent DNA polymerase in the pox-

virus virion permits a unique two-stage uncoating process
    D. Single-stranded RNA viruses of negative polarity contain one or more virion-associated transcriptases
    E. Viral penetration of a cell by phagocytosis is often described as viropexis
17. For an enveloped icosahedral herpesvirus, which of the following descriptions of events in productive infection is **unlikely**?
    A. Adsorption—electrostatic interaction with cellular receptors
    B. Penetration—by fusion with the plasma membrane
    C. Uncoating—may involve lysosomes
    D. Maturation—one segment involves assembly of capsomers
    E. Release—involves final maturation by budding from the plasma membrane
18. Posttranslational cleavage to produce viral structural and nonstructural proteins occurs during infection with:
    A. Papovaviruses
    B. Adenoviruses
    C. Herpesviruses
    D. Picornaviruses
    E. Paramyxoviruses
19. For a naked icosahedral virus, which of the following descriptions of events in productive infection is **unlikely**?
    A. Adsorption—electrostatic interaction with cellular receptors
    B. Penetration—by phagocytosis
    C. Uncoating—may involve lysosomes
    D. Maturation—involves assembly of capsomers
    E. Release—involves budding from the plasma membrane
20. Which of the following virus families is characterized as having a virion-associated transcriptase?
    A. Rhabdoviridae
    B. Picornaviridae
    C. Papovaviridae
    D. Adenoviridae
    E. Togaviridae
21. Genetic reassortment is:
    A. Important in intragenic recombination of double-stranded DNA viruses
    B. Responsible for complementation in mixed infections
    C. A genetic interaction of principal importance to viral families with segmented genomes
    D. Prevalent in parainfluenza and respiratory syncytial virus infections
    E. Responsible for mosaic capsids in mixed infections of poliovirus type 1 and type 3
22. If two viruses infect the same cell and transcapsidated

particles are produced that have the genome of one virus and the capsid of the other virus, this interaction is referred to as:

  A. Genetic reassortment
  B. Cross reactivation
  C. Recombination
  D. Phenotypic masking
  E. Multiplicity reactivation

23. Genetic reassortment accounts for unusually high recombination frequencies with:
  A. Adenovirus and herpesvirus
  B. Papovavirus and herpesvirus
  C. Parainfluenza and respiratory syncytial virus
  D. Reovirus, bunyavirus, and influenza virus
  E. Rhabdovirus

24. The sharing of functional viral gene products at the nonpermissive temperature by viruses that have mutations in different genes is referred to as:
  A. Complementation
  B. Recombination
  C. Cross reactivation
  D. Multiplicity reactivation
  E. None of the above

25. All of the following statements correctly describe phenotypic mixing **except:**
  A. Phenotypic mixing is a form of complementation
  B. Mosaic capsids containing antigenic epitopes of closely related viruses often result from phenotypic mixing
  C. The genome of a phenotypically mixed particle is that of a stable recombinant virus
  D. Phenotypically mixed particles may be neutralized by sera directed against two different viral serotypes
  E. Each mosaic capsid resulting from phenotypic mixing forms capsids homologous to a single parental genotype on replication

26. Which virus-disease relationship is *incorrectly* stated?
  A. Parainfluenza virus type 3—pneumonitis in infants
  B. Mumps virus—unilateral orchitis
  C. Measles virus—encephalomyelitis without sequelae
  D. Parainfluenza virus type 2—croup in children less than 3 years of age
  E. Respiratory syncytial virus—the major cause of bronchiolitis and pneumonitis in children under 6 months of age

For each numbered phrase, select the one lettered heading that is more closely associated with it. *Each lettered choice may be used once, more than once, or not at all.*
  A. Mumps virus
  B. Rubella virus
  C. Measles (rubeola) virus
  D. Influenza virus

  E. Parainfluenza virus type I
  F. Respiratory syncytial virus

27. Individuals previously infected with this virus develop a slow virus disease known as subacute sclerosing panencephalitis

28. This virus infection of children 6 months to 3 years of age is the most common cause of laryngotracheobronchitis (croup)

For each numbered phrase, select the *one* lettered heading that is most closely associated with it. *Each lettered choice may be used once, more than once, or not at all.*
  A. Mumps virus
  B. Measles virus
  C. Respiratory syncytial virus
  D. Poliovirus
  E. Herpes simplex virus
  F. Hepatitis B virus

29. A live attenuated Edmonston B vaccine is used in monovalent form and in combinations for active immunization

30. A live virus vaccine is *not* currently in use for this RNA virus

31. A recombinant vaccine produced in yeast contains the purified surface protein of this virus

32. A virus whose oral trivalent live vaccine establishes intestinal immunity to reinfection

33. Which of the following viruses is associated with epidemic gastroenteritis in school-aged children and adults?
  A. Rotavirus
  B. Poliovirus
  C. La Crosse agent
  D. Norwalk agent
  E. Group B coxsackieviruses

34. Which of the following viruses are the most frequent etiologic agents of common colds?
  A. Echoviruses
  B. Adenoviruses
  C. Coronaviruses
  D. Rhinoviruses
  E. Parainfluenza virus type 1

35. All of the following statements about poliovirus infections are correct **except:**
  A. Virus is predominantly shed from the body and transmitted in respiratory droplets
  B. Most occur as inapparent subclinical infections
  C. Persistent viremia favors CNS involvement
  D. Spinal poliomyelitis involves the anterior horn cells of the spinal cord
  E. Capsid proteins are derived by posttranslational cleavage of a large precursor protein

36. All of the following are typical manifestations of type A coxsackieviruses **except:**
  A. Hand-foot-and-mouth disease

B. Herpangina

C. Pleurodynia (Bornholm disease)

D. Aseptic meningitis

E. Summer febrile illness

37. The immune response elicited by Salk's inactivated polio vaccine is deficient in specific:
    A. Duodenal secretory IgA
    B. Serum IgA
    C. Serum IgM
    D. Serum IgG
    E. None of the above

38. All of the following are typical manifestations of type β coxsackieviruses **except:**
    A. Bornholm disease
    B. Myocarditis or pericarditis
    C. General disease of the newborn
    D. Aseptic meningitis
    E. Herpangina

39. All of the following are true statements about poliovirus structure and replication **except:**
    A. A 22 amino acid protein, Vpg, is covalently attached to the 5' end of the genome
    B. An RNA complementary to genome RNA must be transcribed to serve as viral mRNA in the infected cell
    C. RNA is translated into one large precursor polyprotein
    D. The precursor polyprotein is subject to posttranslational cleavage to yield viral structural proteins
    E. The 3' end of the viral genome encodes an RNA-dependent RNA polymerase

40. All of the following statements correctly describe negative-strand RNA viruses **except:**
    A. Negative-strand RNA viruses do not contain an RNA-dependent RNA polymerase
    B. The genome of a negative-strand RNA virus is of opposite polarity to viral mRNA
    C. Mammalian cells infected by negative-strand RNA viruses do not contain RNA-dependent RNA polymerase
    D. The viral nucleic acid *itself* is not infectious
    E. Negative-strand virus groups have both segmented genomes and nonsegmented genomes

41. Which encephalitis virus is a bunyavirus that utilizes rabbits and small mammals (*not* wild birds) as reservoirs?
    A. St. Louis encephalitis virus
    B. La Crosse virus
    C. Venezuelan equine encephalitis virus
    D. Colorado tick fever virus
    E. Lassa fever virus

42. All of the following statements correctly describe flaviviruses **except:**
    A. Hepatitis C virus is a flavivirus

B. Flaviviruses bud from the plasma membrane while alpha viruses bud from intracytoplasmic membranes

C. Flavivirus genome expression is significantly different from that of togaviruses, to warrant the separate family designation, flaviviridae

D. Dengue fever virus causes bonebreak fever and a secondary exposure shock syndrome

E. Yellow fever virus is a prototype for flaviviruses producing hemorrhagic fever

43. Which of the following agents is a major cause of nonbacterial infantile diarrhea?
    A. Human reovirus
    B. Bluetongue virus
    C. Human rotavirus
    D. Colorado tick fever virus
    E. Group B coxsackievirus

44. All of the following are characteristic of reoviruses **except:**
    A. They strongly induce interferon
    B. They have a virion-associated RNA-dependent RNA polymerase
    C. They have a double-stranded RNA genome
    D. They are transmitted by respiratory droplets
    E. Each genome segment encodes a single viral protein

For each numbered phrase, select the one lettered heading that is most closely associated with it. *Each lettered choice may be used once, more than once, or not at all.*

A. Hepatitis A virus
B. Hepatitis B virus
C. Hepatitis C virus
D. Hepatitis D virus
E. Hepatitis E virus

45. This flavivirus causes posttansfusion hepatitis in HB$_s$Ag ($-$) patients

46. This water-borne virus is associated with enterically transmitted non-A, non-B hepatitis outbreaks principally outside the United States

47. This virus is associated with acute self-limiting infections, low mortality, and fecal-oral transmission

48. A genetically engineered vaccine prevents this virus from infections leading to either chronic carrier states or chronic active liver disease

49. This virus is a defective RNA virus found in HB$_s$Ag ($+$) patients

50. Hepatitis A virus is *most often* transmitted by:
    A. Sexual contact
    B. Contaminated food
    C. Blood transfusion
    D. Shared needles
    E. Air-borne droplets

51. During the incubation period of an HBV infection, which of the following viral diagnostic markers is

most abundant in blood and is commonly used for diagnosis?
A. Viral DNA polymerase
B. HB$_c$Ag
C. HB$_s$Ag
D. Anti-HB$_c$
E. Anti-HBs

52. Which of the following diagnostic markers persists in the bloodstream of HBV chronically infected individuals and is utilized as a measure of increased infectivity and persistent infection?
A. HB$_c$Ag
B. HB$_e$Ag
C. Anti-HB$_c$
D. Anti-HB$_s$
E. Delta antigen

53. All of the following statements about hepatitis viruses are true **except**:
A. Current acute HAV infection is best diagnosed by the presence of IgM anti-HAV antigen
B. Hepatitis A virus infections are *often* associated with arthralgias, arthritis, and immune complex diseases
C. Hepatitis B virus is associated with primary hepatocellular carcinoma
D. Hepatitis C virus is the leading cause of post-transfusion hepatitis (PTH) producing the highest frequency of chronic disease
E. Hepatitis D virus infection only exists as a coinfection or superinfection of HB$_s$Ag (+) individuals

54. A hepatitis virus uncoats its DNA genome to transcribe a (+) strand RNA (the pregenome). The pregenome is encapsidated in immature cores and then reverse transcribed by a polymerase that possesses both RNA- and DNA-directed DNA polymerase activity to produce a double-stranded DNA genome with a single-stranded gap. Which of the following is characterized by this unique replication?
A. Hepatitis D virus
B. Hepatitis C virus
C. Hepatitis E virus
D. Hepatitis A virus
E. Hepatitis B virus

55. The promoter or enhancer insertion hypotheses have been put forth to explain:
A. The generation of new recombinant viruses
B. The transformation of cells by viruses possessing oncogenes
C. The transformation of cells by oncogenes from human tumor cells
D. The induction of leukemias by viruses that lack oncogenes
E. The similarity of cellular and retroviral oncogenes

56. Which of the following mechanisms explains transformation of cells by DNA tumor viruses such as simian virus 40, oncogenic adenoviruses, and human papilloma virus type 16?
A. Translocation of cellular oncogenes leads to heightened expression of a c-onc
B. Point mutation occurs, resulting in an activated c-onc
C. Insertional activation of a c-onc occurs following integration of the viral genome into cellular DNA
D. Viral oncogene products expressed early in infection interact and interfere with the normal function of tumor suppressor gene products such as p53 or RB p110
E. Viral oncogene products act as transcription transactivators for c-oncs

57. All of the following DNA viruses that infect humans are associated with human cancers **except**:
A. Human papilloma viruses
B. Adenoviruses
C. Epstein-Barr virus
D. Herpes simplex type II
E. Hepatitis B virus

58. The retroviral oncogenes (v-oncs) of sarcoma and acute leukemia viruses are known to be:
A. Unrelated to proto-oncogenes in cells
B. Identical in sequence to cellular proto-oncogenes
C. Present in the endogenous retroviral genomes of many species
D. Present in defective retroviral genomes that require helper viruses for replication
E. Transactivators of transcription similar to the HTLV-1 *tax* genes

59. All of the following manifestations or findings are associated with HIV-1 infection **except**:
A. Altered T$_4$ helper/T$_8$ suppressor lymphocyte ratios (T$_4$/T$_8$<1)
B. Enhanced mitogen response to PHA and enhanced lymphokine (interleukin II) production
C. Kaposi's sarcoma
D. *Pneumocystis carinii* pneumonia
E. Increased serum IgG levels

60. Human immunodeficiency virus (HIV-1) differs from typical RNA tumor viruses in all of the following ways **except** that:
A. It is a lentivirus with homology to visna virus
B. It encodes a viral protease, reverse transcriptase, and integrase
C. It encodes a positive transactivator of its own transcription (*tat* gene product)
D. It is a cytocidal virus rather than a transforming focus-forming virus
E. It enters cells using transmembrane gp41-mediated membrane fusion rather than receptor-mediated endocytosis

61. All of the following drugs and their recommended uses are appropriately matched **except**:
    A. Acyclovir (Zovirax)—treatment of cytomegalovirus pneumonia in immunosuppressed patients
    B. 5-Azidothymidine (AZT; Zidovudine, Retrovir)—treatment of AIDS patients with *Pneumocystis carinii* pneumonia
    C. Ganciclovir—treatment of cytomegalovirus-infected AIDS patients
    D. Ketoconazole, fluconazole—AIDS-associated esophageal candidiasis
    E. Acyclovir (Zovirax)—daily prophylactic treatment of patients at high risk of genital herpes recurrence for up to 1 year

62. All of the following statements concerning the AIDS retrovirus, i.e., human immunodeficiency virus (HIV-1) are correct **except**:
    A. There is appreciable antigenic diversity in the envelope glycoprotein (gp120) of the virus
    B. Screening tests for antibodies are useful to prevent transmission of HIV through transfused blood
    C. HIV infection involves the CD4 receptor protein on the surface of helper T cells
    D. HIV has a special mechanism for control of expression of its genes, i.e., the transactivation of transcription *(tat)* gene
    E. The presence of circulating antibodies that neutralize HIV is evidence that an individual is protected against HIV-induced disease

63. Which of the following human immunodeficiency virus type 1 (HIV-1) genes is considered to be a *differential regulator*, acting through an antirepression mechanism to prevent repression of the synthesis of large structural proteins by a sequence known as CRS, thus stimulating the production of HIV structural proteins while also reducing the synthesis of regulatory HIV gene products?
    A. VIF
    B. REV
    C. NEF
    D. TAT
    E. TAR

Associate A, the viral agents, through E with the characteristics listed in items 64 through 70. Each lettered choice may be used once, more than once, or not at all.
    A. Herpes simplex type 1
    B. Herpes simplex type 2
    C. Varicella-zoster virus
    D. Cytomegalovirus
    E. Epstein-Barr virus

64. Vulvovaginitis
65. Infection of B lymphocytes
66. Latent in the dorsal root ganglia
67. Venereal disease
68. Burkitt's lymphoma
69. Fetal malformation, birth defects
70. Heterophil-positive

71. Which syndrome is **not** associated with adenovirus infection?
    A. Keratoconjunctivitis
    B. Pharyngoconjunctival fever
    C. Acute respiratory disease
    D. Pharyngitis
    E. Heterophil-negative mononucleosis

72. Which of the following viral agents is **not** associated with the "common cold" syndrome?
    A. Rhinovirus
    B. Parainfluenza
    C. Coronavirus
    D. Variola
    E. Adenovirus

73. Appropriate postexposure prophylaxis for rabies requires all of the following **except**:
    A. Both passive and active immunization
    B. Washing of the wound with soap and water
    C. Multiple immunizations using human diploid-cell vaccine
    D. Injection of rabies immunoglobulin into the wound area
    E. Use of live attenuated virus

74. An acute febrile illness of about 3 days' duration characterized by a rash and lymphadenopathy that affects children and young adults:
    A. Infectious mononucleosis
    B. Mumps
    C. Rubella
    D. Measles
    E. Parainfluenza

75. All of the following are true for human papilloma viruses **except**:
    A. Are double-stranded DNA viruses
    B. Induce tumors in their natural hosts
    C. Are ether sensitive with a lipoprotein envelope
    D. Cannot be readily isolated and grown in culture
    E. May contain transforming genes

76. Rubella vaccine has been inadvertently used in pregnant females, resulting in:
    A. Fetal infection without congenital malformations
    B. Severe malformations and death of the fetus
    C. Induction of subacute sclerosing panencephalitis after many years
    D. Induction of progressive multifocal leukoencephalopathy
    E. Photophobia and high fever

77. Which of the following is **least likely** to be the cause of influenza epidemics?
    A. Point mutations
    B. Genetic recombination

C. Changes in population immunity
D. Changes in viral core proteins
E. Alteration of hemagglutinins

78. The major cause of serious lower respiratory infection in infants and children is:
    A. Adenovirus
    B. Respiratory syncytial virus
    C. Parainfluenza viruses
    D. Rhinoviruses
    E. Coronavirus

79. The presence of low levels of IgG but not IgM antibodies to rubella virus in the newborn suggests:
    A. Congenital infection
    B. Autoimmune disease
    C. Persistent infection
    D. Presence of maternal antibodies
    E. Susceptibility to rubella virus infection

80. In addition to their antiviral properties, interferons can alter a number of other host-cell functions. All of the following are affected by the addition of exogenous interferons **except**:
    A. Cell growth
    B. Natural killer (NK) cell activity
    C. Enhancement of macrophage functions
    D. Binding of antibody to viruses
    E. Increased expression of cell-surface (HLA) antigens

81. In a localized virus infection at a mucosal surface, which one of the following statements **most** likely applies?
    A. T cells probably play a major role in the host response
    B. Protection against reinfection of the mucosal surface usually correlates best with local IgA antibody titers
    C. Serum antibody is the most important factor in combating these infections
    D. Natural killer (NK) cells probably play a role in host response since they are found in the secretory sites during a virus infection
    E. Macrophages represent one of the key elements of mucosal surface immunity

82. All of the following are properties of influenza virus type A **except** that the virus:
    A. Contains double-stranded DNA
    B. Has multiple segments of single-stranded RNA
    C. Contains an RNA-dependent RNA polymerase
    D. Readily induces interferon
    E. Is capable of releasing sialic acid residues from cell surfaces

83. A fourfold or greater increase in antibody titer measured by an appropriate available viral diagnostic test, and performed on serum collected at the time of disease onset and 14 days later, would:

A. Be highly suggestive for the presence of the disease in question
B. Indicate previous infection with the disease in question
C. Have to be accompanied by the isolation of the virus in question to be diagnostic
D. Not be sufficient for diagnosis
E. Not be informative since the serum specimens were not collected at a proper interval of time

84. Which of the following viruses is **most** likely to be acquired through casual contact with an infected individual?
    A. Influenza virus
    B. Herpesvirus
    C. Cytomegalovirus
    D. Human immunodeficiency virus
    E. California encephalitis virus

85. Live enteric-coated adenovirus vaccine against types 4 and 7 is **most** useful for which population?
    A. Institutionalized children
    B. Military recruits
    C. Schoolteachers
    D. Pediatric nurses
    E. Nursing home patients

86. Influenza virus pandemics occur because of:
    A. The appearance of a new susceptible population (infants) in the interpandemic interval
    B. Defective immunocompetence of individuals at risk
    C. Shifts in the antigenicity of viral hemagglutinin
    D. Shift in the antigenicity of viral nucleoproteins
    E. Waning immunity in the elderly

87. All of the following are true about "T" antigens **except**:
    A. They are induced by DNA viruses
    B. They may be found in the nucleus or occasionally in the cytoplasm
    C. They have not been isolated or purified
    D. They may bind specific antioncogenes
    E. They may associate with host oncogenes or proto-oncogenes

Answers

1. D Viruses replicate using their own genetic material and a number of different replication strategies. Binary fission is not employed.
2. C Hexons are not found at vertices of icosahedral viruses. The presence of a penton or fivefold symmetry arrangement of identical capsomers is characteristic of icosahedral structure.
3. G

4. C
5. B
6. F
7. H
8. E
9. A
10. D
11. I
12. D In most cases, neutralizing antibodies are directed against epitopes in the exterior viral spike glycoproteins such as the influenza hemagglutinin or the HIV-1 gp 120.
13. B The Rhabdoviridae possess helical symmetry, not icosahedral.
14. B The herpesvirus genome contains repeat sequences referred to as terminal redundancy; however, the match is incorrect because the repeats are not inverted sequences as found in adenoviruses.
15. D The poxviruses are classically noted as the only cytoplasmic DNA viruses. All other DNA viruses replicate in the nucleus. Orthomyxoviruses such as influenza uniquely have a nuclear phase of replication unlike all other (-) single-stranded RNA viruses.
16. C The unique two-stage uncoating of poxviruses depends on new transcription; therefore, the enzyme responsible is a DNA-dependent RNA polymerase.
17. E Herpesviruses uniquely bud from the nuclear membrane, not the plasma membrane.
18. D Proteolytic cleavage of polyprotein precursors is characteristic of picornaviruses and retroviruses. Therefore, "picornaviruses" is the only correct choice.
19. E Naked icosahedral viruses are released by cell lysis and not by a budding process.
20. A The Rhabdoviridae are the only (-) single-stranded RNA virus family that can be chosen. The other (+) single-stranded RNA virus families do not have virion-associated transcriptases.
21. C Only viruses with segmented genomes undergo genetic reassortment.
22. D Phenotypic masking is a form of complementation or gene product interaction without genotypic changes. Other choices are all nucleic acid interactions that alter genotype.
23. D Only viruses such as reovirus, bunyavirus, and influenza virus with segmented genomes are involved in genetic reassortment.
24. A Only complementation involves gene product sharing.
25. C Phenotypic mixing does not involve a stable or heritable change in the parental viral genome.
26. C Measles encephalitis is potentially a very severe disease often associated with sequelae.
27. C

28. E
29. B Measles attenuated vaccine is available in monovalent form and in combination with rubella (MR) or in addition with mumps virus (MMR).
30. C Due to various problems, neither an inactivated nor a live attenuated vaccine has been licensed for respiratory syncytial virus.
31. F Hepatitis B virus vaccine was the first vaccine produced by genetic engineering. The surface antigen (HB$_s$Ag) was produced in yeast to yield a purified protein subunit vaccine.
32. D Poliovirus is a trivalent live vaccine (OPV) and as a live vaccine it induces secretory intestinal immunity.
33. D Norwalk agent, a probable calicivirus, causes adult diarrhea while rotavirus causes infantile diarrhea.
34. D The rhinoviruses are the most frequent agents of common colds. Coronaviruses also cause colds but they are second in frequency as compared to rhinoviruses.
35. A Poliovirus is transmitted by the fecal-oral route, not by respiratory droplets.
36. C Pleurodynia (Bornholm disease) is a manifestation of type B coxsackieviruses.
37. A The Salk inactivated polio vaccine produces a good humoral response in serum to protect against CNS disease; however, the production of nasal or duodenal secretory IgA is deficient, allowing for poliovirus infection of the intestine.
38. E Herpangina, a vesicular disease of the posterior oral cavity, is the most typical type A coxsackievirus manifestation.
39. B Poliovirus is the prototype for (+) single-stranded RNA viruses. Removal of the terminal Vpg protein allows the genome to act directly as a message. Therefore, the statement is false because a (-) strand is not needed or used as a viral mRNA.
40. A One of the principal characteristics of (-) strand RNA viruses is an absolute requirement for at least one RNA-dependent RNA polymerase to produce a complementary (+) strand message.
41. B The La Crosse virus (agent) is the principal disease-causing member of the California encephalitis virus antigenic complex. These viruses are bunyaviruses.
42. B The statement is wrong because it reverses the contrasting viral budding patterns. Flaviviruses bud from intracytoplasmic or vesicular membranes, *not* the alpha togaviruses.
43. C The number one cause of nonbacterial infantile diarrhea is rotavirus. An enzyme assay (rotazyme) is used to detect antigen for diagnosis.
44. D Reoviruses are ubiquitous in sewage and are transmitted by the fecal-oral route.

45. C
46. E
47. A
48. B
49. D
50. B Hepatitis A virus is principally transmitted by the fecal-oral route (contaminated food, unwashed hands). Blood-associated transmission is rare and homosexual-associated transmission may be fecal-oral in nature.
51. C Hb_sAg, the surface antigen, occurs in blood during the incubation period and it represents a standard test that is available. Viral DNA polymerase is harder to detect and not routinely used. Other markers listed are not present in blood during the incubation period.
52. B HB_eAg persistence is prognostic of chronic infection, heightened infectivity of blood, and poor outcome. While delta antigen may also be a negative prognostic indicator, it only occurs in persons coinfected or superinfected with HDV; therefore, it does not apply generally to all HBV chronic infections.
53. B Hepatitis B virus is typically associated with extrahepatic complications. The statement applies to HBV, not HAV.
54. E The only hepatitis virus that has reverse transcriptase activity is HBV.
55. D These theories were designed to explain tumor or leukemia induction by viruses that lack oncogenes. They rely on the importance of viral regulatory elements in LTRs rather than v-oncs.
56. D The discovery of tumor suppressor genes led to the understanding that a number of DNA tumor virus oncogenes transform cells by altering or inducing a *lack* or *deficit* in normal cellular growth control.
57. B Adenoviruses produce tumors in hamsters; however, oncogenicity has never been documented in humans.
58. D The acute or transforming retroviruses have acquired v-oncs through an exchange process of recombination that in all cases (except Rous sarcoma virus) have resulted in a loss of viral gene sequences as an exchange for c-onc sequences. Defective sarcoma and acute leukemia viral genomes are the consequence of this process.
59. B This statement is false because all mediated immune responses (mitogen response, skin test, cytokine production, etc.) are diminished by HIV-1 infection-induced AIDS.
60. B All retroviruses encode a protease, reverse transcriptase and integrase. These genes are not unique to HIV-1.
61. A Ganciclovir, not acyclovir, is recommended for cytomegalovirus (CMV) infections in AIDS patients. Acyclovir is not effective against CMV.
62. E Neutralizing antibodies have been detected in AIDS patients and the presence of naturally occurring neutralizing antibodies is not indicative of protection against disease. The value of vaccine-induced neutralizing antibodies is still in question.
63. B The Rev protein is thought to be involved in both antirepression and inhibited splicing of the mRNAs for large HIV-1 structural proteins. Rev protein favors virion production rather than regulatory viral gene products.
64. B Herpes simplex type 2 virus is usually associated with genital herpes.
65. E Epstein-Barr virus replicates in B cells.
66. C Varicella-zoster virus may persist in the dorsal root ganglia.
67. B Herpes simplex type 2 is considered a venereal disease virus.
68. E Burkitt's lymphoma is believed to be causally related to Epstein-Barr virus.
69. D Cytomegalovirus readily passes through the placenta and can cause fetal infection.
70. E Epstein-Barr virus infection results in the generation of heterophil antibodies.
71. E Heterophil-negative mononucleosis is associated with cytomegalovirus.
72. D Variola is the causal agent of smallpox.
73. E A live, attenuated vaccine for rabies is not available for human use.
74. C Rubella can be characterized as a mild disease of 3-day duration associated with rash and lymph node involvement.
75. C The human papilloma virus is a naked icosahedral virus without an envelope.
76. A Rubella vaccine may occasionally result in fetal infection but does not appear to cause deformities.
77. D Influenza core proteins do not readily change and are not associated with epidemics
78. B Respiratory syncytial virus is a major cause of death in infants.
79. D Low levels of IgG suggest presence of maternal antibodies; increasing levels of IgG or the presence of any IgM antibodies to rubella virus found in a newborn suggest fetal infection.
80. D Interferon does not affect binding of antibodies to viruses.
81. B IgA antibodies are the most important immunoglobulins at the mucosal surface.
82. A Influenza virus is an RNA virus.
83. A Fourfold increases in specific antibody generally indicate an ongoing infection.
84. A Influenza virus is readily transmitted by aerosols.

85. B Military recruits are susceptible to acute respiratory diseases caused by adenoviruses.
86. C The hemagglutinin represents the major source of antigenic variations.
87. C Many of the T antigens have been isolated and purified.

Suggested Reading

Belshe, R. B. *Textbook of Human Virology* (2nd ed.). St. Louis: Mosby–Year Book, 1991.

Dulbecco, R., and Ginsberg, H. S. *Virology* (2nd ed.). Philadelphia: Lippincott, 1988.

Evans, A. S. *Viral Infections of Humans, Epidemiology and Control* (3rd ed.). New York: Plenum, 1991.

Fields, B. N., and Knipe, D. M. *Fields Virology* (2nd ed.). New York: Raven, 1990.

Gorbach, S. L., Bartlett, J. G., and Blacklow, N. R. *Infectious Diseases*. Philadelphia: Saunders, 1992.

Hoeprich, P. D., and Jordan, M. C. *Infectious Diseases* (4th ed.). Philadelphia: Lippincott, 1989.

Joklik, W. K., Willett, H. P., Amos, D. B., and Willfert, C. M. *Zinsser Microbiology* (20th ed.). Norwalk, CT: Appleton & Lange, 1992.

Mandell, G. L., Bennett, J. E., and Dolin R. *Principles and Practice of Infectious Diseases* (4th ed.). New York: Churchill Livingstone, 1994.

Webster, R. G., and Granoff, A. *Encyclopedia of Virology*. San Diego: Academic, 1994.

White, D. O., and Fenner F. *Medical Virology* (4th ed.). San Diego: Academic, 1994.

Mycology

W. LaJean Chaffin

Superficial and Cutaneous Mycoses

Members of the kingdom Fungi are nonphotosynthetic, nonmotile eucaryotes that include yeasts, molds, rusts, and mushrooms. Fungi obtain nutrients by absorption and almost all fungi are aerobic. About 150 of the more than 100,000 fungal species are considered to be primary human pathogens. However, in the setting of the immunocompromised host the list of opportunistic fungi is increasing.

Fungi reproduce by spores, which may be formed sexually or asexually. Spores can germinate to produce different morphologic forms such as single-celled yeasts and multicelled molds, which are the forms most often encountered among human pathogens. Such forms may not be mutually exclusive as the growth form of some fungi may differ with the growth conditions. Reproductive structures may be simple or complex and have historically been very important in fungal identification. These structures are maintained by a rigid cell wall, which is composed primarily of polysaccharide that is external to the cell membrane. The plasma membrane of fungi contains ergosterol rather than the cholesterol found in mammalian membranes and this difference has been exploited in antifungal therapy.

Fungi can cause allergic, toxic, and infectious disease in humans. Several classification schemes for fungal infections have been employed. None are completely satisfactory, since particular fungi may cause more than one type of infection. The classifications used in this section are superficial and cutaneous mycoses, subcutaneous mycoses, systemic mycoses, and opportunistic mycoses. With each of these classifications, some of the general characteristics of the infections and their etiologic agents are noted.

Superficial Mycoses

With superficial fungal infections, there is generally no cellular response. The site of infection is so superficial and the infection so innocuous that a response is not elicited. Frequently professional help is sought for cosmetic reasons.

Piedra

There are two superficial infections of the external hair shaft known as piedra. Black piedra, caused by *Piedraia hortae*, is an infection in which black, hard nodules are formed on the hair shaft. This infection is encountered most frequently outside the United States. In some areas of the world, the infection may be encouraged for cosmetic purposes. In white piedra, caused by *Trichosporon beigelii*, soft, light-colored nodules form on the hair shaft. This infection is found in temperate and tropical climates occasionally including the southern United States. A few cases of opportunistic systemic trichosporosis have been reported. Differences in isolates from opportunistic infection and piedra differ sufficiently that they may eventually be placed in different taxa. Infection can be diagnosed by direct examination of the hair and nodules. In black piedra, hyphal strands are often aligned along the periphery of mature nodules, and the center of the mass resembles organized tissue with areas in which asci are produced. In white piedra, the mass of intertwined hyphae of the nodule often fragment into arthroconidia. Nodules may be removed by cutting the hair.

Tinea Nigra

Tinea nigra is a superficial, chronic, and asymptomatic infection of the stratum corneum. The infection is frequently found on the palm of the hand. Infected areas are characterized by brownish color, which is often darker at the edges of the macule. The infection is caused by *Exophiala werneckii (Phaeoannellomyces werneckii)*, a dematiaceous fungus. The infection is found in temperate and tropical climates. In the United States, it is encountered occasionally along the Gulf Coast. The infection is found primarily in teenage girls. Because infection may resemble melanoma or other types of skin cancer, a diagnosis of a fungal etiology is important. Skin scrapings examined for

Mycology

fungal elements reveal pigmented hyphae. Treatment with keratolytic agents such as solutions of salicylic acid or sulfur have been used, as well as, more recently, topical imidazoles such as miconazole.

Pityriasis Versicolor

Pityriasis versicolor (tinea versicolor) is a chronic, mild, asymptomatic infection of the stratum corneum. Lesions are sharply delineated, noninflammatory, and covered with furfuraceous scales. The term *versicolor* is particularly appropriate, since color of the lesion varies according to the normal skin pigmentation, exposure to sunlight, and severity of infection. Lesions occur more often on the upper body, face, neck, arms, and shoulders and may be singular, multiple, coalesced, or very large. The etiologic agent, *Malassezia furfur* (*Pityrosporum obiculare*), is part of the normal microbial flora of the skin and scalp. The organism is lipophilic, requiring lipids for growth. The reasons for a change from normal flora status to a pathogenic agent are not clear. The infection is found worldwide, and some tropical areas may have a 50 percent infection rate. Diagnosis is made by examining a potassium hydroxide (KOH) preparation of skin scrapings. Lesions contain both short hyphal elements and spherical cells, and this observation is virtually pathognomonic. Since the organism can be cultured from uninfected skin, culture identification is not diagnostic, and clinical signs are more important. Selenium sulfide, sodium thiosulfate (odor may be objectionable), miconazole, and other agents have been effective in treatment. Cure is often slow, and recurrence of infection is frequent.

Fungemia due to *M. furfur* has been reported in a small but increasing number of cases in infants and adults who receive intravascular lipid therapy. Generally infection resolves with catheter removal. The organism has also been implicated in seborrheic dermatitis. Treatments such as ketoconazole shampoo that affect the fungus improve the condition.

Cutaneous Mycoses

Infections of the skin caused by fungi are known collectively as dermatomycoses. The vast majority of such infections are caused by a related group of fungi known as dermatophytes and are specifically known as dermatophytoses. Skin infection with yeasts of the genus *Candida* are also encountered and are discussed in the section on opportunistic mycoses. Some of the fungi capable of causing systemic infection may produce cutaneous lesions following dissemination from the primary pulmonary infection. There are also a few case reports of these fungi causing primary cutaneous infections. These agents of systemic infections are discussed in the section on systemic

mycoses. In addition, a few cases of isolation of other fungi from cutaneous infections have been reported.

Dermatophytoses

Infections

Dermatophytes infect keratinized tissue (i.e., skin, hair, nails). Dermatophyte infections are among the most prevalent infections and annoy millions each year. Such infections may account for 5 to 10 percent of visits to dermatologists. Infections can occur from head to foot, with clinical types designated by body location (Table 6-1). The organisms colonize keratinized tissue. Hyphae are found only in the superficial epidermis, hair, and nails in most infections and rarely invade living tissue. Little is known about the initial interactions of the organism and host. Manifestations of infection may be slight, for example, scaling or minimal erythema, or more severe, such as inflammatory and allergic reactions in kerion formation. The reaction is dependent on the host, strain, and species of infecting organism. The nomenclature of these infections is derived from Roman times, when the agents were associated with insects, and consequently the term *tinea* (small insect larvae) was used as a general description. The Greeks had previously described the circular appearance of lesions with the term *herpes*, and subsequently the English term *ringworm* combined both Roman and Greek meanings. The incidence of infection is unknown, since many infections are treated with nonprescription drugs and are not brought to the attention of the health care community. Tinea pedis is the most common infection, occurring in millions of individuals. It may be considered a penalty for civilizations that wear shoes. Tinea pedis, tinea cruris, and tinea unguium are the most common infections among those patients with significant skin pathology. At one time, tinea capitis, in its epidemic form, was a major infection among children.

Disease-Producing Organisms

The three anamorphic or asexually reproducing genera of dermatophytes are *Trichophyton*, *Microsporum*, and *Epidermophyton*. The first two genera include several infectious species. There is a total of about 40 anamorphic species of dermatophytes. The teleomorphs, or sexually reproductive states, of *Microsporum* and *Trichophyton* species belong to the genus *Arthroderma*. The anamorphic species are not isolated with equal frequency from infection, and they do not have a uniform worldwide distribution. Eleven species account for most infections, and in the United States, five species are most commonly isolated from patients who seek medical attention. Some species are associated more frequently with certain clinical types of infection than others and are more often isolated from

Table 6-1 Common Dermatophytoses in the United States[a]

Species	Frequency[b]	Tinea capitis, epidemic	Tinea capitis, nonepidemic	Tinea barbae	Tinea corporis	Tinea cruris	Tinea pedis	Tinea manus	Tinea unguium	Anthropophilic	Zoophilic	Geophilic	Wood's lamp	Endothrix	Ectothrix
		Common clinical syndromes								Habitat			Hair infection		
Microsporum audouinii	7	X[c]								X			+		X
Microsporum canis	5		X[c]		X						X		+		X
Microsporum gypseum	6		X									X	−		X
Trichophyton tonsurans	2	X[d]								X			−	X	
Trichophyton mentagrophytes	3		X	X	X	X	X	X	X	X	X		−		X
Trichophyton rubrum	1				X	X	X	X	X	X			−		
Epidermophyton floccosum	4					X	X	X	X	X			−		

[a]This table lists the seven most frequently isolated dermatophyte species in the United States and the clinical infections with which they are most commonly associated.
[b]Frequency of laboratory isolation from patients seeking medical attention. Species ranked ≤ 6 were less than 1%. (From J. T. Sinski and K. Flouras. *Mycopathologia* 85:97–120, 1984.)
[c]"Gray-patch" ringworm; infection with *M. canis* is more inflammatory.
[d]Black-dot ringworm.

infections in some parts of the world (Table 6-1). Some species have as their natural habitat a soil environment (geophilic species), while others have animals (zoophilic species) or humans (anthropophilic species) as their main habitat. Infections may be initiated by organisms transferred from their normal habitat to the host by contact. Tissue shed from lesions, such as skin scales or hair, may remain on combs, chairs, carpets, around swimming pools, and so on, and subsequently be transferred to a new host. Infections with anthropophilic species tend to be milder and more chronic than infections with other species. In a recent survey in the United States, it was reported that the most common laboratory isolates from humans, in decreasing order of frequency, were *Trichophyton rubrum*, *Trichophyton tonsurans*, *Trichophyton mentagrophytes*, *Epidermophyton floccosum*, *Microsporum canis*, and *Microsporum gypseum*. These species are ubiquitous species found worldwide. Some infections are generally restricted to regions in which the causative organism is endemic. Tinea barbae, for example, is an infection of the bearded areas of the skin of men. Since the causative agents are generally acquired from animals, the infection usually occurs in rural areas. Tinea favosa (favus) is primarily found in regions in which *Trichophyton schoenleinii*, the most common etiologic agent, is endemic. The largest of these areas is around the Mediterranean Sea. The appearance of the yellowish, cup-shaped crusts called *scutula* gives favus

its name. With time, scarring occurs. Tinea imbricata occurs on Pacific Ocean islands where *Trichophyton concentricum* is found.

Laboratory Diagnosis

A diagnosis of a fungal etiology based on morphology of individual lesions and their body location is not always sufficient, since several other skin infections can closely resemble fungal infections. A differential diagnosis of a fungal etiology can generally be determined by additional examination. Some species that infect hair fluoresce under ultraviolet light (Wood's lamp). The infection of the hair shaft may also show arthroconidia outside the shaft (ectothrix) or inside the shaft (endothrix). For infections of skin or nails, a scraping is digested in KOH and examined for the presence of hyaline hyphal elements that are not pigmented. Calcofluor white is also a useful and easy stain for obtaining fluorescent fungi. Species identification requires culture. Culture identification is based primarily on the appearance of the colony and the microscopic appearance of the asexual reproductive conidia. While all of these species grow as molds, they have distinctive features. The reverse of colonies of some species may be pigmented (e.g., red or yellow) and the tops may be fluffy or velvety, white or pigmented. These characteristics combined with the microscopic morphology generally permit an identi-

Mycology

fication. Generally, species of *Trichophyton* are distinguished microscopically by their microconidia. These single-celled conidia have some differences in shape and location. *Epidermophyton floccosum* and species of *Microsporum* are distinguished by their macroconidia. The multicelled macroconidia of *Microsporum* have several distinctive shapes, vary in the number of cells in each macroconidium, and vary in the extent of their production by the species. The macroconidium of *E. floccosum* also has its own distinctive shape. There are several reasons to make a correct diagnosis of etiology. For example, if the source of the zoophilic species is the family pet, infections are likely to recur if the pet is not properly treated.

Treatment

Generally, dermatophyte infections are treated with topical drugs, most of which are available without prescription. Nonprescription products include Whitfield's ointment and preparations that contain undecylenic acid, tolnaftate, and the azoles micronazole and clotrimazole. Prescription preparations include those containing haloprogin, ciclopirox olamine, the azoles econazole or ketoconazole, or the allylamines naftifine and terbinifine. None of the triazoles, fluconazole, intraconazole, or terconazole, have been approved in the United States for cutaneous infections. Tolnaftate and the allylamines appear to inhibit squalene 2,3-epoxidase, an essential enzyme in ergosterol biosynthesis. The azoles inhibit ergosterol biosynthesis at a later step, a cytochrome P-450–dependent demethylation, in conversion of lanosterol to ergosterol. Some azoles may also cause direct physical damage to a fungal cell. Ciclopirox olamine treatment depletes intracellular amino acids and ions probably through inhibition of transport of these substances into the cell. One drug, griseofulvin, which is administered orally, appears to deposit at the base of the stratum corneum and subsequently reaches the infected region. This drug may be considered for particularly chronic infections. Ketoconazole is also an orally administered drug that may be useful in infections that do not respond to topical applications. With tinea pedis (athlete's foot), antibacterial compounds may be required on occasion to reduce secondary bacterial infection.

Virulence Factors, Physiology, Host Response

Dermatophytes show an evolution toward parasitism, as some species develop ways to reduce host response and develop keratinases to utilize the host keratin better. The response of the host to infection is to the metabolites produced by the fungi rather than to the organisms per se, which rarely invade living tissue. In experimental infections, there is a suggestion that host response leads to increased epidermopoiesis, which would increase the rate of shedding of keratin and reduce dermatophyte growth into new keratin. Increased formation of keratin in the area of a lesion could also account for observations of local immunity to reinfection. The growth of the organisms is inhibited at 37°C, which is one factor that helps limit infection to surface areas. A serum factor, probably unsaturated transferrin, also appears to limit infections to the skin. In the case of tinea capitis in the epidemic form, the formation of fatty acids of the scalp after puberty appears to limit this infection to the prepubertal years. Allergic reactions to dermatophyte antigens can cause sterile eruptions, dermatophytids, at other sites, such as on the hands of patients with tinea pedis.

Subcutaneous Mycoses

General Characteristics

Subcutaneous mycoses are found worldwide. In certain areas, some of the infections are endemic. In most of these infections, several species of fungi can cause the same clinical syndrome. The species implicated in these infections are common soil saprophytes. However, one agent may be commonly isolated from a particular infection in a given area. The organisms have no mechanism to invade tissue and must be introduced by some method of traumatic implantation. Frequently, this will take the form of a puncture wound from a thorn, twig, or nail contaminated with the fungus, or the fungus will be subsequently introduced into the unclosed wound. Generally, if a disease develops, it is localized to this site. The course of infection is usually slow and may continue over a period of years.

Sporotrichosis

Manifestation, Etiology, and Epidemiology

Sporotrichosis, caused by *Sporothrix schenckii*, is characterized in its cutaneous lymphatic form by a lesion that begins as a movable nodule and subsequently becomes necrotic. If it is untreated, new lesions appear along the lymphatic draining the area. This pattern is virtually pathognomonic for this form of sporotrichosis (aspects of cutaneous lesions of some bacterial diseases may be similar). In endemic areas, such as parts of Mexico, these lesions are frequently on the legs. In the United States, the infection is particularly associated with gardeners and those involved with horticulture and is sometimes referred to as the rose gardener syndrome. Very rarely does dissemination occur to other body sites. About 75 percent of cases reported in literature surveys are of this type. In endemic areas, another cutaneous form, a nonlymphatic or "fixed" form, may be seen. Single lesions, which do not spread, are often found on the face, neck, or finger. Finally, there is a noncutaneous form of systemic infection that may be on the increase. This is a pulmonary opportunistic infection associated with urban hospitals. It is seldom diagnosed and is often found in chronic alcoholics. Infection is initiated following inhalation of fungal conidia.

S. schenckii is the only etiologic agent of this infection. The organism is found worldwide as an inhabitant of soil and decaying vegetation. Infection can occur in all age groups. About 75 percent of the patients are men. However, this bias probably results from increased exposure.

Laboratory Diagnosis

As previously noted for the lymphatic form, the appearance of lesions along a lymphatic is very characteristic; however, an unequivocal diagnosis requires isolation and culture identification. Material removed from such lesions can be directly examined for cigar-shaped yeast cells. Stains such as calcofluor white and fluorescent antibodies may be useful. However, the number of organisms is often too few for reliable observation, and material should be submitted for fungal culture. The organism is thermally dimorphic. In soil or at room temperature, it grows as a mold with distinctive conidia that are produced in a pattern often described as a daisy head. At 37°C, the organism grows as a budding yeast. Serologic methods are not important in diagnosis.

Treatment

Potassium iodide (KI) has proved an effective therapeutic agent, which can be administered orally in milk or applied topically. The mode of action of KI is unknown, and it is ineffective in vitro. Amphotericin B may be used in relapses of the lymphatic form or in disseminated and pulmonary infections.

Mycetoma (Maduromycosis, Madura Foot)

Manifestation, Etiology, and Epidemiology

Mycetoma occurs as a localized swollen lesion, usually on the hand or foot. Lesions contain suppurating abscesses and multiple sinus tracts that drain exudates with granules containing microorganisms. There are two distinct groups of organisms capable of causing this infection, fungi and actinomycetes. Twenty-one species of fungi, many of which are dematiaceous, have been isolated from cases of mycetoma. Mycetoma infections with fungal etiologies are classified as eumycotic mycetomas, or eumycetomas. In the United States, the dematiaceous *Pseudallescheria boydii* is the most commonly isolated agent in the few reported cases. Other species that have been isolated from eumycetomas are listed in Table 6-2, as are several species of actinomycetes associated with actinomycetoma (see Chap. 4,

Table 6-2 Etiology of Mycetoma

Eumycotic mycetoma	Actinomycotic mycetoma
Acremonium falciforme	*Actinomadura madurae*
Acremonium kiliense	*Actinomadura pelletieri*
Acremonium recifei	*Actinomyces israelii*
Aspergillus nidulans	*Nocardia asteroides*
Corynespora cassicola	*Nocardia otitidiscaviarum*
Curvularia lunata	*Nocardiopsis dassonvillei*
Cylindrocarpon destructans	*Streptomyces somaliensis*
Exophiala jeanselmei	
Fusarium moniliforme	
Fusarium solani var. coeruleum	
Fusarium solani var. minus	
Leptosphaeria senegalensis	
Leptosphaeria tompkinsii	
Madurella grisea	
Madurella mycetomatis	
Neotestudina rosatii	
Polycytella hominis	
Pseudallescheria boydii	
Pseudochaetosphaeronema larense	
Pyrenochaeta romeroi	

under Actinomycetes). The disease is similar regardless of the agent, although infections associated with a bacterial etiology tend to be more severe.

Most of the agents have been isolated in widely separated areas of the world, although some agents show some geographic preference. The disease is found worldwide, and in some areas it occurs commonly. Areas of high endemicity include the Sudan and Mexico.

Laboratory Diagnosis

In diagnosis, the bacterial or fungal etiology must be distinguished. Granules obtained from the draining sinuses are examined for their gross physical characteristics of size and color. Microscopic examination of the width of the organisms generally differentiates between the two major etiologies, with fungi having filaments greater than 1 μm and bacteria filaments less than 1 μm. Organisms from the granules can be cultured and the colonial morphology and conidial formation used to identify the fungi. Bacterial species are identified using colony morphology, cell-wall composition, and physiologic characteristics.

Treatment

The response of eumycetoma to antifungal therapy has been disappointing. Topical nystatin and KI, amphotericin

Mycology

B, and azole compounds have been used with variable success. The agents are often resistant to the drugs and drugs may not penetrate to the sites of infection. Surgical excision of small lesions or even amputation in advanced cases may be indicated. With actinomycotic mycetomas, antibacterial antibiotics such as sulfonamides are often effective. These are discussed in Chap. 4, under Actinomycetes.

Other Subcutaneous Infections Associated with Dematiaceous Fungi

The nomenclature of subcutaneous infections (other than mycetoma) associated with dematiaceous fungi and the taxonomy of the causative agents have been in flux. Until recently, many of these infections were grouped under the terms *chromoblastomycosis* or *chromomycosis*. More recently, the term *chromoblastomycosis* has been used to denote a specific infection and *phaeohyphomycosis* to denote a heterogeneous group of other infections.

Chromoblastomycosis
Manifestations, Etiology, and Epidemiology

This subcutaneous infection is manifest as lesions that begin as small, scaly papules at the site of inoculation and gradually, over a period of time (which may be many years), develop into verrucous, ulcerated, and crusted lesions. Very rarely, infection disseminates to the central nervous system, which appears to be a preferred site in these cases. Lesions most frequently occur on the lower legs and feet. A number of species have been isolated from these infections, including *Fonsecaea pedrosoi*, *Fonsecaea compacta*, and *Phialophora verrucosa*.

The organisms occur in soil worldwide, with infection encountered with greater frequency in tropical areas. They are among the common fungi found in rotting wood and decaying vegetation. Disease is encountered most frequently in the 30- to 50-year-old age group. Infection is more frequent in men than women, which probably, at least to some extent, reflects greater exposure.

Laboratory Diagnosis

Examination of tissue from a lesion of chromoblastomycosis generally reveals characteristic pigmented sclerotic bodies. These structures are round to polyhedral, thick-walled forms that have cross divisions. Hyphae may also be present. Culture is required to identify the etiologic agent specifically. The colonial morphology, growth rate, and microscopic morphology of conidial production are characteristic of the species.

Treatment

In early stages of infection, wide and deep surgical excision has been successful treatment. Many antifungal drugs have been tried, with variable results. Relapse, resistance, and partial cure are common.

Phaeohyphomycosis

Phaeohyphomycosis infections are heterogeneous and range from superficial lesions to deep-seated infections. The terminology used to describe these infections often include a description of the site of infection as well as the etiologic agents. The agents of subcutaneous phaeohyphomycosis include *Exophiala jeanselmei* and *E. dermatitidis*. These infections may result in formation of subcutaneous cysts. Tissue removed from such lesions contains pigmented fungal elements, hyphae, and yeastlike cells. Positive identification involves examination of colonial morphology of the etiologic agent and its conidia. In cases of subcutaneous cyst formation, surgical excision has been successful.

As noted, the terminology used to describe these infections includes a description of the tissue affected. Among the deep-seated infections is cerebral phaeohyphomycosis, which may be increasing in frequency. *Fonsecaea pedrosoi*, *E. dermatitidis*, and *Cladosporium trichoides* have been isolated from these infections. Cases have been reported more frequently in men than women. These infections are generally fatal.

Other Subcutaneous Infections
Entomophthoromycosis (Subcutaneous Zygomycosis)

These subcutaneous infections can be considered a subclass of zygomycosis, and the subclass is divided into two types, entomophthoromycosis conidiobolae and entomophthoromycosis basidiobolae. Another subclass, mucormycosis, which is histopathologically and clinically distinct, is discussed in the section on opportunistic mycoses. The subcutaneous infections of entomophthoromycosis are chronic inflammatory or granulomatous diseases.

Entomophthoromycosis Conidiobolae (Rhinoentomophthoromycosis)

Entomophthoromycosis conidiobolae is an uncommon mycosis that has been diagnosed primarily in adults. Most cases occur in Africa, and most are in men. Nasal polyps develop, and the infection extends into other areas of the body accompanied by edema. The extending mass is palpable. Spread to subcutaneous facial tissue sometimes occurs. The etiologic agent is *Conidiobolus coronatus* or

Table 6-3 Systemic Mycoses

Infection	Etiologic agent	Growth form in nature or at 25°C	Tissue form	Culture morphology used in identification
Blastomycosis	*Blastomyces dermatitidis*	Mold	Yeast	Yeast: broad base attachment of bud to parent cell
Coccidioidomycosis	*Coccidioides immitis*	Mold	Spherule (sporangium)	Mold: arthroconidia produced in alternate cells
Cryptococcosis	*Cryptococcus neoformans*	Yeast (may have minimum capsule)	Yeast: encapsulated	Yeast: encapsulated
Histoplasmosis	*Histoplasma capsulatum*	Mold	Yeast	Mold: tuberculate macroconidia
Paracoccidioidomycosis	*Paracoccidioides brasiliensis*	Mold	Yeast	Yeast: multiple buds attached to parent cell

rarely *Conidiobolus incongruus*. Treatment has included iodides, amphotericin B, ketoconazole, and surgery.

Entomophthoromycosis Basidiobolae (Subcutaneous Phycomycosis)

Entomophthoromycosis basidiobolae is a chronic, self-limiting mycosis diagnosed primarily in young men (less than 20 years of age) in Africa, India, and Indonesia. Infection begins as a subcutaneous nodule that increases in size. With time, a large firm mass forms on the trunk or limb. The etiologic agent, *Basidiobolus ranarum (haptosporus)*, has been isolated from decaying vegetation and from the intestinal tract of beetles, frogs, and lizards. The prognosis is good. Potassium iodide has been used successfully and spontaneous resolutions have been noted.

Lobomycosis (Jorge Lobo's Disease)

Lobomycosis is an uncommon infection. Several hundred cases have been reported in the Americas, the vast majority from South America. The etiologic agent is *Loboa loboi*, which has not been successfully cultured. The infection is chronic and localized in the skin but may spread peripherally by autoinoculation. The lesion is sometimes verrucous and ulcerated. Lesions may develop over an extended period of time. The organism appears in tissue as single cells or chains of globose, or lemon-shaped cells about 9 μm in size. Surgical treatment is generally recommended, especially for single, early lesions. The course of the infection is slow and may persist for 20 to 30 years. There is no evidence of spontaneous healing.

Rhinosporidiosis

Rhinosporidiosis is a chronic, granulomatous infection in which polyps form on the face, particularly in the nasal area. More than 2000 cases have been diagnosed, primarily in India and Sri Lanka. The occupations and activities of

patients suggest that the organism may have a natural aquatic or perhaps soil habitat. However, infection has been noted in many areas including the United States. The etiologic agent is *Rhinosporidium seeberi*, which has not been cultured. In tissue, it develops a large 6- to 300-μm spherical sporangium that, when mature, is filled with endospores. On lysis, these endospores then repeat the developmental sequence.

Systemic Mycoses

General Characteristics

There is a group of fungi that are capable of initiating a systemic infection in a normal, healthy individual. These infections originate as primary pulmonary infections following inhalation of the fungi. Most of these infections are asymptomatic or subclinical; however, the infection may be symptomatic or progress to disseminated disease. The symptomatic and disseminated infections generally occur in a characteristic susceptible subpopulation unless individuals are exposed to large inocula. The infections tend to occur in endemic areas. Epidemiologic surveys, where appropriate immunologic skin test reagents are available, show that as much as 90 percent of the total population has a history of infection. For some of these infections, there appears to be immunity to reinfection. Most of the causative organisms are thermally dimorphic, having different forms in their saprobic habitat and in tissue. Some characteristics of the various fungi are summarized in Table 6-3.

Coccidioidomycosis

Manifestation, Etiology, and Epidemiology

Coccidioides immitis is the etiologic agent of coccidioidomycosis. The disease is an inapparent or benign respiratory infection in approximately 60 percent of infected individuals, but in some it produces mildly severe respiratory symptoms. Less than 20 percent of infected persons have allergic responses. In 5 to 10 percent of symptomatic patients, a benign, chronic pulmonary form develops in which thin-walled lung cavities or granulomas are left. In about 1 to 50 percent of patients, depending on background, a progressive pulmonary infection or disseminated infection develops that may occur in meninges, skin, or bone, or may be generalized. These cases follow either a rapid or insidious course and are potentially fatal. Disseminated infections may have periods of remission and exacerbation.

Coccidioides immitis is generally found in a particular ecologic niche known as the Lower Sonoran Life Zone. These areas are characterized by low rainfall and high summer temperatures and have a characteristic flora and fauna. In the United States, the areas include the San Joaquin Valley of California and along the border of Mexico. Additional areas are located in Central Mexico and South America. *Coccidioides immitis* lives in soil as a mold. During a wet period, the mold proliferates, and during dry periods, alternate cells of some of the hyphae form thick-walled, barrel-shaped arthroconidia that withstand the dry conditions. These arthroconidia may be stirred up when the top layer of soil is disturbed (e.g., by wind, archaeologic excavation) and inhaled. In lungs, the arthroconidia swell to form a spherical structure in which many nuclei accumulate. These nuclei are subsequently surrounded by a cell wall to form endospores contained in a spherule (sporangium). Upon lysis, each of the released endospores forms a new spherule.

Almost all individuals who inhale the arthroconidia become infected, and epidemiologic studies show a 90 percent infection rate in the highly endemic areas and a 50 to 70 percent rate in other endemic areas. The benign pulmonary form of infection with allergic reactions is found most often among white women. Disseminated infections occur most frequently in men, and among these, men with pigmented skin are commonly victims (e.g., Filipinos, blacks). Women in the third trimester of pregnancy and immunocompromised individuals including patients with acquired immunodeficiency syndrome (AIDS) are also susceptible to disseminated infection. Recovery from infection appears to confer a permanent immunity to reinfection.

Laboratory Diagnosis

In endemic areas, coccidioidomycosis may be known by other names, such as valley fever. It is estimated that about 100,000 new cases occur each year in the United States and cause significant morbidity. Outside the endemic areas, a case history that includes information about travel into endemic areas may be useful in suggesting a fungal etiology for a respiratory infection of unknown cause. The infection must be distinguished from other respiratory infections. While pulmonary x-ray may reveal patterns associated with coccidioidomycosis, these patterns are not exclusive. Sputum, pus, and biopsy material need to be examined directly for the presence of sporangia or spherules. Such evidence is sufficient for a tentative diagnosis. Specimens are cultured, and in 1 to 2 weeks, a white mold producing arthroconidia, which must be examined with care in the clinical laboratory, is diagnostic. A deoxyribonucleic acid (DNA) probe is also available for identification. It can be used on relatively young cultures before sufficient growth occurs for morphologic examination of sporulation or for application of the exoantigen test. There are several serologic tests that can be used in diagnosis and culture identification (exoantigen). A skin test reveals past or present infection. Other tests have been developed in which the titer of the reaction may differentiate disseminated and pulmonary infection and that can be used to follow the course of infection.

Treatment

No therapy is required for the majority of infections, which are inapparent or subclinical. For most symptomatic infections, nonspecific supportive therapy is all that is needed. However, the concern is to determine which of the symptomatic patients are likely to have more serious illness and may need antifungal therapy. Amphotericin B is the primary drug for therapy. Ketoconazole is a suitable alternative for non–life-threatening infections.

Pathogenesis and Virulence

Fungal virulence factors and host response are incompletely defined but several observations are relevant. Phagosome-lysosome fusion is inhibited in macrophages ingesting arthroconidia and endospores and these particles are not killed intracellularily. Wall-associated proteinases may be important in liberating endospores from spherules, a step essential in propagation of the microbe. Human sex hormones stimulate in vitro spherule growth, and hormonal levels in pregnant women may in particular contribute to susceptibility. Suppression of T-cell response has been noted in disseminated disease. Immune complexes are detectable in patient sera and may contribute to immune suppression and local inflammatory reactions.

Histoplasmosis
Manifestation, Etiology, and Epidemiology

Histoplasmosis is caused by *Histoplasma capsulatum*. The fungus is an intracellular parasite of cells of the reticuloendothelial system. It is a very common infection with worldwide distribution. There are many presentations of infection. Pulmonary infections range from asymptomatic or subclinical (95%) to severe with a variety of nonspecific symptoms including nonproductive cough, night sweats, and general malaise. Even in infections that run a benign course, transient dissemination occurs as a result of involvement of the reticuloendothelial system. The only evidence of such dissemination may be histopathology with lesions, for example, in the spleen. There are more serious forms of infection that may be considered opportunistic, since susceptible individuals usually have a predisposing factor. Symptomatic disseminated infection occurs in about 1 of every 100,000 to 150,000 cases. In some of these cases, there may be a severe, progressive dissemination resulting in infection of the spleen, liver, oral mucosa, and so on. There is a fulminant form of infection among infants and among immunocompromised adults including AIDS patients that develops very rapidly. The most common disseminated form in adults is a mildly chronic disease in which an oropharyngeal ulcer develops in many patients. There is also a chronic progressive form of the disease in which infections occur in cavitary lesions in the lungs. Resolution of all of these infections provide a certain degree of immunity to reinfection. A form of the disease encountered primarily in Africa is associated with a variant strain of the species, *H. capsulatum* var. *duboisii*. The infection is similar to classic histoplasmosis in that yeasts are found primarily inside cells, but African histoplasmosis differs in that most lesions are cutaneous, subcutaneous, or osseous and are rarely pulmonary. In addition, the yeast cells are much larger than those of variety *capsulatum*.

Histoplasma capsulatum occurs worldwide, but there are endemic areas. Infections have been reported in at least 60 countries. In the United States, the endemic area, in broad terms, is the eastern half of the country. The organism grows well in soil with a high nitrogen content and is generally associated with bird and bat guano. In the United States, the organism is frequently associated with the roosting areas of starlings, which are gregarious birds. Epidemics may be associated with disturbances of soil, particularly in roosting areas. In soil, the organism grows as a mold, producing both macroconidia (10 μm in diameter) and microconidia (3 μm in diameter). Because of their size, it is probably the microconidia that are inhaled and initiate infection.

In highly endemic areas of the United States, epidemiologic survey suggests a history of infection in 80 to 90 percent of the population. Some estimates indicate that 500,000 new cases occur each year, with 4000 requiring hospitalization. In children, symptomatic infections show no sexual bias. Among adults, approximately 75 percent of the symptomatic pulmonary infections occur in men. The mildly chronic form of infection is the most common

complication in adults, and about 75 percent of these cases occur in men. Symptomatic disseminated infection occurs more frequently in males. Among patients with AIDS the frequency may be 15 percent in endemic areas and some hospitals have reported a higher frequency. Many of these infections are thought to occur from reactivation.

Laboratory Diagnosis

The symptoms of infection are very similar to those of tuberculosis, and this is one of the major infections that must be considered in making a differential diagnosis. A case history revealing that the patient has been exposed to soil aerosols suggests a source of air-borne conidia. A direct microscopic examination of cells from sputum, blood, urine, or biopsy may reveal the intracellular yeasts. However, sputum is often negative and less useful in diagnosing histoplasmosis than other fungal infections. Specimens should be cultured. The organism is thermally dimorphic. It grows as a mold at room temperature, and the macroconidia, which are large and echinate with spiky protrusions on the surface, are particularly distinctive in identification. The organism is slow growing, and cultures are generally held 12 weeks before discarding. The hyphal form may be converted to the yeast form. DNA probe and exoantigen tests are also available for *H. capsulatum*. Inoculation of mice, which are susceptible to infection, can be used as an aid to isolate the organism from patient specimens. Serologic tests are an additional aid in diagnosis. The changes in serum titers may be useful in diagnosis and in determining the course of infection.

Treatment

As with other systemic infections, symptomatic pulmonary infection may require supportive therapy. Antifungal therapy is generally used with acute primary pulmonary infections and certainly required for disseminated progressive infections. Amphotericin B is the preferred chemotherapeutic agent. The imidazole compound ketoconazole is an alternative therapy, particularly for non–life-threatening infections. The role of newer azoles is not known. Maintenance therapy in AIDS patients is indicated. Surgical excision may be recommended for pulmonary lesions.

Pathogenesis and Virulence

In a murine model, strains unable to undergo the mycelial-yeast morphogenesis were unable to establish infection. Yeast cells phagocytized by neutrophils are killed while those phagocytized by macrophages survive and multiply. In naive macrophages the yeast cells do not elicit an oxidative burst, but immune T cells or lymphokines are able to activate macrophages that inhibit the growth of fungi they engulf. In a murine model fungal antigen appears to elicit a suppression of the cell-mediated immune response.

Blastomycosis

Manifestation, Etiology, and Epidemiology

Blastomyces dermatitidis is the etiologic agent of blastomycosis. Localized outbreaks provide evidence for asymptomatic infection and spontaneous recovery from symptomatic pulmonary infection. Cases of clinical pulmonary infection have been reported and by analogy with coccidioidomycosis and histoplasmosis most infections are probably subclinical. Most cases brought to medical attention are of two types: unresolving pulmonary infection that frequently leads to generalized dissemination, with skin, bones, genitourinary tract, and central nervous system as the most common sites, or chronic cutaneous infection. Cutaneous lesions are the most common manifestation of extrapulmonary infection. Lesions are most common on exposed surfaces such as face and hand. Lesions begin as a nodule, which subsequently ulcerates and spreads slowly.

Knowledge of the geographic distribution of the organism is based on case reports, originating primarily from North America, and the disease, therefore, was previously called North American blastomycosis. In the United States, infections are reported primarily from the eastern half of the country with localized areas of greater endemicity. The infection is also known now to be endemic in widespread areas of Africa. The natural habitat of the organism is unknown. Since it appears that infection follows the pattern of other systemic fungal infections, the habitat is presumed to be the soil or vegetation. The organism grows as a mold, producing conidia that appear to be inhaled to initiate infection.

As noted, the lack of a skin test limits the epidemiologic information to symptomatic cases. It is known, however, that all ages are affected, with a slight preponderance in the 30- to 60-year age group. Symptomatic infections are reported to occur more frequently among men. However, in epidemics in which several individuals show a common infection history, this bias is not apparent.

Laboratory Diagnosis

The infection must be differentiated from other mycoses, tuberculosis, and other infections. Material removed from lesions is examined for the characteristic yeasts, which are relatively large (8–25 μm in diameter) and thick walled, and have a broad neck or base between the parent yeast cell and the developing bud. In culture, the organism is thermally dimorphic. It grows as a mold at room temperature, where it produces rather indistinctive conidia. The organ-

ism can be converted to the yeast form. The broad-based budding yeasts that characterize this species are very distinctive and useful in identification. DNA probe and exoantigen tests are also available for *B. dermatitidis*. Serologic tests may be useful in establishing a diagnosis but are not as well developed or specific as those previously discussed.

Treatment

Amphotericin B is generally the drug of choice for severe infection. A less toxic and also less effective drug that is used in some cases is 2-hydroxystilbamidine isethionate. Ketoconazole and newer azoles may also be considered particularly for less severe infection.

Pathogenesis and Virulence

In a murine model, morphogenesis from hyphal to yeast form was necessary to establish infection. The fungus produces a chemotactic factor for polymorphonuclear (PMN) lymphocytes whose presence stimulates fungal growth, although macrophage can phagocytize and kill the microbe. Also, in animal models, the fungus induces specific T suppressor cells that block cellular immune response.

Paracoccidioidomycosis (South American Blastomycosis)

Manifestation, Etiology, and Epidemiology

Paracoccidioidomycosis is a chronic, sometimes fatal mycosis that begins with primary pulmonary infections and disseminates to mucosal surfaces, including the gingiva, where it produces ulcerations. The etiologic agent is *Paracoccidioides brasiliensis*. The infection in many individuals is probably asymptomatic or subclinical and self-limiting or may become latent. Most clinical cases can be broadly classified into two types. One type, chronic progressive infection, generally arises from a latent or quiescent lesion and includes more than 90 percent of cases. Some cases are restricted to pulmonary lesions but most have disseminated infections although pulmonary symptoms may also be present. The site of dissemination is most frequently the oropharyngeal mucosa and gingiva, followed by lymph nodes and skin. Internal lesions have also been noted in virtually every organ. A small number of acute/subacute progressive pulmonary cases in children and young adults have been reported.

The infection occurs in Central and South America, although it has not been reported from several countries in these areas. There are regions of increased endemicity in Brazil, Colombia, Venezuela, Argentina, and Paraguay.

Although the ecology of the organism has not been fully described, it is presumed to grow as a mold in a soil environment. The mold form may produce various conidia, none of which are characteristic of the species.

Epidemiologic skin testing shows a positive response rate of 5 to 25 percent, which is somewhat lower in urban environments. Distribution is equal among men and women. Symptomatic disease occurs most often in the 30- to 50-year age group. Most patients are men (80–90%), and many are rural workers.

Laboratory Diagnosis

For diagnosis, material recovered from a lesion or from sputum is directly examined for the presence of the distinctive budding form of the organism. A large yeast cell (about 30 μm in diameter) is capable of producing more than one bud at a time. The buds are connected to the parent cell by a narrow neck, which results in a distinctive appearance. This distinctive picture has been described as "pilot's wheel." The organism is thermally dimorphic. At room temperature, it grows as a mold with sparse production of conidia. The organism may be converted to the yeast form. The very distinctive form of yeast growth is useful for identification. Serologic tests are useful for both diagnosis and prognosis.

Treatment

Ketoconazole is considered by many to be the drug of choice for all but the most serious manifestations. Amphotericin B has previously proved an effective treatment but has greater toxicity and requires an inpatient setting. Also, sulfonamides, such as sulfadiazine, have proved beneficial in an outpatient population. Even with compliance and long-term therapy, relapses have been noted.

Pathogenesis and Virulence

Recent laboratory studies attribute the sexual bias among patients with clinical manifestations to hormonal interactions between the host and fungus. The fungus has estrogen but not androgen receptors. Estrogen inhibits the conversion of the mycelial form, which is inhaled, to the yeast form that is present in infection. The higher estrogen levels in women are thought to reduce the ability of the organism to convert to the form associated with infection. Morphogenesis from hyphal to yeast form in the animal model is required for infection. The fungus induces specific T suppressor cells that block immune response. A role for natural killer (NK) cells in natural resistance to infection has been suggested.

Cryptococcosis

Manifestation, Etiology, and Epidemiology

Cryptococcosis is caused by *Cryptococcus neoformans* var. *neoformans* and var. *gattii*. Most infections are diagnosed as central nervous system (CNS) infections. Cryptococcal meningitis is the most common form, although meningoencephalitis and expanding cryptococcoma are also encountered. The pulmonary form of infection is rarely diagnosed. The absence of a good immunologic test has prevented the determination of the incidence of exposure. However, the frequent incidental finding of cryptococcal lesions in routine autopsies and similarities to other systemic fungal infections suggest that there are many asymptomatic or subclinical infections. Most cases are diagnosed as disseminated infections. In addition to the most common CNS site, infection may also disseminate to skin, bone, or other sites.

The *C. neoformans* var. *neoformans* occurs worldwide and grows well in a high-nitrogen environment. It is frequently found in environments associated with pigeon guano and debris, where it is a major inhabitant. The organism does not infect pigeons but survives passage through the gastrointestinal tract of the bird. Replication of the organisms results in high population densities in the fecal material, and the cells remain viable for 1 to 2 years. The organism is an encapsulated yeast although in its natural habitat the capsule is usually small. In a desiccated environment, the organism is frequently only 1 μm in diameter, small enough to be inhaled into alveolar spaces. While isolations of var. *neoformans* are worldwide, isolations of var. *gattii* are from tropical and subtropical areas. *Cryptococcus neoformans* var. *gattii* has been isolated from *Eucalyptus camaldulensis* (red gum), which is the only known environmental source. Isolations from *E. camaldulensis* have been reported from Australia and San Francisco. The red gum has been exported from Australia to other locations and may have resulted in the concomitant export of the fungus.

In the United States, 200 to 300 cases of CNS infection are diagnosed each year in the non-AIDS population. A significant portion of these cases are fatal, even with diagnosis and treatment. Infection is infrequent before puberty, and there is no relationship to age (although most patients are 30–60 years old) or occupation. It has been estimated that 15,000 subclinical cryptococcal respiratory infections occur each year in New York City. Among diagnosed cases, men predominate by a ratio of 3 : 1. Disseminated disease occurs in both apparently normal individuals and in patients with another underlying disease, such as Hodgkin's disease, leukemia, or lymphosarcoma. The incidence of this opportunistic dissemination is probably increasing. Cryptococcosis occurs in about 7 to 8 percent of patients with AIDS and is the fourth most common life-threatening infection in this population. The frequent occurrence of cryptococcosis in this group has significantly changed the proportion of total cases that are opportunistic. Since most of the AIDS patients in the United States are men, the ratio of men to women with disease has also increased. Isolates from AIDS patients are virtually all var. *neoformans*. AIDS patients generally are diagnosed with cryptococcosis after dissemination to the brain and may have prior or concomitant pulmonary infections.

Laboratory Diagnosis

The diagnosis of a fungal etiology is based on direct examination and culture of specimens from patients. Sputum and spinal fluid from suspected cases should be examined directly. Since the organism is heavily encapsulated, it shows up well with a background of India ink on a microscopic slide. However, the scarcity of yeasts may require concentration of the specimen to increase the probability of finding yeast cells on the slide. In addition, material removed from lesions can be stained to highlight fungal particles. When cultured, the presence of the capsule, production of phenol oxidase (resulting in formation of brown pigment on selective media), and biochemical tests are used for identification. DNA probes are also available for this purpose. Serologic tests to detect antigenic material found in the capsule may be both diagnostic and prognostic.

Treatment

Both amphotericin B and 5-fluorocytosine have been successfully used in treatment. However, some strains may be resistant to 5-fluorocytosine or become resistant during therapy. Generally, a combined therapy of amphotericin B and 5-fluorocytosine is recommended. The AIDS patient with cryptococcosis presents treatment difficulties. Even when initial treatment appears useful, relapse is frequent and cure doubtful. Maintenance therapy is indicated in this population and fluconazole has been extensively used.

Pathogenesis and Virulence

Both the phenol oxidase production and capsule formation (an antiphagocytic structure) have been shown to be factors that promote virulence. The ability to grow at 37°C is also a virulence factor. Cryptococcal cells activate the alternative complement pathway, which results in deposition of complement fragments on the capsular surface. Human neutrophils and monocytes phagocytize and kill opsonized yeast cells. A role for NK cells in host defense has also been suggested. A cascade of specific T suppressor cells induced by the fungus has also been demonstrated in mice.

Drugs for Treatment

The number of drugs available for treatment of systemic fungal infections is small, and each has its limitations. Following is a description of several that are commonly used.

Amphotericin B

Amphotericin B is one of a group of polyene antibiotics that can be administered for systemic infections. The drug affects the course of infection by interacting with both the host and the fungus. The nature of the interaction with the host is not well described but appears to result in an increased activity of host defenses. The drug interacts with sterols in the fungal cell membrane. The interaction is enhanced when the sterol is ergosterol, which is the major sterol present in the plasma membranes of fungi. The drug affects membrane permeability. In sufficient doses, it makes the membrane leaky so that vital metabolites are lost from the fungal cell. The compound can also react with the cholesterol of mammalian plasma membranes, and this interaction may account for its toxicity. The drug must be administered intravenously. Almost all patients who receive a full course of the drug have some adverse reaction. Beyond a certain concentration, permanent damage may occur to the kidneys. Another polyene that is used for topical application is nystatin. In some cases, this drug has been delivered as an aerosol for pulmonary infections.

Azoles

Miconazole and ketoconazole, imidazole drugs, and fluconazole and itraconazole, triazole drugs, are available for therapy. For systemic infections, miconazole must be administered intravenously, while ketoconazole and the more recent fluconazole and intraconazole can be administered orally. The drugs appear to be fungistatic rather than fungicidal. They interfere with membrane function of fungi in one or more ways, including interference with the synthesis of ergosterol. Azoles bind to a cytocrome P-450 and interfere with alpha-14 demethylation of lanosterol in the biosynthesis of ergosterol, the normal fungal membrane sterol. Both the loss of ergosterol and the accumulated alpha-14 methyl sterols affect normal membrane function. Overall, they appear to affect the fungal cell membrane. In general, these drugs seem to be less toxic to the host than amphotericin B. However, some side effects, such as liver dysfunction (seen occasionally), are caused by ketoconazole.

5-Fluorocytosine

5-Fluorocytosine is a nucleic acid analogue that is incorporated into ribonucleic acid (RNA) and affects protein synthesis. It has a limited range of susceptible organisms.

Within a population of susceptible organisms, some isolates are resistant or may develop resistance during the course of therapy. For some usages, combination therapy of amphotericin B and 5-fluorocytosine has been recommended. The drug can be administered orally and is relatively nontoxic, but side effects occur occasionally.

Opportunistic Mycoses

General Characteristics

Fungi that cause opportunistic infections are ubiquitous. They are of low virulence and are unable to establish infections in healthy individuals. The severity of the infection is, in part, determined by the severity of the defect in the normal host defense. Treatment of the underlying condition as well as the fungus is important in controlling the infection. The number of individuals at risk for opportunistic infection is increasing. Various medical procedures for treatment of other conditions increase the number of compromised patients and the severity of the abridgment of normal host defenses, for example, in the use of immunosuppressive drugs administered to patients receiving organ transplants. Compromised patients may also be more susceptible to the severe forms of infections that occur in healthy individuals. There is an ever-increasing list of organisms, including fungi, implicated as agents responsible for opportunistic infection. The ubiquitous nature of these opportunistic pathogens means that they are common in the environment and that compromised patients are frequently exposed to them. Table 6-4 lists some of the more important opportunistic species.

Candidiasis

Manifestation, Etiology, and Epidemiology

Candidiasis is an acute, chronic superficial or disseminated mycosis with a variety of manifestations. The most frequently isolated etiologic agent is *Candida albicans*, and studies of the infectious agent of candidiasis generally focus on this species. However, several other species are isolated from candidal infections with some frequency, and these include *Candida guilliermondii*, *C. krusei*, *C. lusitania*, *C. parapsilosis*, *C. pseudotropicalis*, *C. stellatoidea*, and *C. tropicalis*.

There are a number of cutaneous and subcutaneous candidal infections, which may be acute, chronic, or superficial. These include oral thrush, in which white patchy, pseudomembranous lesions form in the mouth. In neonates, this infection often occurs when colonization with *Candida* precedes colonization with the normal bacterial flora. Nearly all patients with AIDS have oral thrush at some time. Intertriginous infections caused by *Candida* are also observed, with lesions that may be well defined and "weepy.'" Several factors may predispose individuals to this type of infection, such as diabetes, obesity, or other conditions that provide a moist environment and some maceration of skin. *Candida* is frequently isolated from diaper rash in infants, particularly when it is severe. Candidal infections of the nails and surrounding tissue are also encountered, and these may be difficult to clear. These infections, particularly on toenails, are found among older patients. Vaginitis with a fungal etiology is also frequently encountered. *Candida albicans* is the primary cause of the approximately 13 million estimated annual cases of mycotic vaginitis in the United States. Frequency is higher among pregnant and human immunodeficiency virus (HIV)-positive women. In general, these infections are not life threatening, although they may cause considerable discomfort to the patient.

Most deep-seated or systemic infections associated with *Candida* species occur in patients with severe underlying disorders. A variety of systemic infections, which may occur in any tissue, have been reported. The kidney is the organ most often involved in systemic disease. Manifestations of infection in a given organ are related to that system. In almost any abnormal chronic respiratory tract infection, *Candida* can be isolated; however, it is difficult to determine the role of the organism in the disease process. In candidal endocarditis, vegetations grow on the heart valves, usually at the site of preexisting damage to the valve. Patients with valvular disease treated with antibiotics, patients undergoing heart surgery, and drug addicts are particularly at risk for *Candida* infections. Species other than *C. albicans* (e.g., *C. parapsilosis*) are freqently isolated from these lesions. Fungemia caused by *Candida* species is encountered with increasing frequency. Indwelling catheters, continuous intravenous infusions, surgery, and other procedures that abridge natural physical barriers are risk factors. In most patients, fungemia is transitory, and the organisms are cleared from the blood. However, in debilitated patients, fungemia may be a prelude to infection in other sites. Leukemic and other cancer patients who are receiving extensive chemotherapy are among the high-risk group.

The third general class of infection caused by *Candida* is chronic mucocutaneous candidiasis. Lesions associated with this disease become warty and in some cases may cover most of the body surface. All infected individuals have some underlying abnormality, such as a thymus defect, hypoparathyroidism, thymoma, or chronic granulomatous disease. Since humoral immunity is usually intact, deficiency of cell-mediated immunity is thought to be critical.

Mycology

Table 6-4   Opportunistic Mycoses

Infection	Etiology (frequent isolate)	Clinical manifestation	Pre-disposing factors	Direct examination of specimen	Culture Identi-fication	Culture Significance	Route of infection
Candidiasis	*Candida (C. albicans)*	1. Cutaneous, mucocu-taneous	Age, moisture, antibiotics, diabetes, etc.	Yeast generally with hyphae and pseudo-hyphae	Germ tube, chlamydo-spore, phys-iologic tests	Sputum not diagnostic; other non-sterile specimens correlate clinical signs; sterile specimen significant	Mostly endogenous
		2. Deep-seated or systemic	Immunosup-pression; catheters, cortico-steroids				
Aspergillosis	*Aspergillus (A. fumigatus)*	1. Allergic	Overwhelm-ing expo-sure, allergy predisposi-tion	In ABA may see fungi	Colonial mor-phology and microscopic appearance of conidial formation	May be con-tamination, repeat culture significant	Inhalation primary
		2. Noninvasive	Cavity, e.g., sinus, pul-monary	Hyphae with acute angle branching			
		3. Invasive	Immunosup-pression, leukemia	Hyphae with acute angle branching		Single culture may be significant in at-risk patient	
Mucormycosis	*Rhizopus Absidia (R. arrhizus)*	1. Rhino-cerebral	Acidotic diabetic	Wide, non-septate hyphae	Colonial mor-phology and microscopic appearance of sporangia	Significant	Inhalation
		2. Thoracic	Leukemia, lymphoma, etc.				
Cryptococcosis (see section on systemic mycoses)	*Cryptococcus C. neoformans*	Meningitis most common	AIDS, lymphoma, Hodgkin's disease	Encapsulated yeast	Encapsulated yeast, bio-chemical tests	Significant	Inhalation

Candida albicans is part of the normal human microbial flora. It can be isolated from a large portion of the healthy population. Administration of antibacterial antibiotics in-creases the frequency of isolation. The organism is also found in most mammals and birds. It is unlikely that *C.*

albicans survives and propagates outside an animal host. As part of the normal flora, the fungus is readily available to initiate infection when host defense becomes impaired. A wide variety of predisposing factors may place individu-als at risk for candidal infections. Natural physiologic states of pregnancy, infancy, and old age predispose to these infections. Underlying conditions that place patients at risk include diabetes mellitus, neutropenia, leukemia, malignancy, and AIDS. Iatrogenic factors that increase risk include immunosuppression, steroid treatment, antibacterial antibiotics, hyperalimentation, and catheters. Nosocomial fungal infections nearly doubled between 1980 and 1990, and included urinary tract infections, surgical wound infections, pneumonia, and fungemia. *Candida* species were the most commonly isolated (78%). Fungemia was more likely than nonfungal bloodstream infections to contribute to death during hospitalization.

Laboratory Diagnosis

For diagnosis of candidal etiology, sputum, pus, or tissue removed from suspected infections is examined directly for the presence of the organism. Of the *Candida* species, *C. albicans* generally is present in the yeast, pseudohyphal, and hyphal forms in lesions. In contrast, when part of the normal flora, generally only the yeast form is observed. Culture is required for identification. *Candida albicans* forms germ tubes (initial step in hyphal growth) and chlamydospores. A battery of physiologic tests is used to identify the various species. Since *C. albicans* may be part of the normal flora, a culture identification is insufficient in itself to implicate the fungus as an etiologic agent of the infection. Isolation from sputum is not significant. Isolation from urine may be significant if the number of organisms per milliliter exceeds a threshold level. Isolation from specimens from cutaneous and mucocutaneous surfaces should confirm clinical observations. Isolations from a sterile site, such as blood, is significant, however, and should be evaluated with respect to the patient's history. No reliable serologic test has been developed.

Treatment

Cutaneous infections are treated with a number of topical agents, including nystatin (a polyene antibiotic), butoconazole, clotrimazole, econazole, ketoconazole, miconazole, and terconazole (azole antibiotics), and gentian violet. Miconazole and ketoconazole preparations for vaginal infections are now available without prescription. Alleviation of the predisposing factor is also useful, such as keeping the infected area dry in some conditions. Although amphotericin B is generally the drug of choice and the mainstay of therapy for systemic infections, miconazole, fluconazole, ketoconazole, and 5-fluorocytosine are also used. Alleviation of the predisposing factor also contributes to control and resolution of deep-seated infections. All the drugs used in treatment of systemic infections are also given to treat chronic mucocutaneous candidiasis, but recent success with ketoconazole has made this the drug of choice for this type of infection.

Pathogenesis and Virulence

In addition to changes in the host that lower defenses and provide conditions that may permit the localized increase in fungal growth or introduction beyond sites of normal colonization, a number of properties of *C. albicans* itself have been proposed and demonstrated to contribute to infection. In vitro and animal studies, while suggesting the contributions of various factors, have also supported the idea that the host-parasite interaction is complex. The contribution of factors may vary by fungal strains as well as host site of infection. Among the factors that have been implicated are the following: (1) the ability to undergo morphogenesis from yeast to hyphal form; (2) the secretion of an aspartyl acid proteinase; (3) the increased expression on hyphal forms of components that interact with host complement factors C3d and iC3b, and others that bind fibrinogen, transferrin, and extracellular matrix components fibronectin, collagen, and laminin; (4) the expression of lectin-like surface components binding to host carbohydrates; and (5) the expression of hydrophobic surface components. Animal studies have shown that *C. albicans* induces immune suppression in the host.

Aspergillosis
Manifestation, Etiology, and Epidemiology

Aspergillosis is caused by several species of *Aspergillus*. *Aspergillus fumigatus* is most commonly responsible, but *Aspergillus flavus, A. niger, A. nidulans*, and *A. terreus* are also involved. Conidia of *Aspergillus* species are among the fungal particles frequently found in the air and, following inhalation, can be a source of antigen and elicit an allergic reaction. The response varies in atopic and nonatopic hosts and may also be dose dependent. Allergic bronchopulmonary aspergillosis is well characterized and the most common allergic response. The organism is sometimes associated with noninvasive colonization. This occurs in nonpulmonary sites, such as in ears, the nasal cavity, and the paranasal sinuses. Symptoms include those of sinusitis and chronic otitis. The organism may also colonize a preexisting pulmonary cavity left by tuberculosis or histoplasmosis infections. The fungus ball of aspergilloma that develops may produce cough, hemoptysis, and fatal hemorrhage in an infected individual, or it may produce no symptoms at all. Invasive disease is seen with increasing frequency in compromised patients and is a serious infection. Pulmonary infection produces symptoms similar to those of other respiratory diseases and sometimes develops from noninvasive colonization. If not detected early, the course of the rapidly necrotizing pneumonia is fatal. In some cases, there are no pulmonary symptoms, and the infection is disseminated to the gastrointestinal tract, liver, kidney, and other tissue.

The organisms are distributed worldwide as inhabitants of soil and decaying vegetation. They grow as molds producing conidia. Although the allergic response to *Aspergillus* antigen is not very different from allergic response to other antigens, the frequency of allergic aspergillosis is now recognized. For some individuals, the source of *Aspergillus* may be the workplace, such as the brewery where workers are exposed to *Aspergillus clavatus*. The nonallergic diseases occur more frequently in adults than children and more often in men than women. As noted, the existence of a cavity provides a potential site for colonization. A number of factors place a patient at risk for invasive aspergillosis, including leukemia, immunosuppression, and corticosteroid treatment.

Laboratory Diagnosis

Diagnosis is based on direct examination and culture of specimens from the patient. For direct examination, material is observed for septate hyphae with acute angle branching. With aspergilloma, depending on the location of the infection, conidia may be present. The organism may also be seen in biopsy material. In culture, the organisms form conidia on specialized structures, which have distinctive formations that differ among species. The colonial morphology and pattern of conidial formation are used in species identification. *Aspergillus* species are common laboratory contaminants; consequently, a positive isolation alone is not usually considered sufficient to establish an etiology. Repeated positive cultures, however, are of significance. In the invasive form of infection, since the course is fairly rapid and the prognosis grave, aggressive efforts to obtain biopsy material, brushings, or washings for direct examination and culture are recommended. Serologic tests for *Aspergillus* antigen successfully detect most cases of allergic bronchopulmonary aspergillosis and aspergilloma but sera from patients with invasive disease are less frequently positive.

Treatment

Allergic aspergillosis is treated as an allergic response. Asymptomatic aspergillomas have been considered benign conditions and as such no treatment is recommended. However, some studies suggest that the condition has potential fatal progression. Symptomatic aspergilloma, or fungus ball, is generally treated with amphotericin B, surgery, or both. Invasive disease is usually treated with amphotericin B as a single agent, given at an accelerated rate. In some cases, the addition of flucytosine to the therapeutic regimen appears to have been beneficial. Imidazole compounds have not proved effective in vitro and are not recommended. More recently, intraconazole has demonstrated in vivo activity

against *Aspergillus*, and limited favorable clinical experiences, if sustained, may lead to approval for treatment of invasive disease.

Pathogenesis and Virulence

Host factors may place individuals at risk for aspergilloma and invasive aspergillosis. Several possible fungal virulence factors have been identified and include extracellular proteinases, such as elastases and collagenases. In animal models, alveolar macrophages from corticosteroid-treated animals were ineffective in killing dormant conidia, probably through lack of phagolysosome fusion. Normal rabbit pulmonary alveolar macrophages were effective in killing in the absence of antibody or complement, and are probably the first line of host defense.

Mucormycosis

Manifestation, Etiology, and Epidemiology

Mucormycosis is associated with several species of *Rhizopus, Absidia, Mucor, Rhizomucor, Mortierella*, and *Cunninghamella* from the order of Mucorales. Mucormycosis can be considered a subclass of zygomycosis. *Rhizopus oryzae (R. arrhizus)* is the most frequent isolate from disease. These infections have a fairly rapid course to a potentially fatal outcome. Rhinocerebral infections begin in the nasal region and often spread to sinuses and brain. The course of infection is about 1 week. Thoracic forms of infection are initiated as primary pulmonary infections with progressive thrombosis and infarction and often spread systemically to other body sites. The course of infection is 1 to 4 weeks. A small number of cutaneous infections at the site of previous trauma have been reported frequently in patients with underlying factors such as diabetes mellitus.

The organisms are distributed worldwide, and they grow as molds in decaying vegetation and animal dung. The rhinocerebral form of infection is generally associated with acidosis, and most patients are acidotic diabetics. The thoracic form is associated with underlying disorders such as leukemia and lymphoma.

Laboratory Diagnosis

Specimens from suspected cases are examined for wide, nonseptate hyphae. However, fungal elements are often scarce and may not be present in a particular mounting. The organism has a tendency to invade blood vessels, and infarctions and necrosis are the main findings in autopsy specimens. Culture identification of species is based on colonial morphology and formation of asexual reproductive sporangia.

Treatment

The combination of surgery to remove or clean infected areas and drug administration is generally used in treatment. Amphotericin B is recommended as the drug of choice, since imidazole compounds have been inconsistently effective. Even with treatment, the fatality rate remains near 50 percent.

Other Opportunistic Mycoses

In the setting of the immunocompromised patient, virtually any fungus may be isolated from cases of infection. Several rare but increasingly recognized infections are noted such as trichosporonosis (associated with *Trichosporon beigelii* discussed previously) and geotrichosis *(Geotrichum candidum)*. Several cases of infection with *Penicillium marneffei* have been reported recently that appear to have originated in southeastern Asia. Several of the cases have occurred in patients with AIDS. Many AIDS patients have opportunistic pneumonia due to *Pneumocystis carinii*. Although *P. carinii* was classified as a protozoan early in this century, the taxonomic position of this organism has been under consideration since it shares morphologic features with both fungi and protozoa. More recent molecular studies show that sequences for several *P. carinii* genes are closely related to genes from fungal species, although the fungal species with greatest relatedness depend on the gene. This organism is discussed in Chap. 7.

Questions

1. Which infection is caused by an organism that is considered to be a component of the normal flora?
   A. Tinea pedis
   B. Tinea barbae
   C. Pityriasis versicolor
   D. Tinea nigra
   E. Tinea capitis
2. Which of the following is the distinctive structure determined by microscopic examination of colonies that is used in identification of species of *Microsporum*?
   A. Microconidia
   B. Arthroconidia
   C. Germ tubes
   D. Sporangia
   E. Macroconidia
3. Material from a suspected case of tinea corporis was treated with KOH and examined microscopically. Which of the following observations would be associated with a positive identification?
   A. Short hyphal sections and round yeast cells
   B. Pigmented hyphae
   C. Pigmented sclerotic bodies
   D. Hyaline hyphae
   E. Encapsulated yeasts
4. Which of the following situations that allow microorganisms to be introduced into the host would **not** result in dermatophyte infections?
   A. A child playing with the family cat
   B. Two children playing together
   C. Inhalation of conidia
   D. Walking barefoot around the swimming pool
   E. Sharing a towel in the locker room after a strenuous game of tennis
5. Which drug used in the treatment of dermatophytoses is administered orally?
   A. Undecylenic acid
   B. Penicillin
   C. Tolnaftate
   D. Griseofulvin
   E. Amphotericin B
6. Fungal cells **do not** contain which of the following:
   A. Nucleus
   B. Endoplasmic reticulum
   C. Chloroplasts
   D. Mitochondria
   E. Golgi
7. The appearance of round yeasts and short hyphal elements in material from a suspected lesion is associated with which of the following infections?
   A. Pityriasis versicolor
   B. Tinea corporis
   C. Blastomycosis
   D. Tinea nigra
   E. Tinea pedis
8. By which route are the agents of subcutaneous mycoses introduced to the host?
   A. Inhalation of conidia
   B. Ingestion
   C. Implantation
   D. Inhalation of droplets containing yeasts
   E. Invasion by normal flora components
9. Potassium iodide is the drug of choice for which of the following infections?
   A. Actinomycosis
   B. Tuberculosis
   C. Sporotrichosis
   D. Histoplasmosis
   E. Leishmaniasis
10. Which of the following organisms has a predilection for the lymphatic system?
    A. *Cryptococcus neoformans*
    B. *Streptomyces griseus*
    C. *Coccidioides immitis*
    D. *Sporothrix schenckii*
    E. *Blastomyces dermatitidis*

Mycology

11. The presence of pigmented sclerotic bodies in material removed from a lesion is characteristic of which of the following infections?
    A. Coccidioidomycosis
    B. Chromoblastomycosis
    C. Mycetoma
    D. Nocardiosis
    E. Contact dermatitis

12. Which fungal infection has been observed in only a very limited number of cases?
    A. Candidiasis
    B. Lobomycosis
    C. Coccidioidomycosis
    D. Tinea pedis
    E. Sporotrichosis

13. A 35-year-old man presented with a lesion on one finger of the right hand. An additional nodule was noted along the inner area and the underlying lymphatic was firm. The patient was employed as a landscape design consultant with a major local nursery. Which of the following would be a likely diagnosis?
    A. Sporotrichosis
    B. Actinomycosis
    C. Herpes
    D. Scalded skin syndrome
    E. Paracoccidioidomycosis

14. Draining sinus tracts are associated with which of the following fungal infections?
    A. Candidiasis
    B. Pityriasis versicolor
    C. Blastomycosis
    D. Phaeohyphomycotic cysts
    E. Eumycetoma

15. Which organism causing systemic disease has a predilection for brain tissue?
    A. *Sporothrix schenckii*
    B. *Cryptococcus neoformans*
    C. *Histoplasma capsulatum*
    D. *Coccidioides immitis*
    E. *Trichophyton mentagrophytes*

16. The form of *Coccidioides immitis* that initiates infections is:
    A. Yeast
    B. Arthroconidia
    C. Chlamydospore
    D. Microconidia
    E. Macroconidia

17. In the United States, the area in which most cases of coccidioidomycosis occur is:
    A. New England
    B. The southwestern part of the country
    C. East of the Mississippi River
    D. The northeastern states
    E. The Gulf Coast

18. In tissue, *Histoplasma capsulatum* is found as:
    A. Intracellular yeasts
    B. Encapsulated yeasts
    C. Spherules
    D. Yeasts with multiple buds
    E. Hyphae

19. *Cryptococcus neoformans* is most likely to be isolated from which of the following sites?
    A. Soil taken from a cornfield in Iowa
    B. Soil taken near a levee on the Mississippi River
    C. A scraping from a support beam of a football stadium used as a roost by pigeons
    D. A bale of cotton shipped from Texas to North Carolina
    E. Hairs removed from a pillow used as a resting place by a cat

20. During culture identification of *Blastomyces dermatitidis*, which of the following structures is most useful?
    A. Yeasts
    B. Hyphae
    C. Germ tubes
    D. Macroconidia
    E. Spherules

21. Which of the following is a site of action for amphotericin B?
    A. Plasma membrane
    B. Oxidative phosphorylation
    C. DNA replication
    D. Protein synthesis
    E. Enzymes involved in folate metabolism

22. Thermally dimorphic fungi:
    A. *Blastomyces dermatitidis, Candida albicans,* and *Coccidioides immitis*
    B. *Sporothrix schenckii, Histoplasma capsulatum,* and *Candida albicans*
    C. *Coccidioides immitis, Histoplasma capsulatum,* and *Rhizopus oryzae*
    D. *Blastomyces dermatitidis, Sporothrix schenkii,* and *Histoplasma capsulatum*
    E. *Coccidioides immitis, Histoplasma capsulatum,* and *Candida albicans*

23. Azole antifungals:
    A. Inhibit incorporation of ergosterol into the plasma membrane
    B. Inhibit a cytochrome P-450 in the biosynthetic pathway of ergosterol
    C. Bind to ergosterol in preference to other sterols
    D. Are incorporated into RNA
    E. Inhibit squalene 2,3-epoxidase in the biosynthetic pathway of ergosterol

24. An examination of sputum for a suspected case of fungal infection may reveal hyphae in which of the following?

A. Histoplasmosis
B. Sporotrichosis
C. Aspergillosis
D. Paracoccidioidomycosis
E. Cryptococcosis

25. Which of the following is the probable source of infection in aspergillosis?
    A. Ingestion
    B. Implantation
    C. Contact with an infected animal
    D. Inhalation
    E. Water used in preparing lemonade

26. How should a positive sputum culture of *Candida albicans* be interpreted?
    A. The patient has candidiasis
    B. The patient does not have candidiasis
    C. The patient may have candidiasis
    D. The patient probably has candidiasis if the isolation can be repeated
    E. The isolate is a contaminant

27. Which morphologic structure **is not** associated with *Candida albicans*?
    A. Yeast
    B. Hyphae
    C. Pseudohyphae
    D. Chlamydospore
    E. Sporangium

28. Which of the following conditions would **not** be considered a predisposing factor for an opportunistic infection?
    A. A previous history of pneumonia
    B. Diabetes
    C. Recipient of corticosteroids
    D. Cancer
    E. Recipient of immunosuppressive drugs

29. Which of the following drugs would be best for treatment of systemic candidiasis?
    A. Potassium iodide
    B. Griseofulvin
    C. Ketoconazole
    D. Penicillin
    E. Sulfonamides

30. Which infection generally has a very rapid course?
    A. Mucormycosis
    B. Mycetoma
    C. Cryptococcosis
    D. Candidiasis
    E. Histoplasmosis

31. Which infection has a single species etiology?
    A. Mycetoma
    B. Candidiasis
    C. Mucormycosis
    D. Paracoccidioidomycosis
    E. Aspergillosis

Answers

1. C *Malassezia furfur*, the agent of pityriasis versicolor, is part of the normal flora of the skin and scalp.

2. E While dermatophytes may form both macroconidia and microconidia, usually one predominates and is more useful in culture identification. Macroconidia are useful in identification of *Microsporum* and *Epidermophyton* species while microconidia are useful for *Trichophyton* species. Arthroconidia, sporangia, and germ tubes are not produced by dermatophytes.

3. D Dermatophytes are not dematiacrous and thus produce hyaline hyphae that may be observed in skin and nail scrapings of positive specimens.

4. C Dermatophytes are transmitted by skin contact with a contaminated source, such as infected hair, skin scale on towel or floor, lesion on an animal, and so forth.

5. D Antibacterial drugs may be used to treat secondary bacterial infections but not the primary fungal infection; therefore, B is not correct.

6. C While fungi are eucaryotes and contain structures such as mitochondria, endoplasmic reticulum, and Golgi, they are nonphotosynthetic and do not have chloroplasts.

7. A Since the agent of pityriasis versicolor is a component of normal skin flora, culture isolation is not very useful while the appearance of lesions and the microscopic observation of yeasts and short hyphae are diagnostic.

8. C The agents of subcutaneous mycoses have no mechanisms to penetrate the barrier of intact skin and are dependent on some trauma to introduce them beyond the skin barrier into subcutaneous tissue.

9. C KI may be used orally or topically for treatment of lymphatic sporotrichosis.

10. D Most cases of sporotrichosis are of the cutaneous lymphatic form where additional lesions may form along the lymphatic, draining the site of the initial lesion. *Cryptococcus neoformans* and *Blastomyces dermatitidis* frequently have clinical manifestations of central nervous system and skin infection, respectively.

11. B While dematiaceous fungi, which may cause tinea nigra, chromoblastomycosis, and eumycetoma, have pigmented structures in culture as well as in infected tissue, sclerotic bodies are particularly associated with chromoblastomycosis.

12. B Lobomycosis is an uncommon mycosis reported in several hundred patients primarily from South America.

13. A Necrotic lesions on hands, arms, and legs are particularly associated with sporotrichosis where additional lesions may appear along the draining lymphatic. The cutaneous and mucosal manifestations of actinomycosis and disseminated paracoccidioidomycosis are different.

14. E The agents of mycetoma, both bacterial and fungal, cause abscess formation in infected tissue. These abscesses may be connected by sinus tracts that may erupt to the surface.

15. B Most cases of cryptococcosis in the United States are diagnosed as disseminated disease of the central nervous system.

16. B Arthroconidia are formed from hyphal cells in response to unfavorable growth conditions and are small enough to be inhaled into the lungs and initiate infection.

17. B The endemic area of coccidioidomycosis is the southwestern US as well as parts of Mexico, Central America, and South America, where the etiologic agent grows in a particular ecological niche, the Lower Sonoran Life Zone. Blastomycosis and histoplasmosis also have endemic areas in the United States, principally east of the Mississippi.

18. A *Histoplasma capsulatum* is an intracellular parasite of the reticuloendothelial system where it grows as a yeast.

19. C Most isolates in the United States are var. *neoformans* associated with bird guano. The var. *gattii* has been isolated from a *Eucalyptus* species.

20. A The conidia produced by the hyphal form are not particularly distinctive, while the yeast form, with its broad base between parent and daughter cell, is distinctive and useful in culture identification.

21. A Amphotericin B binds preferentially to ergosterol, which is the sterol of fungal plasma membranes and disturbs the normal function and integrity of the cell.

22. D *Coccidioides immitis, Histoplasma capsulatum, Blastomyces dermatitidis, Paracoccidioides brasiliensis,* and *Sporothrix schenckii* are thermally dimorphic fungi. *Candida albicans* is dimorphic but not thermally dimorphic.

23. B Azoles inhibit a cytochrome P-450–dependent alpha-14 demethylation of lanosterol. Allylamines and tolnaftate inhibit squalene 2,3-epoxidase at an earlier step in biosynthesis.

24. C Hyphae may be observed in sputum specimens from cases of aspergillosis and mucormycosis. However, they are not always detected in specimens, even from positive cases.

25. D Aspergilli are common soil microbes and prolific producers of conidia, which may become aerosolized and subsequently inhaled.

26. C *Candida albicans* is a component of the normal flora and may be found in the oral cavity. Thus it is likely to be isolated from any sputum culture whether or not the patient has candidiasis.

27. E *Candida albicans* does not form sporangia.

28. A A previous episode of pneumonia does predispose an individual to subsequent candidal infection while all the other current conditions are predisposing factors.

29. C While amphotericin B is generally the drug of choice in serious infections, azole drugs such as ketoconazole can also be used.

30. A Mucormycosis can be a rapidly fatal disease with a course of 1 to 4 weeks if untreated.

31. D *Paracoccidioides brasiliensis* is the sole etiology of paracoccidioidomycosis. A number of infections may have one of several etiologies, although in some diseases such as candidiasis, a single species (i.e., *C. albicans*) is isolated most frequently.

Selected Reading

Baron, S. (ed.). *Medical Microbiology* (3rd ed.). New York: Churchill Livingstone, 1991.

Boyd, R. F., and Hoerl, G. B. *Basic Medical Microbiology* (5th ed.). Boston: Little, Brown and Company, 1995.

Davis, B. D., Dulbecco, R., Eisen, H. N., and Ginsberg, H. S. *Microbiology* (4th ed.). Philadelphia: Lippincott, 1990.

Joklik, W. K., Willett, H. P., Amos, D. B., and Wilfert, C. M. *Zinsser Microbiology* (20th ed.). Norwalk, CT: Appleton & Lange, 1992.

Kwon-Chung, K. J., and Bennett, J. E. *Medical Mycology*. Malvern, PA: Lea & Febiger, 1992.

Schaechter, M., Medoff, G., and Eisenstein, B. I. (eds.). *Mechanisms of Microbial Disease* (2nd ed.). Baltimore: Williams & Wilkins, 1993.

Sherris, J. C. (ed.). *Medical Microbiology: An Introduction to Infectious Diseases* (2nd ed.). New York: Elsevier, 1990.

Volk, W. A., Benjamin, D. C., Kadner, R. J., and Parsons, J. T. *Essentials of Medical Microbiology* (4th ed.). Philadelphia: Lippincott, 1991.

Parasitology

Danny B. Pence

Lumen Protozoa

Previously one phylum of all single-celled animals, protozoa are now considered as several phyla, including Sarcomastigorpha (amebae and flagellates), Apicomplexa (tissue parasites like malaria and coccidia with complicated life cycles involving sexual reproduction), and Ciliophora (ciliates). Species from all three of these phyla occur as lumen parasites of the gastrointestinal or genitourinary tracts. They are among the most common human infections, having a worldwide distribution. Some are very important opportunistic infections in patients with acquired immunodeficiency syndrome.

Amebiasis (Entamebiasis)

Epidemiology

Trophozoites of *Entamoeba histolytica* asexually reproduce in the lumen and mucosal tissue of the large intestine; cysts are resistant infective stages passed in feces and ingested in contaminated food and drink. Humans are the only reservoir. There are many more asymptomatic carriers than clinical cases. Up to 3 percent of the United States population may be infected, but only 3000 to 4000 clinical cases are reported annually.

Pathogenesis

Lesions result from receptor-mediated adherence of amebae to host target cells, contact-dependent host-cell killing through release of enzymes and cytotoxins and subsequent cytophagocytosis. Trophozoites invade the submucosa of the large intestine and undergo massive proliferation. Ulcerative colitis is the basic lesion. Secondary bacterial infections are common; complications include hemorrhage and perforation. In fewer than 10 percent of the clinical cases, metastatic amebae may cause liver abscesses; rarely, they cause lung, brain, pericardial, or perianal cutaneous lesions. Proliferation of the nest of metastatic trophozoites enlarges the liver lesion, resulting in necrotic areas with amebae at the leading edge of the abscess. Amebic liver abscess may heal with therapy, or rupture and disseminate if untreated.

Clinical Correlations

Infection versus disease must be determined in patients with *E. histolytica*. Usually, chronic cyst passers are asymptomatic. In clinical cases of intestinal amebiasis, there is an early phase of diarrhea with mucus and blood, which alternates with periods of constipation; this may progress to a secondary phase with severe diarrhea, dysentery, increase in the number of neutrophils (neutrophilia), emaciation, and anemia. Ameboma, an obstructive granulomatous lesion that may be misdiagnosed as carcinoma, occurs in fewer than 5 percent of patients with intestinal amebiasis. An amebic liver abscess is usually in the right lobe of the liver (elevated right hemidiaphragm on radiography). There is a history of amebic dysentery, weight loss, fever, and neutrophilia.

Diagnosis

Many infections are undiagnosed. Clinical cases are misdiagnosed because entamebiasis is not considered or *E. histolytica* is confused with several other nonpathogenic amebae that infect humans *(Entamoeba hartmanni, Entamoeba coli, Iodamoeba bütschleii,* and *Endolimax nana)*. Intestinal amebiasis is diagnosed by examining nuclear morphology of the cyst in stained fecal smears. Amebic liver abscess is diagnosed by culture of aspirated material and serologic tests (indirect hemagglutination assay, enzyme-linked immunosorbent assay).

Treatment

Metronidazole (Flagyl) is the most often used drug for all forms of amebiasis, but it is contraindicated during pregnancy. Emetine hydrochloride is an alternative in amebic dysentery, but it is cardiotoxic. Chloroquine is often used concurrently with metronidazole as a tissue amebicide for amebic liver abscess.

Giardiasis

Epidemiology

This is a flagellate infection with *Giardia duodenalis (G. lamblia)*. Trophozoites asexually reproduce on the surface mucosa of the small intestine; cysts are the resistant infective stages passed in the feces. Giardiasis is an unconfirmed zoonosis, possibly reservoired by beavers, dogs, cattle, and other mammals. Infection results from ingestion of cysts in food and water. Once mostly occurring in developing countries of the tropics, thousands of cases are now seen each year in North America and Europe. Small epidemics may occur.

Pathogenesis

Trophozoites mechanically damage intestinal mucosal cells by attaching to their surface with a pair of sucker-like disks, but they do not invade deeply into the mucosa. There may be shorting of the microvilli and some inflammation of the crypts in acute cases. Altered epithelial function leading to malabsorption may occur in chronic cases. Often, the minor pathologic lesions do not coincide with the severity of the clinical symptoms.

Clinical Correlations

Giardiasis is often asymptomatic. Clinical cases occur most frequently in children. Acute cases present with epigastric pain, nausea, diarrhea, and flatulence. Chronic cases may persist for many months, with alternating periods of diarrhea and constipation, weight loss, malabsorption with an excessive amount of fat in the feces, hypoprotein-emia, hypogammaglobulinemia, and vitamin deficiencies.

Diagnosis

Cysts in stained fecal smears are diagnostic when observed, but often they are released irregularly in the feces. Finding trophozoites in duodenal fluids or biopsies and serologic testing (enzyme-linked immunosorbent assay, indirect fluorescent antibody test) may be helpful.

Treatment

Metronidazole is the drug of choice for giardiasis.

Cryptosporidiasis

Epidemiology

Cryptosporidium muris is a coccidian parasite that undergoes asexual and sexual reproduction on the intestinal mucosal cell surface. The oocyst is the infective stage released in the feces. Rodents and many other mammals are reservoir hosts. In immunocompetent persons this is an asymptomatic to benign, mild, self-limiting infection. It is a common cause of protracted diarrhea or severe dysentery in the immunocompromised patient and a significant mortality factor in patients with acquired immunodeficiency syndrome.

Pathogenesis

Massive proliferation by asexual and sexual reproduction of partially embedded organisms on the mucosal surface of the small intestine causing alterations to the brush border and cell surface is the presumed mechanism of pathogenicity. The severe clinical manifestations seen in immunodeficient patients do not match the minor lesions produced by the parasites.

Clinical Correlations

Symptomatic infections in normal individuals involve a self-limiting diarrhea, sometimes with abdominal pain, anorexia, fever, nausea, and mild weight loss. Immunocompromised individuals may have severe protracted diarrhea with from 6 to 25 stools per day, massive fluid losses, weakness, and profound weight loss.

Diagnosis

The minute oocysts can be seen in fresh fecal smears; special stains and phase contrast microscopy are useful in their differentiation from yeasts and other protozoa. Duodenal biopsy may reveal parasites on the mucosal surface. An enzyme-linked immunosorbent assay test is available.

Treatment

Spiramycin has been used as a treatment.

Trichomoniasis

Epidemiology

Trichomonas vaginalis is a sexually transmitted flagellate that lives in the male and female genital tracts. The trophozoite reproduces asexually and is the infective stage; there is no cyst stage. This is one of the most common sexually transmitted diseases; the incidence in women in the United States is estimated to be as high as 25 percent. It is transmitted by coitus. There are many asymptomatic male and female carriers.

Pathogenicity

The exact mechanism of pathogenicity is unknown. Infection establishes when the acidity of vaginal secretions are reduced. Trophozoites do not invade tissue and no known toxins are released. Clinical cases present with intracellular edema and neutrophilia in the vaginal mucosa, hyperemia and petechial hemorrhage of the vaginal wall, a purulent exudate over the lesions, and often a concurrent bacterial or yeast infection, or both. The infection is usually asymptomatic in men; prostatitis and urethritis can occur.

Clinical Correlations

Vaginitis, vulva pruritus, a profuse and irritating (burning, itching, chafing) discharge, and increased frequency of urination or possibly dysuria are common clinical symptoms. Chronic symptomatic trichomoniasis in men results in a thin discharge with dysuria and nocturia.

Diagnosis

Fresh wet preparations of vaginal secretions and prostatic fluid demonstrate motile trichomonads. Flagellates can be seen in Papanicolaou's stained smears.

Treatment

Metronidazole is the usual treatment.

Other Lumen Protozoa

Balantidiasis caused by *Balantidium coli*, a large ciliate that also occurs in domestic pigs, is unproven as a zoonosis. Human infections are often asymptomatic. Although worldwide in distribution and rare, most clinical cases are probably of human origin. Small epidemics have occurred in mental institutions. The life cycle is direct with cysts and trophozoites in the large intestine; cysts are the infective stage. The large trophozoites are chiefly lumen dwellers, but they may release hyaluronidase to facilitate invasion of the large-intestinal mucosa, where they multiply asexually. Following establishment of concurrent bacterial infections, they cause ulcerative lesions similar to those of amebiasis. Extraintestinal lesions are very rare. Clinical cases present with intermittent bloody diarrhea and constipation, fever, anorexia, and neutrophilia. Infection is diagnosed by finding trophozoites or cysts in a fresh unstained fecal smear. Treatment utilizes paromomycin or oxytetracycline.

Isosporidiasis is an infection most commonly caused by *Isospora belli*, a coccidian parasite. Once considered a rare human infection, there are presently increasing numbers of cases of opportunistic infections in patients with acquired immunodeficiency syndrome. The parasite undergoes sexual and asexual reproduction within the small-intestinal mucosal cells, resulting in their lysis. In immunocompetent individuals infection is often asymptomatic, but mild to severe gastrointestinal distress with dysentery is re-

ported. Infection may produce severe chronic diarrhea similar to cryptosporidiosis in immunocompromised patients. Oocysts in a fresh unstained fecal smear are diagnostic. Trimethoprim-sulfamethoxazole is an effective treatment.

Dientamebiasis is an infection with *Dientamoeba fragilis*, a binucleate flagellated trophozoite that lives in the crypts of the small intestine. The exact mechanism of transmission is unknown since there is no cyst stage, but it appears that trophozoites may be transmitted in pinworn eggs. The infection is most common in children in the tropics. Many infections are asymptomatic, but a bloody diarrhea with flatulence, abdominal pain, weakness and weight loss can occur. Diagnosis is difficult because trophozoites quickly undergo cytolysis once the feces is passed. Treatment is with iodoquinol or paromomycin.

Blood Protozoa

Protozoa that occur as intra- and extracellular parasites in the blood vascular system are represented by hemoflagellates (trypanosome and leishmanial infections) in the phylum Sarcomastigorpha and Haemosporidia (malaria) in the phylum Apicomplexa. All are transmitted by arthropod vectors and are most common in the warmer, wetter climates. Malaria is a leading cause of mortality in the world's population.

American Trypanosomiasis (Chagas' Disease)

Epidemiology

Trypanosoma cruzi is a zoonosis reservoired in opossums, armadillos, rodents, dogs, and many other mammals. It is transmitted through the feces of blood-sucking reduviid bugs (*Triatoma* spp., *Rhodnius* spp., etc.) (Fig. 7-1); organisms are inoculated at the site of the bite or into the conjunctiva. Chagas' disease is prevalent in rural areas of Latin America where humans live near vectors and reservoir hosts. It is a major cause of cardiovascular disease in endemic areas of tropical America; there are estimates of 35 to 45 million human cases.

Pathogenesis

Asexual reproduction of amastigotes at the portal of entry evokes a localized inflammatory response (chagoma) and regional lymphadenitis (Fig. 7-1). Trypomastigotes are released into the bloodstream and are disseminated to every organ and tissue of the body. This is the acute febrile phase of infection, with parasitemia, malaise, lymph node

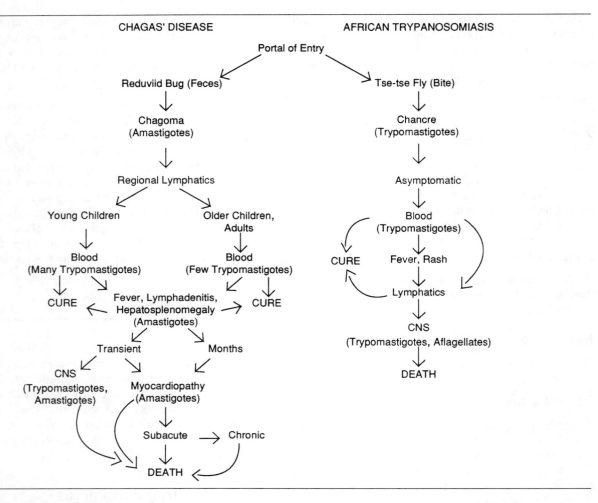

Fig. 7-1 Pathogenesis of trypanosomiases.

inflammation (lymphadenitis), and spleen and liver enlargement (hepatosplenomegaly). As amastigotes become established and undergo massive asexual reproduction as intracellular parasites, the chronic phase of infection begins. Cytolysis of infected cells, release of toxic products, and damage to the parasympathetic nervous system results in inflammation of the heart muscle (myocarditis), encephalitis, and/or dilation of the tubular organs.

Clinical Correlations

Usually, disease is more severe in younger children. Acute Chagas' disease often begins with a unilateral conjunctivitis and edema of the face (Romaña's sign) at the site of inoculation, local lymph vessel inflammation, parasitemia, and fever. This is followed by general lymphadenopathy, hepatosplenomegaly, and increased heart rate in mild cases, or myocardial insufficiency, circulatory collapse, hypotension, meningoencephalitis, and electrocardiographic changes in more severe cases. Subsequently, there may be complete resolution of symptoms, death, or development of the chronic stage. Myocardiopathy characterized by diffuse myocarditis resulting in progressive myocardial insufficiency and leading to eventual cardiac failure is the most common form of chronic Chagas' disease; extremely dilated esophagus and colon or encephalitis are infrequent latent manifestations.

Diagnosis

Trypomastigotes may be seen on stained blood smears during acute febrile periods. Chronic infections can be serologically diagnosed by an enzyme-linked immunosorbent assay.

Treatment

Treatment is largely supportive. Nifurtimox has been moderately successful in acute to early chronic cases.

African Trypanosomiasis (African Sleeping Sickness)

Epidemiology

Trypomastigotes of *Trypanosoma brucei gambiense* and *T. brucei rhodesiense*, the agents of west and east African sleeping sickness, respectively, reproduce asexually in the peripheral bloodstream, lymphatics, and cerebrospinal fluid. Cryptic aflagellate forms may proliferate in the chorioid plexus. Tsetse flies (*Glossina* spp.) are obligate vectors that transmit the organism among reservoir animal or human hosts (Fig. 7-1). African trypanosomiasis is limited to the range of its vectors in central Africa. East African trypanosomiasis is a sporatic zoonosis reservoired by many mammals (antelopes, wart hogs, buffalo); asymptomatic human carriers are not important to the transmission of infection. West African trypanosomiasis is not a zoonosis; chronic asymptomatic carriers maintain the infection.

Pathogenesis

Antigenic variability is the mechanism by which trypomastigotes evade the host immune system; they are able to change surface antigens by turning off one gene coding for the variate surface glycoprotein and turning on another. Thus, by the time the host immune system can mount an effective immune response against one surface coat antigen, the organism changes its antigenic structure and begins another massive asexual reproductive proliferation in an essentially immunologically naive host. With each successive wave of infection the patient becomes more debilitated, illustrating the typical pattern of progressive disease seen in African sleeping sickness. The acute phase of infection is a series of successive high parasitemias with endarteritis and lymphadenopathy as the trypomastigotes invade the lymphatics (Fig. 7-1). The chronic phase follows invasion of the central nervous system where massive proliferation of trypomastigotes cause a progressive encephalomyelopathy that eventually results in death of the patient.

Clinical Correlations

Onset is abrupt and acute in nonnative Africans; it is slower in native Africans. An ulcer (trypanosomal chancre) may occur at the site of the tsetse fly bite. Initially, there is a succession of several parasitemias manifested as febrile attacks followed by an afebrile period of several weeks. As trypomastigotes proliferate in the lymphatic system there is progressive lymphadenopathy, especially enlargement of the posterior cervical nodes (Winterbottom's sign). A circinate rash, mononucleosis, edema, headache, and/or neuralgic pain may develop. After a variable period (days to years) the chronic central nervous system phase devel-

ops, with tremors and signs of meningoencephalitis and/or meningomyelitis (headache, delusions, hysteria, mania, apathy, lethargy); this slowly progresses to the sleeping sickness stage, an almost continual somnolent state with ultimate coma, marasmus, and wasting death. East African trypanosomiasis is usually a more acute disease, with higher parasitemias, minimal lymphatic involvement, and early invasion of the central nervous system. West African sleeping sickness tends to be a more chronic disease with lower parasitemias, severe lymphadenopathy, and latent central nervous system involvement.

Diagnosis

Trypomastigotes in stained thin blood smears during the acute phase of infection and serology (indirect fluorescent antibody test, enzyme-linked immunosorbent assay) are used for diagnosis. There is an indirect hemagglutination assay card test for field diagnosis.

Treatment

Difluromethylornathine in combination with suramine is the treatment of choice.

Leishmaniases

Epidemiology

The leishmaniases are infections with intracellular amastigotes of *Leishmania* spp. that are transmitted among animal and human reservoir hosts by the bite of obligate sand fly (*Phlebotomus* spp., *Lutzomyia* spp., and *Psychodopygus* spp.) vectors (Fig. 7-2). They cause cutaneous (*L. tropica, L. aethiopica, L. major, L. mexicana*), mucocutaneous (*L. braziliensis*), and visceral (*L. donovani*) disease; collectively, *Leishmania* spp. have a worldwide distribution in the subtropics and tropics. They are mostly rural zoonoses that utilize rodents, sloths, dogs, and many other mammal reservoirs.

Pathogenesis

In cutaneous leishmaniasis, intracellular amastigotes reproduce in macrophages and epithelial cells of the small-vessel walls at the site of the sand fly bite (Fig. 7-2). A microabscess develops, leading to an epithelioid cell granuloma with ischemia. This is followed by focal necrosis, ulceration, and a secondary pyogenic infection. The lesion progresses to a few centimeters before it begins slow healing with scarring. There is permanent immunity to subsequent infection. In mucocutaneous leishmaniasis, an initial skin lesion is followed by lymphatic spread to the nasal-oral region. Here, amastigotes induce invasive destructive lesions of the soft tissues that do not spontaneously heal, persist for years, and ultimately result in

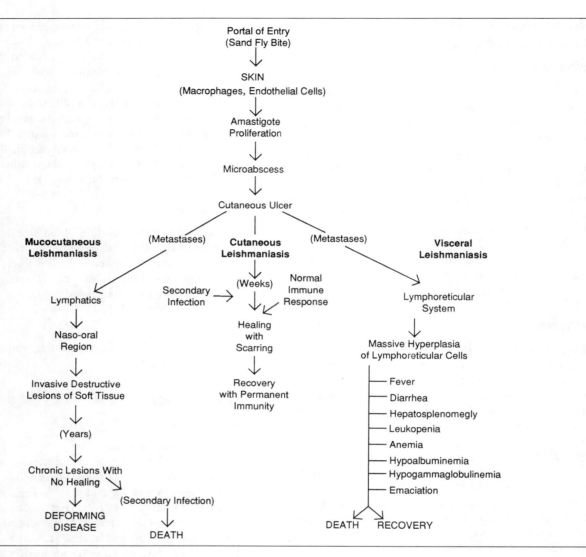

Fig. 7-2 Pathogenesis of leishmaniases.

deforming lesions. An initial skin lesion is usually absent in visceral leishmaniasis, but amastigotes are disseminated to all tissues of the lymphoreticular system from the site of inoculation by the sand fly. They undergo massive asexual proliferation, resulting in extensive hyperplasia of cells in the liver, spleen, lymph nodes, and bone marrow.

Clinical Correlations

Single to multiple dry crusting to wet (secondary bacterial infection) ulcerative skin lesions a few centimeters in diameter that heal with scarring after a few weeks to months characterizes cutaneous leishmaniasis. Following initial cutaneous lesions elsewhere, there develop deforming nasal-oral lesions of long duration (years) that do not heal spontaneously in mucocutaneous leishmaniasis. Eventu-

ally, ulceration results in partial to complete loss of all soft parts of the nose, lips, and soft palate. In visceral leishmaniasis, onset may be gradual, with abdominal swelling without pain, or acute, with fever and diarrhea. Ultimately, all cases manifest high fever followed by hepatosplenomegaly, progressive leukopenia and anemia, hypoalbuminemia, hypergammaglobulinemia, emaciation, and eventual death in untreated patients.

Diagnosis

Amastigotes in stained skin lesion biopsy smears (cutaneous and mucocutaneous leishmaniasis) and bone marrow smears (visceral leishmaniasis) confirm the diagnosis. Also, indirect fluorescent antibody and enzyme-linked immunosorbent assay tests are available.

Treatment

Cutaneous leishmaniasis often is untreated. Antimony sodium gluconate (Pentostam) is an effective treatment for this and all other forms of leishmaniasis.

Malaria

Epidemiology

Malaria is an infection with asexually reproducing intra-erythrocytic *Plasmodium falciparum, P. vivax, P. ovale,* or *P. malariae.* Sexual reproduction occurs in the obligate mosquito (*Anopheles* spp.) vector. Once an individual has been infected by the mosquito bite, a primary exoerythrocytic cycle of asexual reproduction (schizogony) occurs in the human liver (Fig. 7-3). The released stages infect erythrocytes and undergo a series of developmental stages

(trophozoites) leading to asexual reproduction (schizogony). Erythrocytic schizogony results in synchronous lysis of large numbers of erythrocytes. Released schizonts reinfect erythrocytes; some undergo the developmental stages, leading to another cycle of erythrocytic schizogony, while others develop to male and female gametocytes, which are infective for mosquitoes. The primary exoerythrocytic cycle of asexual reproduction is not repeated in *P. falciparum* infections, whereas it is continuous in *P. vivax, P. ovale,* and *P. malariae* infections. Malaria is not a zoonosis and transmission depends largely on the bionomics of the vectors. Malaria is worldwide in distribution between 45°N and 40°S latitudes. An estimated 4 percent of the world's population is infected (150,000,000 cases) with a 1 percent mortality (1,500,000 deaths/year). No vaccine is available; control programs are based on insecticide spraying for mosquitoes and chemoprophylaxis with antimalarial drugs.

Fig. 7-3 Pathogenesis of malaria.

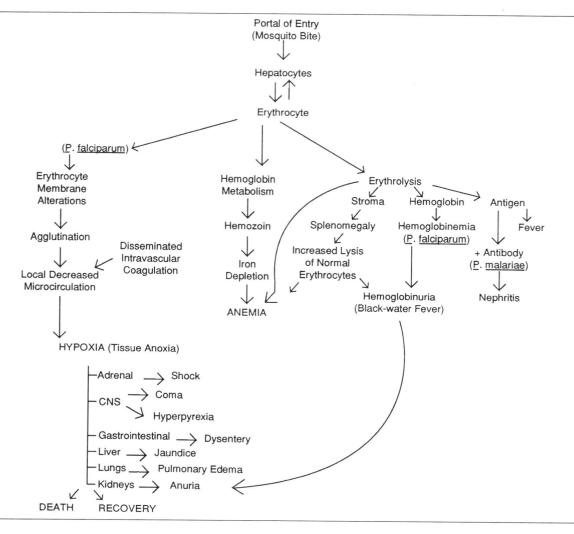

Pathogenesis

Malignant (*P. falciparum*) and benign (all others) forms of malaria are based on species differences in life histories, pathology, and treatment. The basic pathogenic mechanism in malaria results from massive, schizogony-induced, synchronous lysis of erythrocytes (basis of the fever cycle in malaria) followed by liberation of parasite metabolites with a host immunologic response to these antigens (complement-mediated lysis of additional uninfected erythrocytes), and formation and disposal of malaria pigment (hemoglobin breakdown products). (Fig. 7-3). Extensive erythrolysis results in anemia and splenomegaly, which is usually more severe in *P. falciparum* because this species infects all erythrocytes irrespective of age; *P. vivax* and *P. ovale* infect mostly reticulocytes and *P. malariae* infects mature erythrocytes. *Plasmodium falciparum* is more pathogenic because it causes electron-dense knobs on the surface of infected erythrocytes, an alteration of surface membranes that causes sludging in the capillaries. Because erythrocytic schizogony occurs almost exclusively in the capillaries, minute hemorrhages and ischemia from vascular plugging lead to tissue anoxia in many organs and tissues. The result may be cerebral malaria with coma and uncontrolled fever, adrenal shock, dysentery, jaundice, pulmonary edema, and/or renal anuria. Because accumulation of malaria pigment is more excessive in *P. falciparum* infections, overreach of the renal threshold for hemoglobin disposal is more frequent and severe; this often leads to renal anoxia, blackwater fever, and death of the patient.

Clinical Correlations

Prodromal symptoms include headache, photophobia, anorexia, nausea, and vomiting. The paroxymal period of acute febrile disease begins with sudden chills followed by the hot stage with restlessness, high fever, severe headache, and muscle pain. After several hours of profuse sweating the febrile period subsides with the patient falling into an exhaustive sleep. The periodicity of the fever cycle is 42 to 72 hours initially, but after a few febrile episodes it usually becomes continuous. Anemia, leukopenia, and splenomegaly develop after several febrile episodes. Asymptomatic infections persist for months to years in untreated cases; these sometimes recrudesce (from subclinical erythrocytic infections) or relapse (from exoerythrocytic infections) to febrile illness following stress. Cerebral malaria begins as a progressively severe headache and is initially afebrile, but the patient soon lapses into a coma and often there is a rapid uncontrolled rise in temperature followed by death. Blackwater fever begins with prostration and severe chills followed by profuse vomiting, jaundice, red-black urine, a rapidly developing anemia, and possibly anuria followed by death.

Diagnosis

Malaria is diagnosed by observing intracellular erythrocytic stages on stained blood smears. Species must be identified for proper treatment.

Treatment

Chloroquine (an erythrocytic schizonticide) in conjunction with primaquine (a tissue schizonticide) is often used to treat infections with *P. vivax, P. ovale,* or *P. malariae.* Because the primary cycle of exoerythrocytic schizogony is not repeated in *P. falciparum* it can be treated effectively with only an erythrocytic schizonticide such as chloroquine. Sulfadoxine and pyrimethamine (Fansidar), quinine, and other drugs are useful in areas of chloroquine-resistant malaria.

Other Hematozoa

Babesiosis is a rare intraerythrocytic infection with *Babesia* spp. Usually, *B. microti*, reservoired in mice and transmitted by Lyme disease ticks (*Ixodes dammini*), is involved in the eastern United States, where cases are becoming more common. Erythrocytic schizogony is not synchronized; most clinical infections are mild and self-limiting, resembling malaria without fever periodicity. Diagnosis is by finding erythrocytic stages on stained blood smears. Babesiosis is treated with clindamycin or quinine.

Tissue Protozoa

Certain tissue-dwelling coccidians such as *Toxoplasma gondii* and *Pneumocystis carinii* recently have become very important infections in immunocompromised patients. Some species of free-living amebae cause fatal cases of meningitis and granulomatous encephalitis; recently, others are reported as the cause of amebic keratitis in contact lens wearers.

Toxoplasmosis
Epidemiology

Toxoplasma gondii is a coccidian with which humans and many other animals may be infected, but the life cycle with sexual reproduction can be completed only in cats. In all other hosts, tachyzoites undergo asexual reproduction during acute infection, disseminating the parasites throughout the body; following the immune response, bradyzoites remain for long periods as nonreproducing intracellular tissue stages in the immunocompetent host. Toxoplasmosis is a major zoonosis. One third to one half of the population in the United States may be infected, with an estimated 3000 to 5000 cases of congenital toxoplasmosis per year. Infection is acquired by ingesting infective oocysts from cat feces, by ingesting uncooked meat or unpasteurized dairy products, by transplacental transmission, or through blood transfusions. Reactivation toxoplasmosis has become an important infection in patients with acquired immunodeficiency syndrome.

Pathogenesis

Bradyzoites occur as intracellular parasites in vacuoles (phagosomes) within host macrophages and other nucleated cells (Fig. 7-4). Since phagosomes with parasites will not fuse with lysosomes, the parasites are not destroyed by host phagocytic cells. This permanently blocked membrane fusion by an unknown mechanism allows the persistence of viable bradyzoites for years as an inapparent infection in the immunocompetent host. Destruction of the host immune system allows reactivation of bradyzoites and recrudescense of acute infection through unrestricted asexual reproduction. Acute toxoplasmosis in the fetus or newborn results from the uncontrolled asexual reproduction by the parasite in a host with an undeveloped immune system. Focal necrosis in many organs and tissues is the principal lesion in acute, recrudescent, and neonatal toxoplasmosis. Neonatal toxoplasmic encephalitis presents with periventricular lesions leading to edema and intracerebral calcification.

Fig. 7-4 Pathogenesis of toxoplasmosis.

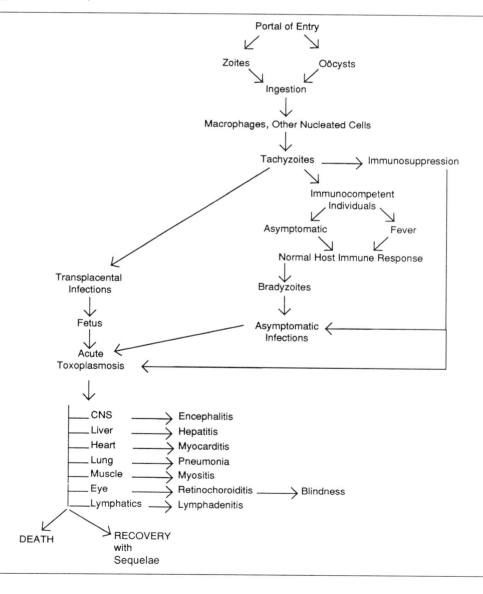

Clinical Correlations

Usually asymptomatic in healthy individuals, acute toxoplasmosis may mimic a mild case of infectious mononucleosis, with chills, fever, headache, myalgic lymphadenitis and extreme fatigue. In 30 to 40 percent of pregnant women, in whom an acute infection develops, transplacental transmission to the fetus occurs. This may result in abortion, prematurity, or neonatal toxoplasmosis with anemia, hepatitis, myocarditis, retinochoroiditis, hydrocephaly and encephalitis, and/or blindness (Fig. 7-4). Pneumonia, myocarditis, myositis, hepatitis, encephalitis, and/or retinochoroiditis are the most common clinical conditions seen in immunocompromised patients.

Diagnosis

Except in patients with acquired immunodeficiency syndrome, for which diagnosis is by clinical symptoms only, serologic tests (indirect fluorescent antibody, indirect hemagglutination assay, enzyme-linked immunosorbent assay) are used in the diagnosis of toxoplasmosis.

Treatment

A pyrimethamine-trisulfapyrimidine combination is the treatment of choice for toxoplasmosis.

Pneumocystosis

Epidemiology

Pneumocystis carinii, a protozoan of undecided taxonomic status, has a direct life cycle with extracellular trophozoites and cysts in the lungs of many species of mammals. It is an opportunistic infection in humans. In about 60 percent of patients with acquired immunodeficiency syndrome, acute pneumocystosis develops (long-term carriers of inactive infections?). Small epidemics have occurred in premature and malnourished children in crowded orphanages and hospitals.

Pathogenesis

Trophozoites line the alveolar walls, blocking gaseous exchange. Although the alveolar septae become thickened with accumulations of lymphocytes, macrophages, and plasma cells, the parasites evoke almost no inflammatory response and, therefore, there is little phagocytosis by tissue macrophages. This results in intraalveolar aggregations of parasites, cellular and necrotic debris, plasma protein, and filopodial processes, which leads to alveolocapillary blockage, oxygen desaturation of the blood, and progressive dyspnea. This is called interstitial plasma cell pneumonia; it is the characteristic lesion of pneumocystosis.

Clinical Correlations

Infections are asymptomatic in immunocompetent individuals. Clinical cases in patients with acquired immunodeficiency syndrome have a slow onset with a dry cough and absence of sputum. A slowly progressive dyspnea leads to cyanosis, which may terminate in death if the infection is untreated. There is usually rapid onset of symptoms after several weeks of administration of immunosuppressive drugs in cases of "transplantation pneumonia." Premature malnourished children manifest symptoms of weakness, progressive dyspnea, extreme tachypnea, cyanosis, and death if the infection is not treated.

Diagnosis

Special stains reveal parasites in percutaneous thoracic needle aspirations or lung tissue biopsies.

Treatment

Trimethoprim-sulfamethoxazole is used for clinical cases; this or aerosolized pentamidine isethionate is used as a chemoprophylactic in patients with acquired immunodeficiency syndrome.

Tissue Amebae

Primary amebic meningoencephalitis (rhinomeningoencephalitis) is a widely distributed but rare infection with the free-living ameba *Naegleria fowleri*, a species with ameboid, cyst, and flagellated stages in the life cycle. Most human infections occur in summer in healthy young persons who have been swimming recently in freshwater streams or reservoirs. Amebae enter the nasal passages and ears, penetrate the cribriform plate into the olfactory bulbs, and invade the brain progressively posteriad to the spinal column. Ameboid trophozoites multiply mostly in the gray matter causing necrosis of the superficial cerebellum and cerebrum. The brain becomes soft and edematous; there is vascular congestion, extensive hemorrhage, and a thin purulent exudate over its surface. Ameboid trophozoites occur in purulent cerebrospinal fluid. Clinical symptoms begin with headache, fever, nausea, and vomiting, which progress to acute signs of meningitis (severe frontal headache, upper respiratory tract disturbances, olfactory disturbances to taste and smell, sore throat, blocked nose). Ultimately, the patient is lethargic, develops a stiff neck, has severe vomiting, and becomes comatose. Most cases are fatal after a clinical course of 3 to 6 days. The infection is diagnosed by finding ameboid trophozoites in cerebrospinal fluid. Amphotericin B and tetracyclines have been used for treatment, but these are of unproven efficacy.

Chronic granulomatous acanthamebic encephalitis is a rare opportunistic infection with *Acanthamoeba* spp., another normally free-living soil and freshwater ameba. Ameboid trophozoites and cysts occur in the central nervous system causing chronic granulomatous encephalitis with areas of focal necrosis. Clinical cases are seen in chronically ill or debilitated immunocompromised patients with no history of contact with freshwater reservoirs or streams. The onset is slow and insidious, leading to a prolonged encephalitis with possible hematogenous spread to the lungs, bone, or skin. Diagnosis is by observing trophozoites and cysts in stained cerebrospinal fluid smears. Sulfadiazine is of possible value in treating this infection.

Acanthamebic keratitis is also an infection with free-living *Acanthamoeba* spp. Numerous cases have recently been reported from North America, Europe, and Australia. The infection occurs in healthy individuals who wear contact lenses, especially the newer flexible types. Amebae occur in commercial washing solutions, tap water, or other water sources, and contaminate the lenses when they are washed. Ameboid trophozoites penetrate the superficial layers of the cornea, producing ulcerative lesions that strongly resemble ocular herpesvirus infections, and may eventually destroy the eye. The clinical course begins with pain and irritation in one or both eyes and progresses with subsequent development of acute inflammatory disease and excruciating pain. Diagnosis is by demonstration of ameboid trophozoites in the eye. This infection can be treated with propamidine isethionate and dibromopropamidine isethionate.

Trematodes (Flukes)

Trematodes are unsegmented flatworms (phylum Platyhelminthes) with an incomplete digestive tract; they have a complicated life history that always includes asexual reproduction in a snail intermediate host. The sexually dimorphic blood flukes cause schistosomiasis, which is a major mortality factor in many tropical areas. Species of hermaphroditic flukes cause liver, lung, and intestinal infections.

Schistosomiasis (Blood Flukes)

Epidemiology

Sexually dimorphic pairs of *Schistosoma* species lie within the abdominal venous plexuses; *S. mansoni* and *S. japonicum* occupy the mesenteric veins and deposit eggs in the intestinal wall while *S. haematobium* is localized in the visceral-pelvic veins and deposits eggs mostly in the urinary bladder wall. Eggs migrate through tissue, escape to the lumen, and are passed in feces or urine. Eggs hatch in fresh water and larvae penetrate a snail and asexually reproduce; infective cercariae are shed back into the water. Humans are infected by cercariae that directly penetrate the intact skin (Fig. 7-5). Following migration through the liver, developing schistosomes localize and mature in abdominal veins. Urinary schistosomiasis (*S. haematobium*) occurs in Africa, the Middle East, and India. Intestinal schistosomiasis occurs in Africa, the Middle East, and Latin America (*S. mansoni*), and in China and Japan (*S. japonicum*). Humans are the primary reservoir for *S. mansoni* and *S. haematobium*; rodents are the reservoir for *S. japonicum*. Approximately one eighth of the world's population is at risk for schistosomiasis, with an estimated 200 to 300 million cases and annual death rate of 500,000 to 1 million persons. Control is difficult because of ethnic and religious practices, fecal and urine contamination of water supplies, expense of chemoprophylactic and therapeutic drugs, no vaccine, and problems with snail control.

Pathogenesis

Adult schistosomes persist in the bloodstream by covering themselves with host antigens or with produced antigens that are so like them that the host antibody-related responses cannot effectively recognize and eliminate them (immunologic camouflage) (Fig. 7-5). Over a period of time female flukes can produce large numbers of eggs. When deposited in the small veins of the intestine or urinary bladder, eggs become walled off; by mechanical and enzymatic action, they migrate through the tissue to reach the lumen of the respective organ. Migrating eggs evoke an intense inflammatory response and if deposited too deeply in the tissue they die and induce formation of a foreign body granuloma. The extent of scarring in the bladder and intestinal wall is both time and density dependent. Likewise, many eggs are swept into portal circulation and become secondarily lodged in the liver, spleen, and lungs. Here, they educe foreign body granulomas, die, and calcify; this leads to extensive fibrosis from scar tissue. The extent of the pathology depends on the species, number of adults in abdominal veins, and duration of the infection. *Schistosoma japonicum* is the most pathogenic species because females lay more eggs and they are deposited in masses.

Clinical Correlations

Early symptoms include cercarial dermatitis, malaise, fever, sweating, lassitude, giant urticariae, abdominal pain, urinary frequency, and/or gastroenteritis. Acute hepatitis may occur as schistosomes migrate through the liver. As adult flukes establish in abdominal veins, acute symptoms of intestinal schistosomiasis include diarrhea or dysentery; with urinary schistosomiasis there is hematuria at the end of micturition. Chronic symptoms occur months to

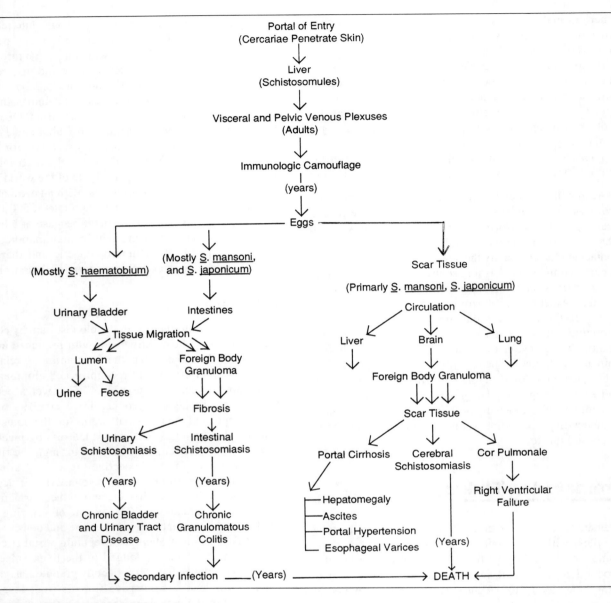

Fig. 7-5 Pathogenesis of schistosomiases.

years later and result from continued insult of migrating eggs through the intestinal or urinary bladder wall plus embolic eggs that lodge in the liver, lungs, and brain. Chronic urinary schistosomiasis presents with polyp formation and fibrosis in the bladder wall, pain, hematuria, contracture, ureter obstruction, secondary bacterial infection, urinary retention, and/or eventual calcification of the bladder wall. Chronic intestinal schistosomiasis resembles granulomatous colitis; there is often intestinal polyposis with bloody diarrhea. Hepatic schistosomiasis with moderate to extensive portal cirrhosis presents with severe hepatomegaly with or without splenomegaly; chronic obstructive liver disease often leads to portal hypertension resulting in esophageal varices and massive ascites. Pulmonary schistosomiasis presents with a nonproductive cough; pseudotubercles formed around embolic eggs result in fibrosis, leading to pulmonary hypertension and possible right ventricular failure (cor pulmonale). Cerebral schistosomiasis is an uncommon chronic form of *S. japonicum* infection; eggs laid in cerebral and spinal cord vasculature cause seizures or myelitis, or both.

Diagnosis

The typical eggs can be observed in urine (*S. haematobium*) or in unstained fecal smears (other species).

Treatment

Praziquantel eliminates adult blood flukes; the egg-induced changes in chronic schistosomiasis are irreversible.

Other Trematodes

Schistosome cercarial dermatitis (swimmer's itch) results from penetration of human skin by cercariae of mammal and bird (especially waterfowl) schistosomes. Schistosomulae persist in the subcutaneous tissues for a short time (1 or 2 days) and then die. Sensitization following repeated exposure leads to increasingly severe dermal lesions; macules form papules with erythema, vesicles, edema, intense pruritus, secondary infection from scratching, and possibly giant urticariae. Diphenhydramine hydrochloride (Benadryl) effectively relieves clinical effects of the allergic response. This zoonosis is most common in the Great Lakes region, Chesapeake Bay area, and parts of the southern United States.

Fascioliasis (sheep liver fluke), caused by *Fasciola hepatica*, is a zoonosis of worldwide distribution and is reservoired by domestic herbivores. It is especially common in France, Algeria, Cuba, Latin America, and other areas where humans eat raw watercress and other aquatic plants on which the cercariae encyst as infective metacercariae. Following ingestion of the flukes, they localize in the bile ducts. Their large size plus the effects of toxic metabolites results in biliary epithelial and ductal connective tissue hyperplasia and partial to total biliary obstruction with possible portal cirrhosis in heavy infections. Severity of disease depends on the number of flukes present. Mild cases present with vomiting and abdominal pain. Symptoms in heavier infections also include fever, chills, jaundice, enlarged tender liver, and eosinophilia. Typical eggs in an unstained fecal smear are diagnostic. Fascioliasis is treated with praziquantel.

Fasciolopsiasis (intestinal fluke), caused by *Fasciolopsis buski*, is a zoonosis reservoired by pigs, dogs, and other mammals in eastern Asia and India. Infection results from ingesting encysted metacercariae on eatable aquatic plants. There are an estimated 10 million cases. Pathogenesis is density dependent, with lesions varying according to the number of flukes in the intestine. The basic lesion results from a large trematode attached to the intestinal mucosa causing mechanical irritation, and leading to inflammation, ulceration, and hemorrhage. Clinical symptoms range from asymptomatic to severe diarrhea, abdominal pain, ascites, facial and abdominal edema, vomiting, and eosinophilia. Death can occur from debilitation and intercurrent infection in severe cases. Typical eggs in an unstained fecal smear are diagnostic. Treatment is with praziquantel.

Paragonimiasis (lung fluke) is a zoonosis with *Paragonimus* spp. reservoired by many different mammals, but especially by wild and domestic cats. Cercariae are released from snails and encyst as infective metacercariae in freshwater crabs and crayfish, which are eaten raw in endemic areas of Africa, Asia, and Latin America. Once ingested, the immature flukes penetrate the intestine and migrate across the diaphragm, where they localize in the lung parenchyma. Here, the basic lesion is an inflammatory and fibrous infiltration forming a cyst wall around paired adult flukes, and causing atrophy and necrosis of adjacent tissues. Eggs infiltrating surrounding tissues educe foreign body granulomas. Early signs of fever and mild cough may progress to paroxysms of coughing with blood-tinged sputum and chest pain. Chronic bronchial inflammation and dilatation, and difficulty in breathing following exertion (dyspnea), may occur in severe cases. Cerebral paragonimiasis is a rare but serious disease caused by migrating flukes that reach the brain and cause convulsive seizures and/or motor and sensory disturbances. Typical eggs can be diagnosed in unstained fecal smears. Praziquantel is the drug of choice for the treatment of paragonimiasis.

Clonorchiasis (Chinese liver fluke), caused by *Clonorchis sinensis*, is a zoonosis with fish-eating mammals (especially cats) as the reservoirs. Cercariae from snails encyst as infective metacercariae on freshwater fish, which are consumed raw in endemic areas of eastern Asia. Immature flukes localize and mature in the distal biliary tree, where they cause bile duct hyperplasia and fibroplasia from mechanical irritation and toxic metabolites. Massive infections can cause portal cirrhosis. Light infections usually are asymptomatic. Heavier infections acquired over time may result in diarrhea and progressive hepatomegaly with associated fever and jaundice. Only in the rare massive infections does massive liver involvement lead to obstructive jaundice, bile duct inflammation and necrosis, liver abscess, and/or retention cysts, which can result in death of the patient. Typical eggs in unstained fecal smears are diagnostic for clonorchiasis. Treatment is with praziquantel.

Several additional trematode infections of more limited distribution infect humans. Echinostomiasis, heterophyiasis, metagonimiasis, gastrodisciasis, and troglotremiasis are intestinal infections. Opisthorchiasis and dicrocoeliasis are liver fluke infections. These diseases will not be discussed here.

Cestodes (Tapeworms)

Cestodes are flatworms (phylum Platyhelminthes) with no digestive tract and a body with many segments (proglottids), each with male and female reproductive organs. Adults are lumen parasites in the small intestine; larvae of some species infect other organs. Life cycles often are

Parasitology

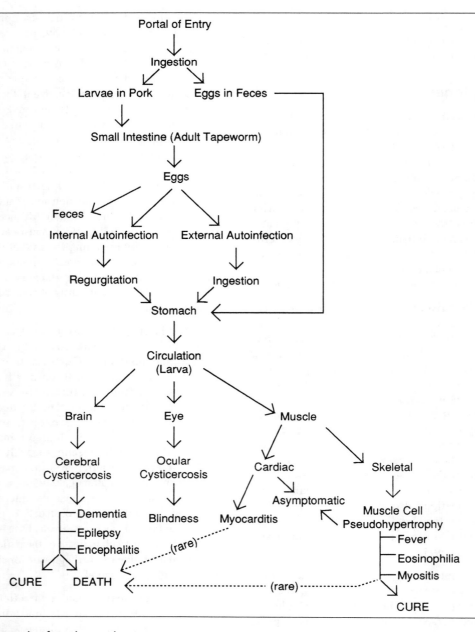

Fig. 7-6 Pathogenesis of cysticercosis.

complicated with one or two invertebrate or vertebrate intermediate hosts. In the United States the most common infections are taeniasis (cysticercosis) and hymenolepiasis.

Taeniasis (Beef and Pork Tapeworm) and Cysticercosis

Epidemiology

Taeniasis is an intestinal infection with the adult tapeworms *Taenia saginata* or *T. solium*. Cysticercosis is a somatic infection with the larval stage of *T. solium*. These

are cosmopolitan but sporadic infections, most common in Latin America, Africa, eastern Asia, the Iberian Peninsula, and Slavic Europe. Humans are the only reservoirs for the adult tapeworms. Infective eggs are passed in feces and ingested by cattle (*T. saginata*) or pigs (*T. solium*), which develop a larval stage (cysticercus) in the musculature. Humans are infected by ingesting the macroscopic cysticerci in raw or poorly cooked beef or pork. By external or internal autoinfection in a patient with taeniasis solium or by ingesting eggs of *T. solium* from an external source, a person can develop cysticercosis (Fig. 7-6).

Pathogenesis

The very large size of the adult tapeworm in the small intestine results in mechanical irritation to the mucosa. Otherwise, there is little pathology in taeniasis. In contrast, cysticercosis is a serious disease, with cysticerci forming space-occupying lesions surrounded by an inflammatory response and a fibrous capsule (Fig. 7-6). Cysticerci ultimately die, leaving a necrotic lesion that eventually caseates and calcifies. In muscle, they cause pseudohypertrophy, and symptoms depend on their location and numbers. In the brain cysticerci may cause noncommunicating hydrocephalus if they localize in the ventricle, acute to chronic meningitis with communicating hydrocephalus if they develop in the subarachnoid cysterns, or seizures and focal neurologic defects if they occur in the parenchyma. Cysticerci in the spinal column, eye, and heart now are reported more frequently than they were in the past.

Clinical Correlations

Taeniasis is usually asymptomatic, except that most patients pass proglottids. There may be increased appetite, vague abdominal discomfort, hunger pains, chronic indigestion, weakness, weight loss, and/or eosinophilia. Cysticercosis may be asymptomatic or present with variable signs, depending on location and number of cysticerci. There may be firm nodules in subcutaneous tissues or muscle pseudohypertrophy with myositis, eosinophilia, and high prolonged fever if cysticerci are numerous. In neurocysticercosis, dead or dying larvae may evoke an intense inflammatory response leading to acute encephalitis. Space-occupying lesions may cause dementia, epileptiform convulsive seizures, mental changes, or other clinical signs of brain tumor. Compression necrosis in the upper brain stem may lead to lethargy, hyperactive tendon reflexes, and visual problems. Ocular cysticercosis results in decreased visual acuity and visual field defects. Myocardial cysticercosis is often asymptomatic, but it may result in mild to severe myocarditis.

Diagnosis

Taeniasis is diagnosed by the typical eggs in unstained fecal smears. The species are differentiated only by examining proglottids passed in the feces. Cysticercosis is diagnosed by radiography or computed tomographic (CT) scan, or serologically (enzyme-linked immunosorbent assay).

Treatment

Praziquantel is used for taeniasis. Cysticerci are surgically removed or can be treated with praziquantel plus dexamethasone (except for ocular cysticercosis).

Hymenolepiasis

Epidemiology

This is an intestinal infection with the adult dwarf tapeworm *Hymenolepis nana* or the rat tapeworm *H. diminuta*. They are cosmopolitan zoonoses; *H. nana* is most common, with an estimated 20 to 30 million cases. Humans are infected with *H. nana* by ingesting eggs in food or drink contaminated with human feces or mouse droppings, and also by ingesting uncooked grain products containing insects (grain beetles) infected with cysticercoid larvae. The entire life cycle of *H. nana* can be completed in the human host, with cysticoid larvae developing from eggs in the small intestine. Internal autoinfections are common and without treatment infections may persist for years. Infection with *H. diminuta* can develop only following ingestion of insect intermediate hosts in uncooked grain products. Often, there are mixed infections of the two species.

Pathogenesis

The small adult tapeworms cause only minor mechanical irritation in the small intestine; they may educe an eosinophilia.

Clinical Correlations

Often, infections are asymptomatic. Complaints may include abdominal pain, diarrhea, headache, dizziness, and anal pruritus.

Diagnosis

The typical eggs in unstained fecal smears are diagnostic.

Treatment

Praziquantel is an effective treatment.

Diphyllobothriasis and Sparganosis

Epidemiology

Diphyllobothriasis is an intestinal infection with the adult of *Diphyllobothrium latum* and related species; sparganosis is a subcutaneous infection with the plerocercoid larvae (spargana) of animal tapeworms related to *D. latum*. Diphyllobothriasis occurs in areas where humans consume raw or poorly cooked fish (northern Europe, Great Lakes region, Latin America, Japan); sparganosis is cosmopolitan but rare. Both infections are zoonoses with fish-eating mammals as reservoirs. Humans acquire diphyllobothriasis from ingesting raw or smoked fish that contains the infective plerocercoid larvae. Sparganosis is acquired as a result of drinking water containing copepods (*Cyclops* spp., etc.) infected with the first-stage procercoid larvae, ingesting raw or poorly cooked meat containing second-stage plerocercoid larvae, or using vertebrate flesh containing plerocercoid larvae as a poultice on an infected wound or eye.

Pathogenesis

The large adult cestode in the small intestine causes mild mechanical irritation and may compete with the host for glucose and amino acids; if located in the proximal part of the jejunum, it may compete for vitamin B_{12} and cause a deficiency. In sparganosis mechanical damage and toxic effects of the larval metabolites cause a massive inflammatory response around the larva in the subcutaneous tissues. The number of lesions and severity of infection depend on the number and location of larvae. Larvae may migrate for some time before they become localized; their death results in a caseous mass without calcification.

Clinical Correlations

Except for passing proglottids, diphyllobothriasis is often asymptomatic, or there may be complaints similar to those of taeniasis. A megaloblastic pernicious type of anemia occurs in some patients. In cases of sparganosis there are initially soft, edematous, and painful subcutaneous nodules without erythema. These may later suppurate as boil-like or acne-like nodular pustules that persist for weeks to months as the larva dies and resorbs. Ocular lesions are very painful, with erythema and edema of the conjunctiva, corneal ulceration, or toxemia, or the spargana may penetrate the cornea and localize in the anterior or posterior chamber of the eye.

Diagnosis

Typical eggs in unstained fecal smears distinguish *D. latum* infections. Diagnosis of sparganosis is difficult and often only possible after surgery.

Treatment

Praziquantel is the drug of choice for both infections. Often spargana are removed surgically.

Other Cestodes

Echinococciasis (hydatidosis) is an infection with the larvae of *Echinococcus* spp. The adult and larval stage (hydatid) of unilocular hydatidosis (*E. granulosus*) are reservoired mostly in domestic dogs and sheep, respectively; reservoirs of the less common multilocular hydatidosis (*E. multilocularis*) and polycystic hydatidosis (*E. vogeli*) are foxes and small rodents, and bush dogs and large rodents, respectively. Unilocular hydatidosis occurs mostly in temperate to subtropical sheep-raising areas of North and South America, Europe, Asia, Africa, and Australia. Multilocular hydatidosis ranges throughout temperate and arctic Eurasia and North America. Polycystic hydatidosis occurs in northern South America. All three forms of hydatids mostly occur in the liver (rarely lung, brain, bone). Unilocular hydatids grow by exogenous budding of scolices (heads) within a single fluid-filled cyst surrounded by a thick laminated membrane. The lesion behaves much like an expanding tumor; the cyst grows slowly for years, sometimes reaching 30 cm in diameter. There is a danger of anaphylaxis if a cyst ruptures. The multilocular hydatid is not delimited by an exterior membrane and grows by exogeneously budding scolices into viable tissue, behaving much like an invasive tumor with necrosis at the center of the lesion. The polycystic hydatid is like a unilocular hydatid with exogenous budding at its surface. Clinical signs depend on the size and location of the hydatid. Eosinophilia is common. Infection with unilocular/polycystic hydatid in the liver may result in indigestion, biliary colic, and jaundice; lung infection may present with cough, breathing difficulty, chest pain, and blood in the sputum. Multilocular hydatid in the liver leads to typical signs of intrahepatic portal tension, including hepatomegaly, jaundice, and ascites. Diagnosis is often difficult; serologic tests (indirect hemagglutination assay and enzyme-linked immunosorbent assay) confirm hydatidosis. Treatment is usually by surgical intervention, but cortisteroids and mebendazole may be useful.

Intestinal Nematodes

Nematodes (roundworms) are a class of slender wormlike organisms in the phylum Aschelminthes. They are covered by an impervious cuticle, have a complete digestive tract, and are sexually dimorphic. There are many free-living and parasitic species. All species that infect the human gastrointestinal tract have direct life cycles. Some of these are the most common of all infections in humans.

Ascariasis (Large Intestinal Roundworm)

Epidemiology

Adults of *Ascaris lumbricoides* occur in the small intestine. Eggs are infective after development in the soil; once ingested, they hatch and larvae undergo a migration through the lungs before localizing and maturing in the small intestine. This is the most common human parasite, infecting one fourth of the world's population (>1 billion people). Humans are the only reservoir and children are most commonly infected.

Pathogenesis

Larvae migrating through the alveolar walls cause mechanical damage and irritation by their metabolic and secretory products. They induce a transient pneumonitis often called verminous pneumonia. The large, muscular adults maintain their position in the intestinal lumen by constant movement, resulting in mechanical irritation to the mucosa; they sometimes migrate to extraintestinal sites (liver, esophagus) or occlude the intestine (if there are large numbers).

Clinical Correlations

Pulmonary ascariasis may be asymptomatic in mild cases; clinical signs in heavier infections include eosinophilia, transient fever, coughing, rales, blood in sputum, and asthmatic attacks in sensitized persons. Intestinal ascariasis is often asymptomatic except for passing worms (light infections). More severe cases may present with vague to colicky epigastric or umbilical pain with symptoms of partial to complete ileocecal obstruction, including fever, malaise, abdominal distention and tenderness, vomiting, and rebound tenderness.

Diagnosis

Typical eggs are seen in unstained fecal smears.

Treatment

Mebendazole (Vermox) is effective against adults and larvae. Surgery may be required in cases of obstruction.

Enterobiasis (Pinworms)
Epidemiology

Enterobius vermicularis is a cosmopolitan colon parasite of humans. Adult females migrate into the perianal area and deposit infective eggs. Children are most frequently infected. Autoinfections from ingestion of eggs or retroinfections by hatched larvae in the perianal region are common. There are many adult asymptomatic carriers. Pinworm is one of the most common parasitic infections.

Pathogenesis

Pinworms are lumen dwellers that usually cause no lesions; sometimes they evoke granulomas by burrowing into the intestinal wall or migrating up the female reproductive tract. Cutaneous irritation in the perianal area results from scratching and secondary bacterial infection. Pinworm appendicitis is rare.

Clinical Correlations

Infection is asymptomatic in adults. In children, cases range from asymptomatic to presenting with intense anal pruritus, anorexia, restlessness, insomnia, and behavorial changes.

Diagnosis

Most cases are diagnosed by mothers observing the small nematodes in the perianal area of their children. Confirmation is by finding eggs in the perianal area by the cellophane tape slide technique.

Treatment

Mebendazole is the drug of choice for pinworms.

Trichuriasis (Whipworm)
Epidemiology

Trichuris trichiuria is a whiplike nematode with its slender anterior extremity embedded into the mucosa and its larger posterior extremity hanging into the lumen of the large intestine. Eggs are infective following development in the soil. This is a common (estimated one eighth of the world's population is infected) and cosmopolitan infection in the warmer wetter climates. Humans are the only reservoir. As with pinworm, there is no pulmonary migration of larvae.

Pathogenesis

The macroscopic adults in the mucosa cause mechanical and other damage, resulting in acute inflammation of the colonic mucosa; heavy infections (thousands of worms) may demonstrate hemorrhage, coagulative necrosis, and catarrhal inflammation. In young children with massive infections, the continual irritation of the rectum due to constant tenesmus and edema may result in brief periods of rectal prolapse with subsequent retention.

Clinical Correlations

Light infections are asymptomatic. Heavier infections may result in epigastric pain, abdominal distention, vomiting, fever, bloody diarrhea, anemia, eosinophilia, and/or rectal prolapse.

Diagnosis

Typical eggs occur in unstained fecal smears.

Treatment

Mebendazole is the usual treatment.

Parasitology

Strongyloidiasis (Intestinal Threadworm)

Epidemiology

Small, threadlike, parthenogenetic females, eggs, and larvae of *Strongyloides stercoralis* infect the mucosa of the small intestine. The life cycle is complicated with a free-living cycle of males and females in the soil. Infection results from direct penetration of the intact skin by microscopic filariform larvae. Gravid females in the small intestine release rhabditiform larvae that are passed in the feces. External and internal autoinfections resulting from molting of rhabditiform to infective filariform larvae are common and result in long-term (many years) infections. Following skin penetration filariform larvae undergo a pulmonary migration before establishing themselves and maturing in the small intestine. Humans are the primary source of infection; dogs and other mammals are possible reservoirs. Strongyloidiasis is of worldwide distribution in the subtropics and tropics.

Pathogenesis

Allergic dermatitis (ground itch) due to hypersensitivity from repeated exposure to larvae may occur. Pneumonitis identical to pulmonary ascariasis is common. Adult females, eggs, and larvae evoke an acute inflammatory response in the intestinal mucosa, resulting in congestion (mild infections) or mucosal necrosis, submucosal inflammation and fibrosis, microhemorrhages, and/or larval dissemination to all parts of the intestine or possibly other organs (heavier infections). Pronounced eosinophilia is usually present. At certain times and by an unknown mechanism, an increased proportion of rhabditiform larvae are transformed to filariform larvae in the intestine. This is hyperinfection syndrome if only the lungs and intestines are involved. Disseminated strongyloidiasis results if numbers of migrating larvae are large enough to involve also the liver, heart, kidneys, pancreas, central nervous system, and so forth; usually, this occurs only in malnourished, debilitated, or immunosuppressed patients.

Clinical Correlations

An intensely pruritic patchy dermatitis on the feet, pneumonitis with an irritative nonproductive cough, and eosinophilia characterize early stages of strongyloidiasis. Intestinal strongyloidiasis cases range from asymptomatic to those with anorexia, nausea, vomiting, severe diarrhea, malabsorption syndrome with excessive fat or blood in the feces, or ulcerative colitis symptoms. Hyperinfection results in fever, acute gastritis, difficulty in breathing and cough, weakness, and rarely death.

Diagnosis

Rhabditiform or filariform larvae, or both, in an unstained fecal smear are diagnostic.

Treatment

Thiabendazole (Mintezol) is the usual treatment.

Hookworm Infection

Epidemiology

Adult hookworms (*Ancylostoma duodenale, Necator americanus*) are small nematodes attached to the mocosa of the small intestine. Eggs are passed in the feces, where they hatch into free-living larvae that ultimately molt to infective filariform larvae. The latter penetrate the intact skin and subsequently undergo a lung migration before localization and maturation in the small intestine. Hookworm distribution is worldwide in the warm and wet subtropics and tropics. Humans are the only reservoir; there are many asymptomatic carriers.

Pathogenesis

Dermatitis results from repeated exposure to larvae. Hookworm pneumonitis is usually less severe than pulmonary ascariasis or strongyloidiasis because larvae are smaller and fewer in number. Adult hookworms attach to the intestinal mucosa by their mouth parts, secrete an anticoagulant, and continually pump blood through their digestive tract as a source for food and oxygen (aerobic pathways of carbohydrate metabolism). Blood loss may reach 0.25 ml per day per worm. Severity of infection with resultant hookworm disease is a density-dependent relationship based on hookworm numbers and the patient's ability to compensate for blood loss. The latter depends on the patient's nutritional and general health status. Hemorrhagic anemia results from failure in the compensatory replacement of iron losses; well-nourished healthy persons with many hookworms may not develop anemia, whereas malnourished and protein-deficient individuals infected with fewer hookworms may be anemic. There is always a negative correlation between hookworm numbers and hemoglobin levels in any population.

Clinical Correlations

Initial signs may include "ground itch" dermatitis and mild pneumonitis. Intestinal manifestations may range from asymptomatic to signs of chronic hookworm disease, including bloody diarrhea, weakness, fatigue, cardiac palpitation, pallor, mild to severe anemia with possible hyperproteinemia, potbellied children with hemoglobin values to 15 percent, and hypereosinophilia.

Diagnosis

Eggs are diagnostic in unstained fecal smears.

Treatment

Mebendazole is the treatment of choice.

Other Gastrointestinal Nematodes

Marine fish are often infected by the larvae of *Anasakis* sp. and related nematodes; adults occur in marine mammals. If these larvae are ingested by humans in raw fish, they cause eosinophilic granulomas in the stomach and intestines. Severe gastroenteritis is the clinical consequence. Surgery is the only treatment for clinical anasakiasis.

Eustrongyloidiasis is an infection with *Eustrongyloides* spp. larvae, which infect the fish commonly used for bait by fishermen. The practice of swallowing bait minnows with beer on fishing trips has resulted in acute gastro-nematodiasis when the large larvae penetrate the stomach wall. Surgical intervention has been necessary in several cases in the eastern United States.

Other nematodiases that affect the human gastrointestinal tract are of limited distribution. Intestinal capillariasis in the Philippines and Thailand, and trichostrongyliasis in Asia, are sporadic infections rarely seen by physicians in North America.

Tissue Nematodes

Tissue-dwelling nematodes represent a heterogeneous group that parasitize many different organs and tissues. These infections evoke a very severe type I hypersensitivity reaction that accounts for the hypereosinophilia and hyper-gammaglobulinemia E as a major host response.

Trichinosis

Epidemiology

Infection with the larvae of *Trichinella spiralis* is a widespread zoonosis in temperate areas, but sporadic in arctic and tropical climates. Pigs and rats are the primary reservoirs, with infective larvae encysted in their musculature. Following ingestion in infected raw pork, larvae mature to adults in the small intestine, reproduce, and release larvae that migrate to skeletal muscle cells and subsequently encyst; encysted larvae may remain viable for years. An estimated 150,000 to 300,000 individuals are infected in the United States, but fewer than 150 clinical cases are seen per year. Most infected pork comes from small rural abatoirs and certain isolated pig farms.

Pathogenesis

Depending on intensity of infection and the host's previous experience with trichinosis, adult nematodes are usually rejected due to a tissue immune response within 50 days after infection. Migrating larvae released by adults in the intestine evoke hypereosinophilia and vasculitis, leading to splinter hemorrhages under the fingernails, periorbital edema around the eyes, and rarely central nervous system involvement. Larval encystment results in destruction of striated muscle cells with inflammation (myositis). Each larva penetrates a skeletal muscle cell, becomes tightly coiled, and causes host-cell necrosis with development of a thick capsule (nurse cell) around the whole complex; the nurse cell calcifies following death of the larva.

Clinical Correlations

Most infections are asymptomatic. In only the heaviest infections are nausea, vomiting, diarrhea, and abdominal pain seen in the first few weeks following ingestion of raw pork. During larval migration there may be fever, circum-orbital edema around the eyes, petechial hemorrhages under the nails, leukocytosis with hypereosinophilia, and hyperglobulinemia E. Larvae entering muscle cells result in mild to severe myositis with painful and pressure-sensitive muscles. Myocarditis, encephalitis, meningitis, pneumonitis, nephritis, and/or death occur only in the most severe cases.

Diagnosis

Trichinosis is diagnosed by finding larvae in muscle biopsies or by serologic testing (enzyme-linked immunosorbent assay).

Treatment

Prednisone plus mebendazole is useful in treating clinical cases.

Lymphatic Filariasis (Bancroftian and Malayan Filariasis)

Epidemiology

Infection with the filariids *Wuchereria bancrofti* or *Brugia malayi* results in small adult nematodes in the lymphatics and microscopic larvae (microfilariae) in the bloodstream. Mosquitoes (*Culex* spp., *Aedes* spp., and *Anopheles* spp., etc.) are vectors (Fig. 7-7). Humans are the only reservoirs for *W. bancrofti*; monkeys, dogs, and other mammals are reservoirs for *B. malayi*. Lymphatic filariasis is endemic in humid areas between 40°N and 30°S latitudes. By an unknown mechanism there is nocturnal periodicity of microfilariae in the peripheral circualtion, with their high-

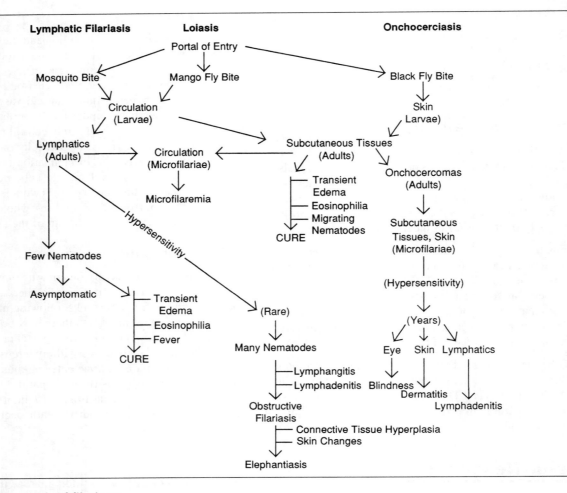

Fig. 7-7 Pathogenesis of filariases.

est densities occurring during the period of greatest activity of night-feeding mosquito vectors.

Pathogenesis

The basic mechanism of pathogenesis results from the inflammatory response educed by adult nematodes in the lymphatics (mostly pelvic and inguinal nodes) (Fig. 7-7). In many individuals, infection results in transient edema and hypereosinophilia with fever and microfilaremia (microfilaria in the bloodstream). In certain sensitized persons, inflammation of the lymph nodes (lymphadenitis) and vessels (lymphangitis) results in fibrosis, followed by lymphedema from diversion of lymph fluid into adjacent tissues. Chronic obstruction follows repeated inflammatory episodes plus connective tissue hyperplasia and results in woody induration of the affected tissue. After many years, there may be massive thickening and verrucous changes in the overlying skin leading to severe elephantiasis of the affected extremity.

Clinical Correlations

In the acute inflammatory period, vague generalized symptoms may be present, plus an urticarial rash, hypereosinophilia, and microfilaremia. Subacute obstructive filariasis presents with signs of lymphangitis, lymphadenitis, inflammation and swelling in the male genitalia, secondary bacterial abscess, and lymphedema. During the chronic obstructive phase, there is usually no microfilaremia; clinical signs include rupture of lymph vessels with lymph fluid in the scrotum, connective tissues, urine, and abdominal cavity. Elephantiasis of affected extremities may be an uncommon late complication.

Diagnosis

Finding typical sheathed microfilaria in stained blood smears is diagnostic during the earlier phases of infection. Chronic filariasis is diagnosed clinically.

Treatment

Diethylcarbamazine (Hetrazan) is used for treatment of lymphatic filariasis.

Onchocerciasis (River Blindness)

Epidemiology

Onchocerciasis (river blindness) results from infection with the long, threadlike *Onchocerca volvulus* adults in subcutaneous nodules (onchocercomas) and microscopic unsheathed microfilariae in the skin. Humans are the only reservoirs of infection. This filariid is transmitted by a black fly (*Simulium* spp.) vector (Fig. 7-7). Onchocerciasis is endemic in Africa and Latin America. Transmission depends on the vector's distribution and its anthropophilic feeding habits.

Pathogenesis

Groups of adults are encapsulated in tough, fibrous subcutaneous granulomas (Fig. 7-7). They release large numbers of microfilariae into the skin and subcutaneous tissues. By continual antigenic stimulation over time, microfilariae cause severe allergic reactions; deposition of tissue immune complexes results in dermal lesions, obstructive lymphangitis, and ocular lesions (possible blindness).

Clinical Correlations

Onchocercomas may appear anywhere on the body. They are painless, or may be hot, edematous, and painful. Onchodermatitis with dermal lesions caused by microfilariae presents as a maculopapular pruritic rash, depigmentation, patchy erythematous dermatitis, papulopustular nodules, or pruritic papular eruptions on one extremity (sowdah). Chronically infected skin loses its elasticity; it becomes atrophied and wrinkled, with possible development of inguinal and femoral hernias, hanging groin, and/or elephantiasis. Chronic lymphatic involvement may include obstructive lymphadenitis and hydrocele in the pelvic region of some patients. Ophthalmologic lesions usually begin as punctate keratitis with microfilariae in the cornea and in the anterior chamber. Corneal opacities coalesce and chronic inflammation of the iris and ciliary body lead to blindness from pupillary occlusion.

Diagnosis

Unsheathed microfilariae are seen in skin-snip biopsies. Serologic tests (indirect fluorescent antibody test, enzyme-linked immunosorbent assay) are available.

Treatment

Ivermectin is the drug of choice for treatment in endemic areas. Periodic nodulectomy is also effective.

Other Tissue Nematodes

Cutaneous larval migrans is not an uncommon infection in the southern United States and Latin America with the larvae of dog and cat hookworms (*Ancylostoma caninum, A. braziliense*). Children are most frequently involved. Microscopic filariform larvae penetrate the skin, cause mechanical trauma, and release excretory and secretory products in the subcutaneous tissues. Larvae wander for several days, evoking an intense inflammatory response before they ultimately die (humans are an unacceptable definitive host). The skin lesion is an erythematous, serpiginous, linear, elevated tunnel that is several centimeters long. There is severe pruritus around the lesion, loss of sleep, secondary bacterial infection from scratching, local edema, hypergammaglobulinemia E, eosinophilia, and possibly verminous pneumonia with eosinophilia, dry cough, and a transient pulmonary infiltrate if large numbers of larvae reach the lungs. Local freezing of lesions kills the larvae and relieves the pruritus. Thiabendazole is used in severe cases.

Visceral larval migrans (toxascariasis) is also a zoonosis reservoired by dogs and cats in the southern United States and other areas where children are exposed to pet feces. Upon ingestion of the eggs of the dog or cat ascarids (*Toxocara canis, T. cati*) the larvae undergo a pulmonary migration. Unable to localize and mature in the human intestine, the microscopic larvae wander in the visceral (usually liver, lungs, heart, brain, and eye) organs for several days before they die and calcify. Wandering larvae cause mechanical damage and release cytotoxic substances, resulting in necrosis, hemorrhage, and inflammation; a foreign body granuloma develops around dead, calcified nematode larvae. Continuous migration of larvae in heavy infections in children who have been repeatedly infected leads to extensive inflammatory tracks and trails in tissue. Clinical symptoms vary according to the intensity of infecting egg dose and location of larvae; the infection often runs a chronic benign course with eosinophilia as the only sign, and is self-limiting in the absence of reinfection. Severe cases present with hypereosinophilia, hepatomegaly with fever and pain, hypergammaglobulinemia, patchy pneumonitis with dry cough, and sometimes lymphadenopathy, retinal detachment, heart failure, or epilepsy. Diagnosis is often by clinical signs alone. Serologic tests (indirect fluorescent antibody test, enzyme-linked immunosorbent assay) are available. Thiabendazole is an effective treatment for severe cases.

Parasitology

Loiasis (African eye worm) is a filariid nematode infection transmitted by blood-feeding mango (deer) flies (*Chrysops* spp.) (Fig. 7-7). It is a possible zoonosis from monkeys. Humans are considered the primary reservoir for *Loa loa*, which is endemic only in central Africa. Following inoculation, it takes one to several years for the immature worms to mature and produce infective microfilariae in the peripheral bloodstream. During this time they wander extensively in the subcutaneous tissues causing hypereosinophilia and transient allergic edema (Calabar swellings). Often the first symptom is when the several centimeter long nematode migrates beneath the conjunctiva or in the skin across the bridge of the nose. The most common lesions are Calabar swellings, which are transient, erythematous, pruritic, edematous areas, especially at the wrists and ankles. This is a common infection in persons returning from travels in Central Africa. Diagnosis is usually based on clinical symptoms, since sheathed microfilariae appear in stained blood smears only after the nematodes mature. Loiasis is treated with Hetrazan.

Mansonelliasis is a form of benign filariasis caused by *Mansonella ozzardi*, *M. perstans* or *M. streptocara*. It is a possible zoonosis from apes and monkeys. Humans are the primary reservoir for infection in endemic areas of Africa and Latin America. Biting midges (*Culidoides* spp.; also, black flies for *M. ozzardi*) are the vectors. *Mansonella ozzardi* adults occur in mesenteries and visceral fat with microfilariae in peripheral blood and skin. Adults of *M. perstans* localize in the peritoneal, pleural, and pericardial cavities; microfilariae are in peripheral blood. Mature *M. streptocara* are in subcutaneous tissues; microfilariae infect the skin. Often, the only clinical sign of any of these infections is hypereosinophilia; vague symptoms of fever, skin rash, transient edema, lymphadenopathy, and/or abdominal pain may occur. Unsheathed microfilariae in skin biopsies or stained blood smears, or both, are diagnostic. Asymptomatic cases are not treated. Hetrazan will eliminate the adult nematodes and larvae.

In the United States, there have been reports of human infections with animal filariids. These include pulmonary lesions resembling those of lung cancer (coin lesions) from the dog heartworm *Dirofilaria immitis*, nodular cutaneous lesions from animal *Dirofilaria* spp., and lymphatic infections of animal *Brugia* spp.

Angiostrongyliasis is infection with *Angiostrongylus cantonensis* (eosinophilic meningitis) or *A. costaricensis* (abdominal angiostrongyliasis). Both are zoonotic infections harbored by wild rats and have land snail or slug intermediate hosts. Humans become infected by ingesting infective larvae in raw snails (*A. cantonensis*) or on uncooked green vegetables (*A. costaricensis*). Eosinophilic meningitis is usually a benign, self-limiting infection resulting

from wandering larvae in the central nervous system. These induce an eosinophilia of the cerebrospinal fluid, sometimes with signs of acute meningitis or meningoencephalitis. It is endemic in southeastern Asia and Oceania including Hawaii. Abdominal angiostrongyliasis in Latin America is often a serious infection, especially in children. Adult nematodes localize in abdominal and mesenteric arterioles where they induce a severe chronic inflammatory response; massive granulomas may result in partial to complete intestinal obstruction. An enzyme-linked immunosorbent assay test is confirmatory for eosinophilic meningitis. Abdominal angiostrongyliasis is usually confirmed at surgery. Thiabendazole may be effective in clinical cases of eosinophilic meningitis. Usually, only surgery is effective in correcting obstructive abdominal angiostrongyliasis.

Dracunculiasis (guinea worm) has been targeted by the World Health Organization for eradication within the next few years. *Dracunculus medinensis* is still endemic in parts of Africa, the Middle East, and India. Humans are the major reservoirs of infection; zoonotic hosts include dogs and other mammals. Infection results from ingestion of water-containing copepods (*Cyclops* spp.) with infective larvae. The large nematodes are localized in the subcutaneous tissues of an extremity in a long, indurated tortuous tunnel. An ulcerative lesion develops in the skin over the female worm and a loop of her prolapsed uterus releases large numbers of larvae when it is exposed to water. The edematous, painful, and often debilitating ulcerative lesion persists for 2 to 3 weeks until release of all the larvae, after which the worm dies and calcifies. Treatment is usually by manual or surgical extraction. Hetrazan, thiabendazole, or metronidazole will eliminate the nematode.

Questions

Directions: Each group of items in this section consists of lettered options followed by a set of numbered items. For each item, select one lettered option that is most closely associated with it. Each lettered option may be selected once, more than once, or not at all.

Questions 1–5: Match each infection with its vector.

    A. Black fly
    B. Mosquito
    C. Reduviid bug
    D. Sand fly
    E. Tsetse fly

1. African trypanosomiasis
2. Chagas' disease
3. Leishmaniasis
4. Malaria
5. Onchocerciasis

Parasitology

Questions 6–10: Match the infection with the stage that is infective for humans.

 A. Cercariae
 B. Cysts
 C. Eggs
 D. Filariform larvae
 E. Microfilariae

6. Amebiasis
7. Ascariasis
8. Giardiasis
9. Schistosomiasis
10. Strongyloidiasis

Questions 11–15: Match the infection with its appropriate drug treatment.

 A. Diethylcarbamazine
 B. Mebendazole
 C. Metronidazole
 D. Praziquantel
 E. Sodium antimony gluconate

11. Ascariasis
12. Leishmaniasis
13. Lymphatic filariasis
14. Vaginal trichomoniasis
15. Taeniasis

Questions 16–20: Match the infection with its associated mechanism of pathogenicity.

 A. Antigenic variability
 B. Blocked phagosome-lysosome fusion
 C. Immunologic camouflage
 D. Invasive exogenous budding
 E. Synchronous erythrocytic schizogony

16. African sleeping sickness
17. Malaria
18. Multilocular hydatidosis
19. Schistosomiasis
20. Toxoplasmosis

Questions 21–25: Match the infection with the primary pathologic lesion.

 A. Interstitial plasma cell pneumonia
 B. Hemorrhagic anemia
 C. Lymphoreticular hyperplasia
 D. Muscle cell pseudohypertrophy
 E. Portal hypertension

21. Hookworm disease
22. Visceral leishmaniasis
23. Pneumocystosis
24. Schistosomiasis
25. Trichinosis

Directions: Each of the numbered items or incomplete statements in this section is followed by answers or by completions of the statement. Select the one lettered answer or completion that is best in each case.

26. A 27-year-old white man returning from a 2-month active military duty in Panama was hospitalized with chills and fever, and a unilateral conjunctivitis with facial edema and regional lymphangitis. Stained thin blood smears revealed extracellular trypomastigotes. What is the most probable diagnosis?
 A. African trypanosomiasis
 B. Babesiosis
 C. Chagas' disease
 D. Malaria
 E. Lymphatic filariasis

27. Opportunistic infections in immunocompromised patients may include all of the following **except**:
 A. Acanthamebic keratitis
 B. Chronic granulomatous acanthamebic encephalitis
 C. Disseminated strongyloidiasis
 D. Protracted cryptosporidiosis
 E. Reactivation toxoplasmosis

28. In a young child from the southeastern United States with a history of recurrent febrile illness, transient pneumonitis, hypereosinophilia, and hepatomegaly, which of the following should always be included in the differential diagnosis?
 A. Amebic liver abscess
 B. Clonorchiasis
 C. Hepatic schistosomiasis
 D. Visceral larval migrans
 E. Unilocular hydatid disease

29. Embolic egg-induced foreign body granulomas are common lesions in which of the following?
 A. Abdominal angiostrongyliasis
 B. Clonorchiasis
 C. Fascioliasis
 D. Hepatic ascariasis
 E. Schistosomiasis

30. Now also used as a chemoprophylactic against pneumocystosis in AIDS patients, clinical pneumocystosis and isosporidiosis are effectively treated with which of the following?
 A. Chloroquine and primaquine
 B. Clindamycin and quinine
 C. Perimethamine and trisulfapyrimidine
 D. Spiramycin and metronidazole
 E. Trimethoprim and sulfamethoxazole

31. Progressive dyspnea resulting from alveolocapillary blockage caused by asexually reproducing trophozoites that fail to evoke a tissue macrophage response describes the pathogenicity of:
 A. Cysticercosis
 B. Paragonimiasis
 C. Pneumocystosis
 D. Pulmonary ascariasis
 E. Pulmonary schistosomiasis

32. Ulcerative colitis describes the intestinal lesions seen in clinical cases of which of the following?
 A. Ascariasis

B. Amebiasis

C. Cryptosporidiasis

D. Giardiasis

E. Enterobiasis

33. Enterobiasis, strongyloidiasis, and hymenolepiasis have which of the following in common?

A. Autoinfection

B. Filariform larvae

C. Nematodes

D. Nonpathogenic

E. Zoonoses

34. Which of the following is a characteristic lesion of children in the tropics with visceral leishmaniasis, malaria, or schistosomiasis?

A. Cor pulmonale

B. Giant urticaria

C. Hemoglobinuria

D. Hepatomegaly

E. Meningoencephalitis

35. Because the primary exoerythrocytic cycle of schizogony is not repeated, it is necessary to treat the infection with only an erythrocytic schizonticidal drug in which of the following?

A. *Leishmania donovani*

B. *Plasmodium falciparum*

C. *Plasmodium vivax*

D. *Plasmodium malariae*

E. *Trypanosoma brucei gambiense*

36. Disseminated intravascular coagulation resulting in decreased microcirculation and tissue anoxia is responsible for the severe renal and cerebral manifestations of:

A. African sleeping sickness

B. Amebic meningoencephalitis

C. Malignant malaria

D. Neonatal toxoplasmosis

E. Urinary schistosomosis

37. A 3-year-old girl was admitted to the hospital with severe emaciation and anemia secondary to a long-term bloody diarrhea. While hospitalized, she experienced several episodes of rectal prolapse. Numerous white worms were seen attached to the surface of the prolapsed rectal mucosa. The patient was successfully treated with mebendazole without further complications. What is the diagnosis?

A. Dwarf tapeworm

B. Hookworm

C. Pinworm

D. Visceral larval migrans

E. Whipworm

38. Initial gastritis followed by hypereosinophilia and vasculitis, and ultimately myositis, are symptoms of clinical cases of which of the following?

A. Cysticercosis

B. Dracunculiasis

C. Sparganosis

D. Trichinosis

E. Visceral larval migrans

39. The infective larval stage in fascioliasis, fasciolopsiasis, clonorchiasis, and paragonimiasis that is encysted on certain plant and animal foods is called which of the following?

A. Cercaria

B. Cysticercoid

C. Filariform

D. Metacercaria

E. Plerocercoid

40. Schistosome cercarial dermatitis, hookworms, cutaneous larval migrans, and strongyloidiasis have which of the following in common?

A. Animal reservoirs

B. Drug treatment

C. Pathogenic mechanism

D. Portal of entry

E. Taxonomic classification

41. Liver (rarely brain and lung) abscess, perianal cutaneous lesions, and ameboma may result secondary to which of the following?

A. Acanthamebiasis

B. Entamebic colitis

C. Balantidiasis

D. Dientamebiasis

E. Negleriasis

42. Finding intraerythrocytic trophozoite, schizont, and gametocyte stages in stained thin blood smears during febrile periods is the usual means for diagnosis of which of the following?

A. African trypanosomiasis

B. American trypanosomiasis

C. Malaria

D. Toxoplasmosis

E. Visceral leishmaniasis

43. Sparganosis, cysticercosis, trichinosis, and toxoplasmosis have which of the following in common?

A. Immunodeficiency

B. Neuropathy

C. Raw meat

D. Transplacental

E. Tapeworms

44. Rhabditiform larvae in unstained fecal smears is the usual diagnostic finding for which of the following?

A. Ascariasis

B. Enterobiasis

C. Hookworm

D. Strongyloidiasis

E. Trichuriasis

45. Hypergammaglobulinemia E and hypereosinophilia are usually seen in infections with which of the following?

A. Hemoflagellates
B. Intestinal cestodes
C. Amebae
D. Malaria
E. Tissue nematodes

Answers

Questions 1–5: There is a specific vector for each of these infections.

1. E
2. C
3. D
4. B
5. A

Questions 6–10: The life history stage that is infective for the human host is specific for each of these infections.

6. B Cysts ingested in food or drink result in entamebiasis.
7. C Eggs ingested in food or drink result in ascariasis.
8. B Infection is by ingestion of cysts in food and water.
9. A Infected freshwater snails shed cercariae that penetrate the intact skin.
10. D Filariform larvae in fecal contaminated soil penetrate the intact skin.

Questions 11–15: Each infection has a specific drug treatment.

11. B This is an effective drug for many luminal nematodiases.
12. E This is used for cutaneous, mucocutaneous, and visceral leishmaniases.
13. A This effectively eliminates microfilariae and adults.
14. C This is the drug of choice for most flagellate infections.
15. D Cestode and trematode infections are treated with this drug.

Questions 16–20: Each phrase represents a unique aspect peculiar to the mechanism of pathogenesis for the respective infection.

16. A This allows successive waves of parasitemia.
17. E This causes the periodic fever cycle due to erythrolysis.
18. D This produces a lesion that resembles an invasive tumor.
19. C Schistosomes survive by confusing the host immune system.
20. B This allows long-term survival of bradyzoites in tissue.

Questions 21–25: Each lesion is specific for the respective infection.

21. B This results from blood-sucking activity in the intestine.

22. C Massive proliferation of amastigotes causes hyperplasia.
23. A Trophozoites block gaseous exchange and evoke little macrophage response; plasma cells accumulate in septae.
24. E This is the result of portal cirrhosis following massive, long-term deposition of embolic eggs.
25. D This lesion results from larvae encysting in muscle cells.

Questions 26–45: These questions have a single best response.

26. C Romaña's sign is a pathognomonic lesion in endemic areas.
27. A This occurs in immunocompetent contact lens wearers.
28. D Transient pneumonitis indicates verminous pneumonia.
29. E This is the primary lesion of schistosomiasis.
30. E This is the treatment of choice for both infections.
31. C Dyspnea and no tissue macrophages to clear the alveolar infiltrate characterize pneumocystosis pathology.
32. B Clinical intestinal amebiasis causes ulcerative lesions.
33. A All three infections are transmitted by external or internal autoinfection, or both.
34. D Only liver enlargement is common to all three infections.
35. B Schizogony only occurs in *Plasmodium* spp.; the liver cycle is continous in *P. vivax, P. ovale,* and *P. malariae.*
36. C Only *P. falciparum* causes the capillary plugging and intracapillary erythrolysis that produces this lesion.
37. E Only in trichuriasis is there sometimes rectal prolapse.
38. D These clinical signs refer to the three phases of larval production, migration, and encystment in trichinosis.
39. D Cercariae released from snails encyst as metacercariae on aquatic plants and animals in all of these infections.
40. D Larvae penetrate the intact skin in all these infections.
41. B These are metastatic lesions of intestinal amebiasis.
42. C These are the intraerythrocytic stages in malaria.
43. C Ingesting raw meat is the common cause of all of these infections.
44. D Eggs are the infective stage for the other nematodes.
45. E Tissue-dwelling nematodes almost always educe a severe type I hypersensitivity reaction.

Parasitology

Suggested Reading

Acha, P. N., and Szyfres, B. *Zoonoses and Communicable Diseases Common to Man and Animals* (2nd ed.). Washington, D. C.: Pan American Health Organization, 1987.

Ash, L. R., and Orihel, T. C. *Atlas of Human Parasitology* (3rd ed.). Chicago: American Society of Clinical Pathologists, 1990.

Bogish, B. J., and Cheng, T. C. *Human Parasitology*. Philadelphia: Saunders, 1990.

Cook, G. C. *Parasitic Disease in Clinical Practice*. London: Springer-Verlag, 1990.

Cotran, R. S., Kumar, V., and Robbins, S. L. *Robbins Pathologic Basis of Disease* (5th ed.). Philadelphia: Saunders, 1994.

Despommier, D. D., and Karapelou, J. W. *Parasite Life Cycles*. New York: Springer-Verlag, 1987.

Katz, M., Despommier, D. D., and Gwadz, R. W. *Parasitic Diseases* (2nd ed.). New York: Springer-Verlag, 1989.

Markell, E. K., Voge, M., and John, D. T. *Medical Parasitology* (7th ed.). Philadelphia: Saunders, 1992.

Warren, K. S., and Mahmoud, A. A. F. *Tropical and Geographic Medicine* (2nd ed.). New York: McGraw-Hill, 1990.

Summation

Thomas C. Butler

Infectious agents localize preferentially in various organs and tissues according to properties of the organisms (tropism) and according to susceptibility of the hosts's organs. The approach to diagnosis of infections is dictated by evidence for localized inflammation or disease in one or another organ system. This section provides a reference to common human infections that occur in specific organ systems. The following tables (8-1 to 8-11) list the major pathogens that are leading causes of infectious diseases in humans.

Table 8-1 Organisms that Cause Clinical Pictures of Meningitis or Encephalitis and Brain Abscess

Meningitis or Encephalitis
  Bacterial
    Streptococcus pneumoniae
    Haemophilus influenzae
    Neisseria meningitidis
    Escherichia coli
    Staphylococcus aureus
    Listeria monocytogenes
    Mycobacterium tuberculosis
    Streptococcus agalactiae, group B
    Leptospira
  Viral
    Enteroviruses, including coxsackieviruses, echoviruses, and polioviruses
    Arboviruses, including equine encephalitis viruses
    Herpes simplex virus
  Fungal
    Cryptococcus neoformans
Brain abscess
  Bacterial
    Staphylococcus aureus
    Proteus species
    Escherichia coli
    Pseudomonas species
    Streptococcus milleri
    Bacteroides species
    Clostridium species
  Fungal
    Cryptococcus neoformans
  Parasitic
    Toxoplasma gondii
    Taenia solium (cysticercosis)

Table 8-2 Organisms that Cause Upper Respiratory Tract Infections

Rhinitis
  Viral
    Rhinoviruses
    Coronaviruses
    Adenoviruses
    Parainfluenza viruses
    Influenza viruses
    Respiratory syncytial virus
Pharyngitis
  Bacterial
    Streptococcus pyogenes, group A
    Neisseria gonorrhoeae
  Viral
    Adenoviruses
    Epstein-Barr virus
Otitis media
  Bacterial
    Streptococcus pneumoniae
    Haemophilus influenzae
    Streptococcus pyogenes, group A
    Moraxella catarrhalis
Sinusitis
  Bacterial
    Streptococcus pneumoniae
    Haemophilus influenzae
    Staphylococcus aureus
    Streptococcus pyogenes, group A
    Moraxella catarrhalis
    Bacteroides species
    Other anaerobes
  Viral
    Rhinoviruses
    Influenza viruses

Table 8-2 (continued).

Gingivitis
  Bacterial
    Bacteroides species
    Actinobacillus species
    Capnocytophaga species
    Fusobacterium species
    Streptococcus species

Table 8-3 Organisms that Cause
Lower Respiratory Tract Infections

Bronchitis
  Viral
    Influenza viruses
    Adenoviruses
  Bacterial
    Streptococcus pneumoniae
    Haemophilus influenzae
    Mycoplasma pneumoniae
Bronchiolitis
  Viral
    Respiratory syncytial virus
    Parainfluenza viruses
    Adenoviruses
    Influenza viruses
  Bacterial
    Mycoplasma pneumoniae
Pneumonia
  Bacterial
    Streptococcus pneumoniae
    Haemophilus influenzae
    Klebsiella pneumoniae
    Staphylococcus aureus
    Moraxella catarrhalis
    Legionella pneumophila
    Pseudomonas aeruginosa
    Mixed anaerobic (aspiration)
  Viral
    Influenza viruses
    Adenoviruses
    Respiratory syncytial virus
    Parainfluenza viruses
  Mycobacterial
    Mycobacterium tuberculosis
  Fungal
    Histoplasma capsulatum
    Aspergillus species
    Coccidioides immitis
  Rickettsial
    Coxiella burnetii (Q fever)
  Parasitic
    Pneumocystis carinii

Table 8-4 Organisms that Cause
Gastrointestinal Tract Infections

Esophagitis
  Fungal
    Candida albicans
  Viral
    Cytomegalovirus
Gastritis
  Bacterial
    Helicobacter pylori
  Viral
    Norwalk virus
Enteritis
  Bacterial
    Escherichia coli
    Salmonella enteritidis
    Salmonella typhi
    Vibrio cholerae
    Campylobacter jejuni
    Yersinia enterocolitica
  Viral
    Rotaviruses
    Enteroviruses
    Intestinal adenoviruses
    Norwalk virus
    Caliciviruses
    Astroviruses
    Cytomegalovirus
  Parasitic
    Giardia lamblia
    Cryptosporidium
    Isospora belli
Colitis
  Bacterial
    Shigella species
    Salmonella species
    Campylobacter jejuni
    Clostridium difficile
    Escherichia coli
  Parasitic
    Entamoeba histolytica
    Schistosoma mansoni

Table 8-5 Organisms that Cause Liver
Infection, Including Hepatitis and Hepatic Abscess

Hepatitis
  Viral
    Hepatitis virus A
    Hepatitis virus B
    Hepatitis virus C
    Epstein-Barr virus
  Bacterial
    Mycobacterium tuberculosis

Mycobacterium avium-intracellulare
Leptospira species
Fungal
   Histoplasma capsulatum
Parasitic
   Schistosoma mansoni
Hepatic abscess
  Bacterial
   Bacteroides fragilis and other anaerobes
   Escherichia coli
   Staphylococcus aureus
  Parasitic
   Entamoeba histolytica

Table 8-6 Organisms that
Cause Infections of the Heart

Endocarditis
  Bacterial
   Streptococcus sanguis, Streptococcus mutans, and other
    viridans streptococci
   Streptococcus (Enterococcus) faecalis
   Staphylococcus aureus
   Staphylococcus epidermidis
   Pseudomonas aeruginosa
  Fungal
   Candida albicans
Myocarditis
  Viral
   Coxsackievirus group B
   Echoviruses
   Polioviruses
   Mumps virus
  Bacterial
   Corynebacterium diphtheriae
   Clostridium perfringens
   Borrelia burgdorferi
  Rickettsial
   Rickettsia tsutsugamushi
Pericarditis
  Viral
   Coxsackievirus group B
   Echoviruses
   Mumps virus
  Bacterial
   Streptococcus pneumoniae
   Staphylococcus aureus
   Haemophilus influenzae
   Neisseria meningitidis

Table 8-7 Organisms that Cause
Urinary Tract Infections

Cystitis
  Bacterial
   Escherichia coli
   Klebsiella pneumoniae
   Enterobacter species
   Staphylococcus saprophyticus
   Proteus species
   Streptococcus faecalis
  Fungal
   Candida albicans
  Viral
   Adenoviruses
  Parasitic
   Schistosoma haematobium
Pyelonephritis
  Bacterial
   Escherichia coli
   Klebsiella pneumoniae
   Enterobacter species
   Proteus species
   Streptococcus faecalis
   Pseudomonas aeruginosa
Fungal
  Candida albicans
Prostatitis
  Bacterial
   Escherichia coli
   Klebsiella pneumoniae
   Enterobacter species
   Proteus species
   Streptococcus faecalis
   Chlamydia trachomatis

Table 8-8 Organisms that
Cause Sexually Transmitted Diseases

Urethritis or genital ulcer
  Bacterial
   Neisseria gonorrhoeae
   Chlamydia trachomatis
   Ureplasma urealyticum
   Haemophilus ducreyi
   Calymmatobacterium granulomatis
   Treponema pallidum
  Viral
   Herpes simplex virus
Vaginitis or cervicitis
  Fungal
   Candida albicans
  Parasitic
   Trichomonas vaginalis
  Bacterial
   Gardnerella vaginalis

Summation

Table 8-8 (continued).

    Neisseria gonorrhoeae
    Chlamydia trachomatis
  Viral
    Herpes simplex virus
Pelvic Inflammatory Disease
  Bacterial
    Neisseria gonorrhoeae
    Chlamydia trachomatis
    Bacteroides fragilis and other anaerobes
Acquired immunodeficiency syndrome
  Viral
    Human immunodeficiency virus 1
    Human immunodeficiency virus 2

Table 8-9 Organisms that Cause
Infections of Skin and Subcutaneous Structures

Pyoderma, cellulitis, or abscesses
  Bacterial
    Staphylococcus aureus
    Streptococcus pyogenes
    Staphylococcus epidermidis
    Pseudomonas aeruginosa
    Clostridium perfringens
    Mixed anaerobes
    Corynebacterium diphtheriae
    Francisella tularensis
    Bacillus anthracis
    Erysipelothrix rhusiopathiae
    Vibrio species
    Pasteurella multocida
    Capnocytophaga canimorsus
    Borrelia burgdorferi (Lyme disease)
    Mycobacterium leprae (leprosy)
    Leishmania species (leishmaniasis)
  Fungal
    Candida albicans
    Aspergillus species
    Sporothrix schenckii
    Tinea species
Vesicles or exanthems
  Viral
    Herpes simplex virus
    Varicella-zoster virus
    Measles virus
    Rubella virus
  Rickettsial
    Rickettsia rickettsii (Rocky Mountain spotted fever)
    Rickettsia typhi (murine typhus)
Lymphadenitis and lymphangitis
  Bacterial
    Staphylococcus aureus
    Streptococcus pyogenes
    Mycobacterium tuberculosis

    Yersinia pestis
    Francisella tularensis
    Chlamydia trachomatis
    Treponema pallidum
  Rickettsial
    Rickettsia rickettsii (Rocky Mountain spotted fever)
    Rochalimaea henselae (cat-scratch disease)
  Fungal
    Histoplasma capsulatum
  Viral
    Epstein-Barr virus
    Cytomegalovirus
    Adenoviruses
    Human immunodeficiency virus 1
    Herpes simplex virus type 2
  Parasitic
    Wucheria bancrofti
    Brugia malayi
    Loa loa
    Onchocerca volvulus
    Toxoplasma gondii
Fasciitis
  Bacterial
    Bacteroides fragilis
    Peptostreptococcus species
    Escherichia coli
    Streptococcus pyogenes
    Staphylococcus aureus
Myositis
  Bacterial
    Staphylococcus aureus
    Clostridium perfringens
    Clostridium septicum
    Peptostreptococcus species
    Bacteroides fragilis
  Viral
    Influenza viruses
    Coxsackievirus group B
  Parasitic
    Trichinella spiralis
    Taenia solium

Table 8-10 Organisms that Cause
Infections of Bones and Joints

Osteomyelitis
  Bacterial
    Staphylococcus aureus
    Escherichia coli
    Klebsiella pneumoniae
    Salmonella enteritidis
    Proteus species
    Pseudomonas aeruginosa
    Mixed anaerobes
    Mycobacterium tuberculosis

Arthritis
   Bacterial
      Staphylococcus aureus
      Haemophilus influenzae
      Streptococcus pneumoniae
      Streptococcus pyogenes
      Neisseria meningitidis
      Neisseria gonorrhoeae
      Mycobacterium tuberculosis
      Escherichia coli
   Viral
      Rubella virus
      Mumps virus
      Hepatitis B virus
Fungal
      Sporothrix schenckii
      Coccidioides immitis

Table 8-11 Organisms that Cause Infections of Blood and Blood Cells

Septicemia
   Bacterial
      Escherichia coli
      Staphylococcus aureus
      Klebsiella pneumoniae
      Pseudomonas aeruginosa

      Streptococcus pneumoniae
      Salmonella typhi (typhoid fever)
      Mycobacterium avium-intracellulare
      Yersinia pestis (plague)
      Borrelia species (relapsing fever)
   Fungal
      Candida albicans
   Viral
      Cytomegalovirus
Erythrocyte infections
   Parasitic
      Plasmodium falciparum
      Plasmodium vivax
      Plasmodium ovale
      Plasmodium malariae
      Babesia microti
Leukocytes
   Viral
      Epstein-Barr virus
      Cytomegalovirus
      Human immunodeficiency virus 1
      Human lymphotropic viruses (oncoviruses)
   Parasitic
      Leishmania donovani (kala azar)
Trypanosomiasis
   Parasitic
      Trypanosoma cruzi (Chagas' disease)
      Trypanosoma brucei (sleeping sickness)

Summation

Index